Gary G. Ferguson, Ph.D.

College of Pharmacy and Health Sciences, Northeast Louisiana University
Monroe, Louisiana

PATHOPHYSIOLOGY
MECHANISMS AND EXPRESSIONS

W.B. SAUNDERS COMPANY   1984
Philadelphia   London   Toronto   Mexico City   Rio de Janeiro   Sydney   Tokyo

W. B. Saunders Company: West Washington Square
Philadelphia, PA 19105

1 St. Anne's Road
Eastbourne, East Sussex BN21 3UN, England

1 Goldthorne Avenue
Toronto, Ontario M8Z 5T9, Canada

Apartado 26370—Cedro 512
Mexico 4, D.F., Mexico

Rua Coronel Cabrita, 8
Sao Cristovao Caixa Postal 21176
Rio de Janeiro, Brazil

9 Waltham Street
Artarmon, N.S.W. 2064, Australia

Ichibancho, Central Bldg., 22-1 Ichibancho
Chiyoda-Ku, Tokyo 102, Japan

Library of Congress Cataloging in Publication Data

Ferguson, Gary G.

Pathophysiology: mechanisms and expressions.

1. Physiology, Pathological.   I. Title. [DNLM: 1. Pathology.   2. Physiology. QZ 4 F352p]

RB113.F37 1984   616.07   83–20195

ISBN 0–7216–3616–0

Pathophysiology   ISBN   0–7216–3616–0

Last digit is the print number: 9   8   7   6   5   4   3   2   1

To my wife
Lois
and daughters
Laurie and Katie
who make it all
worthwhile.

Preface

Pathophysiology: Mechanisms and Expressions developed as an outgrowth of my two-semester course called "Disease Pathogenesis and Therapy" at the College of Pharmacy and Health Sciences, Northeast Louisiana University. During the past several years I searched for a book that could provide the essentials of pathophysiology without the detailed treatment given by most medical school pathology texts. I was interested in how pathologic principles *apply* to human diseases and how they could be used as an aid to learning.

The purpose of my writing this textbook was to give the health science student a concise, readable book that would cover the disease processes common to many diseases and to show the relationship between the process and the clinical illness. The text covers the more common diseases with respect to cause, development, symptoms, signs, laboratory findings, treatment, and prognosis. The major goal, however, was not to discuss as many diseases as possible, but to show the principles of disease development via disease processes. Many diseases have interconnecting threads of pathology that become apparent when the processes of disease development are understood. Whenever possible, the major disease process responsible for a clinical disease is identified and its relevance to the disease in question and other diseases is demonstrated. This format should provide, for the student, a continuity that otherwise might be missing. The inclusion of general coverage of the *treatment* of common diseases makes this book somewhat unique among pathophysiology texts.

The book is divided into two major sections. The first section deals with the mechanisms of pathogenicity, i.e., what goes wrong with the human organism to cause clinical disease. Included in this section are the major disease processes, terms describing disease processes, factors contributing to disease, and some discussion of normal functions for comparison. The second section consists of representative diseases affecting the various body systems. Here, knowledge about disease processes is applied toward an understanding of particular diseases. The emphasis is on showing the similarities among diseases, when possible, through common disease processes.

The text requires only a modest background in the life sciences. Great effort has been made to define terms that might be unfamiliar and to avoid language that is unnecessarily technical. Much of the mystery surrounding disease disappears when complicated-sounding language is revealed for what it is. Thus, the statement "cholelithiasis is the major etiologic factor in cholecystitis" means that gallstones are the most common cause of gallbladder inflammation!

As an aid to students who wish to pursue the subject further, I have provided questions at the end of each chapter that I consider to be thought-provoking. The separate Study Guide gives the answers to these questions and also contains 37 case studies covering diseases of most body systems. Pertinent additional readings are also listed at the conclusion of each chapter.

I hope that *Pathophysiology: Mechanisms and Expressions* will succeed in presenting this fascinating subject to the reader in an interesting and useful way.

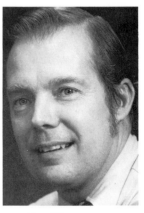

Gary G. Ferguson

Acknowledgments

Among the many things an author learns in writing a book is that the finished product represents the combined ideas and efforts of dozens of people. Numerous friends and colleagues have provided helpful suggestions during the planning and writing of the manuscript. I would especially like to thank Dr. August M. Hochenedel and Professor Beverly Jarrell of the Department of Dental Hygiene, Northeast Louisiana University, for their careful evaluation of Chapter 19, Diseases of the Oral Cavity. In addition, my father, Dr. N. M. Ferguson; my brother, Mike Ferguson; and Marilyn Gottlieb, all of whom have written books, provided many helpful hints and comments during the planning of the outline for the book.

I was extremely fortunate to have been associated with the W. B. Saunders Company for the publication of *Pathophysiology: Mechanisms and Expressions.* In his role as editor, Mr. Baxter Venable went far beyond the call of duty in helping me in many ways, and was ably assisted in this by Mrs. Debra Vickery. I would also like to acknowledge the expert work of Ms. Carol Robins Wolf, Copy Editorial Department; Mr. Bill Donnelly, Design Department; and Mrs. Margaret Shaw, Illustration Department, along with the many others I've not yet had the pleasure of knowing.

Contents

INTRODUCTION

Pathophysiology is defined as the changes in physiologic function seen in disease. It is a derangement of the normal life processes of sufficient magnitude that clinical disease results. The term *disease* means sufficient departure from the normal for *signs* and *symptoms* to be produced. Often it is difficult to determine what the limits of normal are; that is, when a function leaves the normal range and enters the area of abnormality.

We humans are much more variable in this regard than are most animal species. Laboratory rats, for example, represent strains of animals inbred for dozens or even hundreds of generations. There is extreme homogeneity with respect to physiologic function. No such situation exists for humans except in extremely remote areas in which intermarriage is the only means of survival. Thus, laboratory values must always be considered with this variability in mind. This makes the task of the clinician more difficult, since it is not always possible to state with certainty that a test result "proves" that a particular disease state exists. For example, if a patient who complains of chronic fatigue has a "borderline" thyroid function test, does this mean that the patient is fatigued *because* the thyroid function is at the bottom end of the normal range? Might it mean that the fatigue is a result of other factors and that the thyroid function is normal for that person? An elusive blend of judgment and experience is required to evaluate the entire situation. This is the "art" rather than the "science" of medicine.

Human variability notwithstanding, it is still possible to determine, in most cases, that sufficient departure from the normal has occurred, i.e., that a disease exists. The health professional can thus make a diagnosis and determine the type of treatment necessary to correct the problem. From personal past experience and from experiences of others, the clinician is often able to predict the prognosis or outcome of the disease state.

Although hundreds of diseases exist, there are common denominators that link many of them together. These are the disease processes forming the basis for the departure from normal physiologic function. For example, rheumatoid arthritis and ulcerative colitis are both chronic inflammatory disorders. Much concerning the pathophysiology of these two seemingly unrelated conditions is similar, although the obvious clinical manifestations are quite different—one affects the joints, and the other affects the large intestine. Likewise, bronchial asthma and allergic conjunctivitis seem, on the surface, quite different. They are in reality different manifestations of the same basic allergic reaction, except that the "shock organ" is the respiratory tract in one case and the eye in the other.

The pathologist, who studies disease processes closely, is like a modern-day Sherlock Holmes. Often arriving at the scene after the "crime" has been committed (pathologic damage has occurred), the pathologist must look carefully for clues to the crime (tissue changes). His solution of the crime may not help the current victim but may prevent others from getting into a similar predicament. For example, a pathologist who autopsies a patient who died from congestive heart failure may find that the heart failed because it had

1

enlarged too much from long-term overwork. High blood pressure, which is generally treatable, caused the heart to overwork and enlarge in this case. The lesson learned is that early detection and treatment of high blood pressure can prevent heart enlargement that may lead to congestive heart failure and death.

Human disease is often the result of interaction of several deleterious factors. Although there are definite disease-causing agents, such as viruses or bacteria, often illness occurs within the setting of old age, debility, or exposure to toxic materials. The tendency toward certain diseases granted by heredity frequently is a major factor in disease development and has been implicated in such common diseases as coronary atherosclerosis and breast cancer. Therefore, the "cause" of a disease should always be examined in the light of any contributing factors present.

Physicians and others who treat human diseases develop a way of arriving at a diagnosis using deductive reasoning. That is, they assemble as many facts as possible concerning the illness in question and then pursue the correct diagnosis by a process of elimination. Symptoms, signs, history, and laboratory findings help the practitioner to eliminate some possibilities and to concentrate on the more likely ones. Additional laboratory tests help to differentiate between closely related conditions. Finally, all possibilities are eliminated except the correct diagnosis.

It is not the aim of this text to train the student to be a diagnostician. Nonetheless, we can all learn to use deductive reasoning and to appreciate the process that goes on in disease diagnosis. This will also help us to understand rational therapy, complications, and prognosis of disease.

Terms in Pathophysiology

Many terms relating to disease processes are used repeatedly in texts and lecture materials. The following list includes a number of common pathophysiologic terms. A few minutes spent learning the definitions of the terms will pay great rewards in ease of understanding of the remainder of the book.

General Terms **Pathology**—study of the nature, cause, and course of disease, which involves changes in tissue structure and function.

Pathophysiology—change in physiologic function seen in disease.

Disease—sufficient departure from the normal for signs and symptoms to be produced. Often a disease has only one cause (e.g., pneumococcal pneumonia, which is caused by infection with one type of bacterial organism).

Syndrome—condition having a defined collection of signs, symptoms, and lesions. Often a syndrome has more than one cause (e.g., epilepsy, which can be caused by brain damage, brain infection, or other factors).

Sign—an abnormality noted by an observer such as a physician (e.g., pupil dilation).

Symptom—an abnormality noted by the patient (e.g., headache).

Lesion—a variation from the normal. Lesions may be anatomic (tumor), physiologic (muscle spasm), or biochemical (phenylketonuria).

Etiology—the theory of the cause of disease.

Pathogenesis—the development of a lesion.

Idiopathic—having no known cause. Most cases of high blood pressure (hypertension) are idiopathic.

Note: Some confusion occurs in the common usage of a few of these terms. *Disease* and *syndrome* are often used interchangeably, even though the exact meanings of the terms are not identical. Sometimes a condition is called a disease when first discovered because it is thought that there is only one cause. When other causes are identified, it may then be called a syndrome. However, the "old" term *disease* may remain. The meanings of *etiology* and *pathogenesis* are also often confused. In a patient who suffers a heart attack (myocardial infarction), the etiology (cause) is often said to be coronary artery deposits (coronary atherosclerosis). The real cause may be an inherited biochemical lesion that results in an overproduction of cholesterol, leading to coronary artery deposits. Thus, coronary atherosclerosis represents the *development* (pathogenesis) of the condition rather than the cause of it.

Common Terms Representing Specific Pathophysiologic Changes

Hyperemia—an increase in circulation to an area of tissue. Hyperemia is a common result of warming a tissue.

Ischemia—a decrease in circulation to an area of tissue. Ischemia of the heart muscle causes chest pain (angina pectoris).

Infarction—death of tissue caused by lack of circulation. In a myocardial infarction, a portion of the heart muscle dies and is replaced with scar tissue.

Thrombus—a blood clot that remains in one place as it develops. In a coronary thrombosis, a clot develops in a coronary artery and usually causes heart damage (myocardial infarction).

Embolus—a blood clot that leaves its site of origin and travels elsewhere in the body through the circulatory system. In a pulmonary embolism, a clot fragment, often from a leg vein, travels through the venous circulation to the heart and enters the pulmonary circulation. It then jams in a smaller pulmonary artery, causing pain and shortness of breath.

Necrosis—death of cells or tissue. In hepatic necrosis, a toxic agent such as chloroform causes death to liver cells and loss of liver function.

Degeneration—deterioration of cells or tissue. In multiple sclerosis, degeneration occurs in the myelin sheath of nerves in the central nervous system.

Regeneration—regrowth of viable tissue. Skin usually regenerates well following a cut or scrape.

Infiltration—invasion of body tissues with abnormal material. In Wilson's disease, large amounts of copper compounds are stored in various body organs and tissues and tissue damage results.

Atrophy—reduced size of an organ or tissue. When cortisonelike drugs are given for extended periods of time, the adrenal cortex may atrophy, since it is no longer required by the body to produce cortisonelike compounds.

Hypertrophy—increased size of an organ or tissue caused by the enlargement of each cell, but not by increasing the number of cells. In cardiac hypertrophy, the heart enlarges because of long-term overwork, often caused by high blood pressure or valve disease.

Hyperplasia—increased size of an organ or tissue caused by the formation of more cells. Under certain conditions, the thyroid gland can undergo hyperplasia and increase its function.

Metaplasia—a change from one type of tissue to another. In squamous metaplasia, the ciliated columnar epithelial cells that line the bronchial system are converted to squamous cells in response to heavy smoking. The squamous cells do not have the cleaning action provided by the cilia in the columnar epithelial cells.

Neoplasia—a perversion of cellular growth both in rate and in type of cell formed. Tumors are examples of neoplastic growth. Usually the cell grows faster than normal and is histologically more primitive. Often, *neoplasia* is used interchangeably with the term *malignant growth*, although technically there are types of neoplasia that are not malignant.

Additional Reading

Chabner, D.: *The Language of Medicine*, Philadelphia, W. B. Saunders Company, 1981.

CHAPTER 1

FACTORS CONTRIBUTING TO DISEASE

Medical thinking a century or more ago stressed the concept of a single cause for each disease. This was probably largely due to the earlier discovery of bacteria as causes of human infection. When it was shown that specific infectious agents could cause specific diseases, there was considerable thought that every disease might have a single cause. Streptococcal infection was identified as the precipitating cause of rheumatic fever, pneumococcal infection was shown to be the major etiologic factor in pneumonia, and even the elusive spirochete *Treponema pallidum* was identified as the cause of syphilis. It must have been satisfying for clinicians at that time to be able to explain the multifaceted pathophysiology of syphilis on the basis of infection with a single pathogenic organism. The concept of "one cause, one disease" was an attractive one, and it was applied to most of the clinical conditions known at that time.

However, some diseases refused to cooperate with the idea of a single cause. Epileptic seizures were noted in individuals with traumatic brain injury, infection, stroke, overhydration, and hyperthermia. It was difficult to assign a single cause to high blood pressure (hypertension), since kidney damage or infection, adrenal tumors, and certain anatomic defects in the circulatory system all were associated with the common denominator of hypertension. It also appeared that some diseases did not have a known cause or could be caused by unknown as well as known factors. Finally, the concept of "one cause, one disease" sifted to its proper level. It certainly applied for some diseases, but not for all.

Modern thinking about disease states recognizes the clear-cut relationship of single cause–disease in many cases. However, there is now a much greater appreciation of the role of multiple factors in disease pathogenesis. Indeed, the term *multifactorial* has come to be used for describing conditions such as coronary artery disease, hypertension, and even some forms of cancer. We talk about "risk factors" that add together to increase the total odds of contracting a particular disease. Thus, an individual with a high cholesterol level, obesity, inactivity, high saturated fat intake, and a heavy cigarette smoking habit probably has a greater risk of heart attack than a person without these risk factors.

It is the aim of modern medicine to identify multiple etiologic factors and to prevent disease through their control. This is often easier and more effective than drastic treatment after a problem develops. It is a better solution for the multiple-risk potential heart attack victim to lower the cholesterol level, lose weight, exercise more, substitute some unsaturated for saturated fat in the diet, and stop smoking than to undergo coronary bypass surgery for severe coronary atherosclerosis. A discussion of some of the well-known etiologic factors follows.

HEREDITY

It was a wise philosopher who first jokingly suggested that we must "select our ancestors carefully" if we are to avoid disease. How wonderful it would be if we could pick only strong, long-lived ancestors, free of heart disease and cancer and with excellent resistance to infection. Unfortunately, many people have a heritage that predisposes them to coronary atherosclerosis, breast cancer, or some other illness, and it is almost "in the cards" that they will eventually develop the disease. Some people from families having a high incidence of diabetes mellitus are doomed to the disease even in spite of taking every precaution to avoid it. They may maintain normal weight, watch their intake of sugar, drink moderately or not at all, and still eventually become diabetic.

Intermarriage

Heredity is a known factor in some diseases. The royal families of Europe who developed hemophilia probably had a spontaneously occurring trait for it that was strengthened by their practice of intermarriage of cousins. The desire to maintain the royal blood line eventually caused a widespread incidence of hemophilia among the males and a decimation of the family members. Likewise, the high incidence of diabetes mellitus among the Australian aborigines is partly attributed to their close-knit existence. By propagating only within the tribe, they ensure that the hereditary tendency toward diabetes mellitus will be strengthened instead of being weakened by dilution with other populations. *Sickle cell trait,* which is thought to have been a beneficial adaptive response of certain African natives to malaria, became a liability through tribal intermarriage. Intermarriage created some offspring with a trait from each parent. These individuals had *sickle cell disease.* Sickle cell disease is a devastating affliction that leads to early death from organ failure or other complications.

Mendel's Law

Diseases that have a strongly hereditary basis often follow Mendel's laws of genetics. A trait or *gene* for the disease is carried on the *chromosome* and alters the development of the individual so that the disease is more likely to occur. If the trait is inherited from only one parent and the corresponding gene from the other parent is normal, the person is said to be *heterozygous* for the disease. If a trait is inherited from each parent, the individual is *homozygous* for the disease. The homozygous person often has a more severe form of the condition than does the heterozygous individual. For example, a person with sickle cell trait (heterozygous) has little or no disability and a normal life expectancy, whereas a person with sickle cell disease (homozygous) has a disabling and life-threatening condition.

Genetic Influence

Genes vary in the degree of influence they have upon the developing individual. *Dominant* genes exert a powerful effect whether the person is homozygous or heterozygous for them. Thus achondroplasia, a form of dwarfism caused by an inherited dominant gene, surfaces even if the individual is heterozygous for it. Huntington's chorea, a degenerative nervous system disorder that afflicted folk singer Woodie Guthrie, is also transmitted by a dominant gene.

Recessive genes may require that the affected person be homozygous for full expression. Phenylketonuria (PKU), in which the affected person fails to metabolize the amino acid phenylalanine, is an example of this. Without the use of a diet low in phenylalanine, a child with PKU will develop brain damage and mental retardation. Fortunately, PKU is easily detected at birth and a preventive diet can be instituted immediately. Albinism is another example of a recessive genetic disorder. The skin, hair and irises fail to pigment completely, and the individual has very light blue eyes, white skin, and pale yellow hair. The cause is a defect in the pigment-producing cells (melanocytes).

Sex-Linked Diseases

Some genetic diseases are classified as *sex-linked*. The gene is usually recessive and located on the X chromosome. Males are affected by the disease, but females carry it to succeeding generations. Hemophilia, previously discussed, is an example of a sex-linked disorder.

Inherited Conditions

Hereditary factors are suspected in a variety of human diseases. For instance, a family history of breast cancer increases the risk of its development in female family members. Also, there is ample evidence to support the role of heredity in some *hyperlipidemias,* conditions in which certain blood fats such as cholesterol are at elevated levels. Hyperlipidemias generally increase the tendency toward atherosclerosis.

Allergy tends to run in families, although the exact manifestation of allergy may vary among family members. One family member has allergic rhinitis (hay fever); another, bronchial asthma; another, hives; and still another, digestive allergies. It is presumed that all have an inherited defect in the body's recognition of substances as safe or harmful. Harmless substances, such as pollen, dust, milk, or chocolate are misread by the body as being potentially threatening. An allergic reaction results as the body responds to these "threats."

Additional Influences

In some cases, it appears that a hereditary tendency toward the disease is aided by additional factors. In diabetes mellitus, it is thought that an inherited tendency toward it may be activated by viral infection or autoimmune reaction. The pancreas, already vulnerable, is damaged by infection or autoimmune reaction (see Chapter 4), and diabetes mellitus appears clinically. This sort of cooperation among etiologic factors is also seen with atherosclerosis, breast cancer, and other disorders. The exact role played by heredity becomes difficult to assess in these cases.

AGING

One of the questionable features of being over 40 years of age is that we join the ranks of what some people call "middle age." Although this is correctly termed as the midpoint of life—perhaps even a little past the middle—we don't *feel* middle-aged and tend to reject this unflattering term. Even worse, we enter the group of people who become vulnerable to most of the serious diseases. As long as we are under 40, we can almost forget about heart attacks and most common forms of cancer, along with a raft of less prevalent conditions. Entering the 40s, we are increasingly aware of our own vulnerability, which we had hardly admitted to before. We see our contemporaries stricken with severe illnesses and silently refigure our chances of escaping, unscathed, into old age.

The process continues as we get older, and we become even more aware of our increasing chance of serious illness. We try to offset this risk by exercising, losing weight, and watching our diet more closely. We buy vitamins and health foods, dress casually, learn new "buzz" words, and try new dance steps. But we know down deep that the aging process is continuing its inexorable march onward.

What is it we fear most about aging? Is it illness itself and the loss of vitality that it may bring? Is it fear of being useless and unwanted? Do we fear that we may become a burden on our loved ones? A study conducted in Vilcabamba, Ecuador, examined a large number of factors relating to aging. In Vilcabamba, one of the few places in the world with a significant number of inhabitants documented to be over 100, such factors as heredity, diet, work habits, and others were carefully investigated.* The results of the study suggested that multiple positive factors were operating in favor of the long-lived citizens. They were descended from hardy European stock, probably thinned out by the difficult journey to South America. There is a high infant mortality rate in Vilcabamba, thus ensuring a healthy survivor population. The air and water are pure, partly as a result of the lack of industrial development. Most work is done by hand, and walking is the universal form of transportation. The diet emphasizes protein, with little sugar or fat intake. Strips of beef fat are sold on the street corner to be eaten sparingly like candy. Consumption of alcohol is modest or nonexistent for most. There is little sense of frustration among the people. They accept what cannot be changed. The community is strongly Catholic and believes firmly in God and in an afterlife. Everyone, even the oldest, feels needed and has a specific job to do. There is great reverence for the aged, much like in the Oriental cultures, and it is felt that wisdom increases with age.

It would appear that the people of Vilcabamba have strong "health factors" operating for them to increase life span, just as risk factors reduce life span. Perhaps we could learn a lesson from this and increase our health factors as well.

Throughout history, humans have been obsessed with the idea of forestalling the inevitable aging process. From Ponce de Leon's search for the "fountain of youth" to the quest for the Romanian youth serum, virtually every society has sought to prolong youth. The fountain of youth was never discovered and the Romanian youth serum turned out to be ordinary procaine, a local anesthetic. Still the hope continues that a drug or potion will delay aging.

Aging causes a gradual deterioration in many body tissues. The process of atherosclerosis, which begins at birth, continues in everyone at various rates. It has often been said that "we are as old as

---

*A later report disputes the authenticity of the "documented" age. See Kent, S.: What is the maximum human lifespan? Geriatrics, 36:123, 1981.

our arteries," since the quality of arterial circulation is of vital importance to body tissues. There is a certain daily attrition of brain cells, which for some creates a path to early senility. A larger number of chromosome breaks and mitotic errors occur in old cells than in younger ones, and the risk of spontaneous tumor formation generally increases with advancing age. With aging, calcium often becomes depleted from the bones and fracture occurs after trivial injury. The elderly person breaks a hip after a fall. Organ function decreases with aging: the heart, liver, kidney, and other vital organs lose some of the capacity they once had.

Exactly why aging is associated with loss of body functions is not clear. Perhaps the body "wears out" through long use, much as a machine does. Maybe long-term exposure to harmful elements in the environment takes its toll. It is well known that sunlight can age the skin prematurely. It is possible that unknown factors have effects on other body tissues as well.

Drug therapy of older patients is somewhat different than for younger ones. Often less of a drug is required, since the machinery for metabolism and excretion of drugs works more slowly. Frequently, unusual reactions to drugs occur. For example, phenobarbital, a drug having sedative properties in young adults, often causes excitation in senior citizens. Older people are often more vulnerable to the central nervous system effects of drugs. Mental confusion or agitation tends to occur as a side effect more frequently in the elderly than in the young. In a sense, the nervous system of the older person is more vulnerable to the undesirable effects of drugs than that of the younger person.

Many drugs are less effective in the elderly because the tissue cannot respond as fully as it once did. Drugs that dilate cranial blood vessels well in children or young adults often fail to work in the elderly, since their cranial arteries may be rigid from atherosclerosis.

The older individual fights disease with the same weapons as the young person, but the swords are duller, the guns less powerful, and the shields more flimsy. A longer period of convalescence is needed, and the chance of complications developing is greater. Major surgery is more often necessary and also riskier. These and the previously mentioned factors add together to make age itself a risk factor in disease development.

DRUGS AND CHEMICALS

We are all aware of the devastating effects of drug abuse on society. Alcohol, an old villain, is still around, as it has been in nearly all cultures. The effects of alcohol abuse on the liver, digestive tract, and central nervous system are well documented. The contribution of alcohol to accidents, violent acts, and low-grade illness resulting in missed work is also without question. We have passed through periods of glue sniffing, widespread abuse of lysergide (LSD), narcotics, phencyclidine (PCP), and marijuana, and now we seem to be in the throes of a cocaine epidemic.

Illicit Drugs

Each type of illicit drug carries its particular risks to the abuser. Glue sniffing, for instance, is often toxic to the liver and central nervous system because of solvents contained in the glue coupled with hypoxia caused by breathing from a closed, glue-containing plastic bag. Lysergide and PCP can cause psychotic reactions and flashback phenomena, in which the hallucinogenic experience is repeated without drug administration.

Narcotics cause inevitable addiction, requiring increasing doses to maintain freedom from withdrawal symptoms. Many narcotic-related health problems also plague the addict, such as hepatitis and endocarditis, which are caused by using contaminated injection equipment. Materials used to dilute (cut) the narcotics may have pharmacologic action or may mechanically obstruct small blood vessels. Strychnine, sometimes used as a heroin diluent, is a potent convulsive drug. Starch, also used to cut heroin, causes small emboli to form in lung capillaries and elsewhere in the body. Marijuana, at the very least, causes respiratory tract irritation and loss of motivation. Cocaine use is frequently associated with escalation of the dose. If the drug is inhaled through the nose (snorted), perforation and deterioration of the nasal septum can occur. Intravenous use of cocaine often causes psychotic symptoms resembling acute paranoid schizophrenia.

Legitimate Drugs

Besides drugs of abuse, legitimate drugs also frequently cause harmful side effects. It is not the purpose of this book to discuss the various side effects of drugs. Nonetheless, drug side effects result in illness, loss of work, hospitalization and even death. The thalidomide tragedy of the 1960s taught us that a drug must be considered unsafe until proven otherwise. Thalidomide, a mild sedative drug used widely in Europe, was found to cause severe birth deformities if taken during pregnancy. Infants were born with missing or greatly shortened and deformed arms and legs (phocomelia). The drug was used in the United States only on an experimental basis and was withdrawn completely when the problem surfaced in Europe. None-theless, some American children were affected during the time the drug was used.

Virtually any tissue of the body can be affected by a harmful drug, but common sites for toxicity include skin, bone marrow, nervous system, cardiovascular system, digestive tract and liver. Therefore, new drugs must be extensively tested in animals before clinical trials with humans are permitted. The Food and Drug Administration (FDA) has the final responsibility for ensuring the safety and efficacy of drug products released to the American public.

Environmental Chemicals

In addition to abused drugs and drugs taken for legitimate medical purposes are chemical agents found in the environment. These are not intended for human use, but human exposure to them occurs, sometimes on a long-term basis. While many chemicals appear harmless even on long-term exposure, others cause pathologic effects to the human system. Included in the harmful group are certain insecticides, chemical solvents, byproducts of rubber and plastic, and compounds formed in food preparation.

Dichlorodiphenyltrichloroethane (DDT) was removed from the American insecticide market when it was found that it easily became stored in body fat and was retained for an extended period of time. Long-term exposure to DDT would, therefore, cause an accumulation in fatty tissue. Likewise, strontium fallout from the atomic testing of the 1950s caused accumulation of the radioactive material in bones. Since the rate of decay of radioactivity with strontium is extremely slow, any material absorbed into the bones is there for life. The long-term effects of radioactive strontium on bone tissues are not known, although some authorities believe that it is a cause of leukemia.

Some chemical solvents used in the dry cleaning industry and in many other industrial applications have been shown to be toxic to the liver. Carbon tetrachloride is a good example of such a solvent. Long-term inhalation of this volatile agent can cause fatty degeneration of the liver and eventual liver failure.

Various rubber and plastic byproducts are also known to be toxic to humans. Beta-naphthylamine, used in the rubber industry, can cause bladder cancer in industrial rubber workers. Vinyl chloride, produced when vinyl wrap material is heated, can cause liver cancer. The risk is greatest to those receiving chronic exposure. Thus, meat wrappers and others who heat-seal vinyl packages may increase their risk of liver cancer.

Originally isolated from coal tar, 3,4 benzpyrene is also formed when meat is broiled at high temperature. This chemical can cause skin cancer if applied repeatedly to mouse skin in the laboratory. The question of whether or not heavy consumption of broiled meat can increase the risk of gastric cancer has not been answered.

Chemical agents often fall into a gray area of risk. Although it can be shown that heavy exposure for long periods causes illness, the effects of light or short-term exposure are not as clear cut. Since we cannot eliminate all exposure to chemicals, we should strive to limit exposure to those agents known to cause disease in animals or humans. It is likely that there are many agents, as yet undiscovered, with potential for human toxicity. Perhaps these will have a bearing on future understanding of the etiology and pathogenesis of diseases that are now poorly understood.

POLLUTANTS   Pollutants may be chemicals, particulate matter, radioactive material, or infectious material. They can be defined as agents that contaminate the air, water, soil, or other aspects of the environment. For example, the exhaust vapors from a plant making a legitimate chemical product could be considered a pollutant. Dust from a sawmill could constitute an airborne pollutant.

We have become accustomed to living with pollution. Even those who are in observatories high in the mountains have difficulty in finding clear nights for stargazing. Water obtained from any source but extremely deep wells contains a variety of chemicals that affect its taste, odor and, occasionally, safety. Food supplies, both plant and animal, contain insecticides and other chemical agents. Some are in the soil that grows the produce or provides forage for the animals, and some are applied intentionally for parasite control or for better growth of the product.

Air pollution is an important contributor to respiratory disease. Emphysema, chronic bronchitis, bronchial asthma, and even lung cancer can be partly attributed to the effects of airborne particulate matter. During periods of heavy smog, the number of attacks of bronchial asthma and emphysema increases dramatically. Besides soot particles from industrial discharge, air also contains lead compounds, sulfur dioxide and carbon monoxide from automobile exhaust. The use of industrial filters, smog control devices, and lead-free gasoline has improved, but not eliminated, the problem.

Of great concern has been the finding that the Mississippi River contains cancer-causing agents (carcinogens) in addition to its usual assortment of pollutants. Whether or not this is important in the development of human cancer is not known at present.

Some "pollutants" may be helpful. High concentrations of fluoride compounds in water from some areas of the country help to protect against dental caries. At these concentrations there seem to be no harmful effects to humans, although the density of the teeth and bones is increased. The teeth show a splotchy gray mottling and some areas of bone appear discolored. Another example of a helpful pollutant is the mold *Penicillium notatum* that grew on Alexander Fleming's petri dish in the late 1920s. By studying the inhibitory effects of the mold on bacterial growth, Fleming deduced that an inhibitory compound was being produced by the mold organism. Fleming named the compound *penicillin!*

RADIATION

Chronic Ingestion of Radium

Concern over the harmful effects of radiation began early in the 20th century with the finding that women who painted the numbers on radium dial watches were likely to develop cancer. The women used radium-containing paint that would glow in the dark and used their lips to put a point on the tips of their tiny brushes. This chronic ingestion of small amounts of radium led to greatly increased incidence of leukemia and osteosarcoma (bone cancer).

Heavy Exposure

Survivors of atomic blasts were found to have delayed illness caused by damage to the bone marrow. Approximately 2 weeks after heavy radiation exposure, the blood count fell rapidly. The damaged marrow failed to replace cells that died as a result of normal aging as well as those killed by the exposure to radiation. Infection, anemia, and bleeding episodes combined to cause death shortly thereafter. The disease is called *aplastic anemia.*

Long-Term Low-Level Exposure

Low-level, chronic radiation exposure is also an etiologic factor in disease. Radiologists, x-ray technicians, and others who absorb small amounts of radiation on a regular basis have an increased risk of leukemia. Presumably the radiation exposure damages the bone marrow's control mechanisms so that white blood cells are formed in excessive numbers at the expense of red blood cells and platelets. Long-term x-ray exposure has also been associated with skin cancer, especially when used for treating chronic skin conditions.

X-ray Treatment

Within the last few years, there has been increasing concern over the possible development of thyroid cancer in individuals previously exposed to x-ray to the oral cavity and upper chest areas. From approximately 1930 until 1960, x-ray treatment was used to shrink enlarged adenoids and thymus gland tissue (located in the upper chest). Although such treatment was effective in causing these tissues to decrease in size, the method failed to shield the patient adequately. X-ray to the upper chest or oral cavity spilled over the thyroid gland. Because the thyroid gland is quite vulnerable to the effects of radiation, the treatment increased the risk of thyroid cancer. A massive effort was made to identify all individuals who received such treatment and to examine them periodically for early signs of thyroid malignancy.

Sunlight   Ultraviolet light, obtained from sunlight or sunlamps, is a known risk factor to the skin. States with a high percentage of sunny days, like Texas, New Mexico, and Arizona, have high rates of skin cancer. Individuals who work outdoors without protective clothing are the most vulnerable. Farmers, ranchers, and construction workers are especially affected by prolonged sun exposure in the course of their work. Ultraviolet light also causes premature aging of the skin, as previously discussed. This is exemplified by the leathery-skinned farmer, cowboy, or sunbather. Conversely, nuns and monks have a very low incidence of skin cancer and maintain youthful-looking skin. Like many other environmental factors, ultraviolet light seems relatively harmless in small doses.

SUMMARY

Multiple etiologic factors appear to be at work in the pathogenesis of many diseases. Heredity, aging, drugs and chemicals, pollution, and exposure to radiation often have a direct effect on disease development. It is the aim of modern medical science to reduce the harmful effects of these and to prevent their interaction in the promotion of human disease.

Questions   1. Is the average city dweller exposed to more, the same amount of, or less air pollution today than 25 years ago? Five years ago?
2. Which industries have made the greatest progress in improving environmental conditions for workers in the past 25 years?
3. What are the pros and cons of nuclear energy as far as the environment and public health are concerned?
4. Suppose a "youth serum" were discovered today. How might it work to retard the aging process?

Additional Reading   Bergman, H. D.: Drug use in the elderly patient. Southern Pharmacy Journal, August 1980, p. 24.
Follow these seven rules and you'll live up to 11 years longer. Pharmacy Times, November 1976, p. 42.
Zimmet, P., et al.: Diabetes mellitus in an urbanized, isolated Polynesian population: The Funafuti survey. Diabetes, 26:1101, 1977.

CHAPTER 2

INFECTION

Infection occurs when a parasitic organism (bacterium, virus, or other) enters the host organism. This discussion is confined to human infection, but it is apparent that other animal species have a similar host-parasite relationship.

The route of entry depends upon the organism and its properties. Many infections begin when the organism enters the oral cavity and/or respiratory tract. Common viral infections that cause cold and flu symptoms start this way. Likewise, rheumatic fever is usually traced to a previous streptococcal infection in the throat ("strep throat"). Bacteria such as shigellae and salmonellae may enter the body through the gastrointestinal tract and cause symptoms of gastroenteritis. Such a condition is often the result of ingestion of contaminated food or water. Intestinal "flu" is thought to be caused by gastrointestinal entry of viruses. Some infections are spread through direct contact via mucous membranes or skin. Syphilis is noteworthy in this regard. With rickettsial infections, a "third party" or *vector* is required to carry the organism to the host. For example, Rocky Mountain spotted fever is carried by a tick found on squirrels or other wild animals. The tick lights on the host and transmits the rickettsial organism to him or her.

For infection to become well established, the infecting organism must multiply within the host. Therefore, conditions must be suitable for organism growth. Tissue conditions such as temperature, moisture content, and quantity of light greatly influence the success or failure of the organism to infect. Spread of the organism occurs directly through the tissues or indirectly via the lymphatic or circulatory systems.

NORMAL BACTERIAL FLORA

In the late 1950s, the term "peaceful coexistence" was coined to describe the relationship between the Soviet Union and the United States. The ending of the Korean war had established the two major powers as being in balance in terms of military strength. Each side had weapons that could cause virtual annihilation of the other. Both countries were reluctant to begin activities that might lead to military confrontation. Thus, by means of peaceful coexistence, both countries not only could survive but also could prosper and even interact positively for educational or cultural purposes.

A similar situation exists between humans and their constant adversaries, the bacteria. The body houses a multitude of different bacterial organisms that theoretically are capable of causing disease but that cause no harm to the host under normal circumstances (Table 2–1). In fact, there are benefits derived from having such "resident" bacteria in or on the body. Organisms in the intestinal tract synthesize vitamin K and supply this element vital to the synthesis of blood clotting factors. Certain bacteria help to digest

Table 2–1. TYPICAL RESIDENT ORGANISMS

Body Area	Common Residents
Skin	Streptococci, Staphylococci, Corynebacteria
Upper respiratory tract and oral cavity	Streptococci, Staphylococci, Neisseriae, Actinomycetes, Bacteroides
Intestinal tract	Lactobacilli, Bacteroides, Coliforms (Escherichia, Klebsiella, Enterobacter, Serratia, and Hafnia)
Vagina	Lactobacilli
Eye	Corynebacteria

milk products to provide nutrition from them. Intestinal bacteria also provide a normal flora that occupies space within the colon (coliforms) and prevents the overgrowth of more harmful microorganisms. Resident bacteria in the vagina help keep harmful organisms at bay.

As long as this balance between host and organism is maintained, both profit from it. The host receives the benefits of specialized functions of the bacteria and is protected from invasion by more harmful organisms. The resident organisms are given a protected environment so that they may prosper without having to compete as strongly with environmental organisms outside the body. They are, after all, trying to survive in a relatively hostile world, as are other living populations, including humans.

If this balance between host and organism is shifted in either direction, problems result. For example, if coliforms from the intestinal tract enter the bladder, they become capable of causing disease (pathogenic). The resulting common bladder infection is frequently due to poor hygiene, in which the urethral opening is contaminated with fecal material containing coliforms. Likewise, a break in the skin allows resident organisms to enter the tissues below and infection results. The same former "friends" are now "enemies" and must be eliminated with drug treatment.

On the other hand, if the normal bacterial population is disturbed and the protection afforded by them is lost, harmful organisms may be allowed to proliferate and cause disease. Thus, the patient who takes a long course of therapy with a "broad-spectrum" antibiotic such as tetracycline may develop a severe infection with yeast organisms (moniliasis, candidiasis). The yeast organisms are normally limited to only token population in the intestinal tract by the large numbers of resident coliforms. The tetracycline drug kills virtually all intestinal bacteria but leaves unaffected yeast organisms that then have a clear field in which to multiply. *Superinfection* with yeast results. Although yeast infection is most often seen as whitish patches in the oral cavity, rectal and vaginal infection can also occur. The infection will persist until the yeast organisms are killed or until a strong normal flora of coliforms, which will inhibit monilial growth, is established. Drugs such as mycostatin (Nystatin) will kill yeast organisms and products such as Lactinex, that contain intestinal bacteria, will re-establish a normal intestinal flora. Peaceful coexistence is thus restored.

If the immunity of the host is reduced or lost, serious consequences result from infection with "normal" resident organisms. Cancer patients taking anticancer drugs, which suppress the body's immune response, suffer from a wide variety of infections not usually seen in normal individuals. Pneumonia results from resident organisms proliferating in the respiratory tract. Systemic blood infection (sepsis) results from overwhelming bacterial invasion, often caused by former intestinal residents. If immunosuppressive drugs are used to block tissue rejection, as in a kidney transplant patient, the body's ability to resist infection from a resident or nonresident organism is greatly decreased and life-threatening infection often results.

MECHANISMS OF PATHOGENICITY

Pathogenicity is defined as the ability of an organism to cause disease. Some viruses, even though they have infected the body, are not pathogenic because the body is not harmed by them. The term *virulence* refers to the *degree* of pathogenicity. An extremely virulent organism causes severe disease when only a small number enter the body.

Whether or not an infecting organism will be pathogenic depends largely upon the number and types of harmful weapons it can use upon the host. Organisms with limited weaponry have low virulence and may even be normal residents (as in normal bacterial flora). An example of such an organism is *Streptococcus viridans*. Organisms that have developed several powerful weapons are quite virulent and often cause life-threatening infections. Such an organism is *Staphylococcus aureus*. Staphylococcal sepsis was usually a lethal infection in the 1940s and 1950s before specific antibiotics were developed for it. It is still a serious infection, even with the excellent drugs and supportive therapy available today. A discussion of common mechanisms of pathogenicity follows.

Toxin Production

Some bacterial organisms produce toxins that cause specific injury to the host. They are chemical substances secreted by the bacteria into the surrounding host tissue. These substances are called *exotoxins* and *endotoxins*.

Exotoxins

Exotoxins are usually proteins having a molecular weight of 10,000 to 900,000. They are most often secreted by gram-positive bacteria, and the bacterial cell is not destroyed in the process. Tetanus toxin, produced by the organism *Clostridium tetani,* is a good example. Other well-known exotoxins include those of diphtheria and botulism. In these cases, the infectious process is almost unimportant, except that it is the means by which toxin is released to the host. The great virulence of these infections comes from the potency of the exotoxin produced. Toxin from *Clostridium botulinum,* the causative agent in botulism, has a median lethal dose in white mice of 5×10^{-5} micrograms (μg). Exotoxins can be inactivated by the use of heat, prolonged storage, chemicals such as formaldehyde, or specific antitoxin preparations.

Endotoxins

Endotoxins are polysaccharide compounds closely associated with the bacterial cell wall. They are usually secreted by gram-negative bacteria, and secretion involves cell wall destruction. Endotoxins are relatively heat-stable and most have a molecular weight of 100,000 to 900,000. They frequently produce fever and other symptoms in man. Bladder infection with *Proteus vulgaris,* for example, causes low-grade fever that is due to endotoxin release. Inactivation of endotoxin occurs partly as a result of adsorption onto circulating white blood cells (leukocytes).

Enzyme Production   Many bacterial organisms produce enzymes that are indirectly harmful to the host. For instance, pathogenic staphylococci often produce *coagulase,* an enzyme that combines with factors in the serum to coagulate plasma. Coagulase also helps to form a protective wall around the infected areas, which impairs body defense mechanisms. This may also hinder the penetration of anti-infective drugs into the infected areas.

Clostridium perfringens, the causative organism in gas gangrene, forms *collagenase,* which destroys collagen, a connective tissue. This allows bacteria to spread more easily into body tissues.

Many streptococci produce *streptokinase,* an enzyme that activates fibrinolysin. Fibrinolysin dissolves small blood clots that would normally restrict the movement of the organism through the tissues.

Tissue spread of infection is also aided by secretion of *hyaluronidase* (produced by many streptococci, staphylococci, and pneumococci). Hyaluronidase dissolves the ground substance of the tissues and literally takes them apart.

Penicillin-resistant staphylococcal organisms such as *S. aureus* produce *penicillinase,* which inactivates most forms of penicillin. The discovery of penicillinase-resistant penicillins, such as oxacillin (Prostaphlin), and cephalosporin drugs, such as cephalothin (Keflin), has greatly aided the drug therapy of staphylococcal infections.

Many microorganisms produce compounds that dissolve red blood cells (erythrocytes) or leukocytes. These substances, called *hemolysins* and *leukocidins,* respectively, cause blockage of circulation with debris from the damaged cells and thus hinder the body's response to infection. *Streptolysin O,* formed by group A hemolytic streptococci is an example (see discussion of rheumatic fever in Chapter 10). Part of the pathogenicity of hemolytic streptococcal infection comes from erythrocyte destruction (hemolysis). Besides streptococci, some staphylococci, pneumococci, and coliforms also produce hemolysins.

Some of the pathogenic effect of virulent organisms may be due to body response to the infection rather than to specific compounds produced by the organism. Thus, in pneumococcal pneumonia, a major part of the harmful effect is caused by the formation of a large quantity of fibrin-containing edema fluid, along with erythrocytes and leukocytes, in the area of infection. This forms a semisolid mass in the lung (consolidation) and retards the healing process. Finally, liquefaction of the mass occurs and the debris is carried away or reabsorbed.

HOST DEFENSES   The battle between man and microbe is an unrelenting one from birth to death. With many organisms, a balance of power is thus established so that the organisms reside in or on, but do not harm, the host. Organisms that are more virulent have developed sophisticated mechanisms of pathogenicity. Host defenses, equally sophisticated, serve to counteract these mechanisms. Among the defenses available to the normal individual are skin, mucous membranes, and surface secretion, fever, leukocyte response, inflammatory response, and specific antibody production.

Skin and Surface Secretion

Normal skin is an excellent barrier to most organisms. The only chinks in the skin's armor are the hair follicles and the glands that produce perspiration and sebum (a waxy material). In these areas, special chemical secretions help to prevent microbial penetration. The acidic pH of normal skin helps to destroy bacteria or retard their growth. *Lysozyme,* an enzyme that dissolves susceptible bacteria, is present on the skin surface. Alterations in skin secretions, which affect pH, greatly change resistance to certain organisms. For example, ringworm (tinea) infection is much less common in adults than in children, primarily because of the increased content of fatty acids in sebaceous secretions that begins at puberty. The same secretions that protect against ringworm infection also increase the risk of infection with *Corynebacterium acnes,* the causative agent for acne.

If the protective barrier of the skin is lost by cutting, burning, or scraping, infection easily results. Likewise, if the keratin layer of the skin is damaged through excessive sweating, infection may result. Skin infections are more common in the summer and in tropical climates in general. Interestingly enough, other body surfaces do not require the degree of integrity that the skin does. Minor injuries to the lining of the oral cavity, esophagus, or stomach rarely result in infection. Even oral surgery is only occasionally accompanied by infection. Underlying tissue seems to help resist infection.

Mucous membranes, which line the oral cavity, respiratory tract, and other body areas, continually secrete a film of mucus that entraps bacteria. The action is similar to that of flypaper. In addition, the film is constantly moving toward body openings for removal. In the respiratory tract and in some other areas, special cells having hairlike projections (cilia) help to move particles and drops of mucus away from closed areas where infection could begin more easily. Organisms are also removed by the normal flow of tears, saliva, and urine. Finally, gastric acid and proteolytic enzymes help to destroy organisms that have somehow passed the first line of defense in the oral cavity. This mechanism is also important for respiratory pathogens that have been coughed up and swallowed.

Fever

Most systemic bacterial infections and some infections with other organisms cause fever. Although fever is sometimes useful in altering the environment of the infecting organisms in an adverse way, this is not always the case. Some organisms grow poorly if the temperature is increased by only a degree or two. Many, however, are relatively unaffected by this change. Fever, therefore, may be an important body defense, or it may be an incidental finding in infection. "Fever therapy" was an early treatment for syphilis and for mental disorders. Infection with malaria was established, and the resulting fever often improved the underlying condition. Interestingly, the only mental patients who were improved by this treatment were those later found to be suffering from syphilis affecting the central nervous system. The syphilis organism, having very specific requirements for growth, was killed by the high temperature.

Endotoxins from bacteria trigger fever production by causing release of *endogenous pyrogens* from damaged leukocytes. Endogenous pyrogens are proteins that have a molecular weight of 10,000 to 20,000 and act on the hypothalamic thermoregulatory center. Body temperature is "reset," much as a furnace thermostat can be reset to a higher temperature. Besides endotoxin production, other situations provoke the release of endogenous pyrogen. These include viral infection, inflammatory reactions, neoplastic growth, and exposure to certain drugs and chemicals.

Leukocyte Response

Normal Leukocyte Count

The leukocyte count is the number of leukocytes per cubic millimeter of blood. In the normal, healthy person, the value is 5000 to 10,000/mm^3. Often a *differential* leukocyte count is performed in addition to a total leukocyte count. In this, the relative percentage of each type of leukocyte is determined. In practice, a random count of 100 leukocytes is made from a blood sample, The number of each cell type is then expressed as per cent (Table 2–2).

Leukocytes consist of *granulocytes*, which include eosinophils, basophils, and neutrophils, and *agranulocytes*, consisting of lymphocytes and monocytes. Granulocytes contain granules in the cytoplasm of the cell, whereas agranulocytes have a relatively clear cytoplasm. Granulocytes exist in two major forms. Immature forms have a nonsegmented nucleus and are termed *bands* or *stabs* (Fig. 2–1), whereas mature granulocytes have a segmented nucleus and are called *segs*.

In practice, only the band forms of *neutrophils* are usually considered, since they represent the vast majority. Since new, immature cells are formed to replace cells that die or are used during infection, knowing the relative proportion of bands versus segs is often helpful. During acute infection, when large numbers of segs are needed, the band population is increased to provide them. This is called a *shift to the left*. Later, as the infection subsides, the relative proportion of segs increases and the proportion of bands decreases *(shift to the right)*. This is a sign of recovery.

The various types of leukocytes have different functions. *Neutrophils* are primarily *phagocytic*. They act by engulfing and digesting organisms and products of infection. Lysozymes and other chemicals within the cell aid in the digestion process. *Eosinophils* are thought to have a phagocytic action against antigen-antibody complexes and are of importance in allergic reactions and in certain types of parasitic infection (e.g., roundworm infestation). *Basophils* are poorly under-

Table 2–2. TYPICAL DIFFERENTIAL LEUKOCYTE COUNT

Type of Leukocyte	Count (%)
Neutrophils (bands—0–5%; segs—40–65%)	40–65
Eosinophils	1–3
Basophils	0–1
Lymphocytes	20–40
Monocytes	4–8

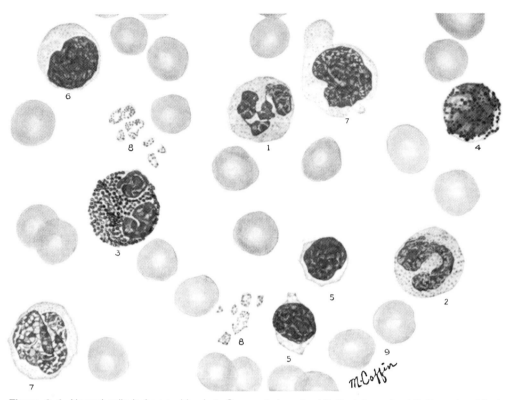

Figure 2–1. Normal cells in human blood. *1,* Segmented neutrophil; *2,* stab neutrophil; *3,* eosinophil; *4,* basophil; *5,* small lymphocyte; *6,* large lymphocyte; *7,* monocyte; *8,* platelet (thrombocyte); *9,* red blood cell (erythrocyte). (From Custer, R. P. (ed.): *An Atlas of the Blood and Bone Marrow,* 2nd ed. Philadelphia, W. B. Saunders Company, 1974.)

stood as to function. *Lymphocytes* are involved in the immune response (see Chapter 4) , which may result from infection. *Monocytes* have a phagocytic action and are largely involved in the cleanup of debris from an infection. *Macrophages* are highly phagocytic cells derived from monocytes and certain other cells. These are found primarily in areas where infection or tissue damage has occurred.

The process of phagocytosis is aided by the formation of *opsonins,* compounds in the blood stream that coat bacteria. Opsonins are often called the "salt and pepper" that makes the organisms more "tasty" to the phagocytic cells (Fig. 2–2).

Leukocytosis
Infection with most bacteria or with certain other organisms results in an increase in the leukocyte count (leukocytosis). Usually the count is between 10,000 and 20,000/mm³. Often there is a shift to the left as an increased number of band forms are released from the bone marrow in response to infection. As previously mentioned, these mature into segmented granulocytes. The response is much like a military operation, in which existing troops are mobilized for action and additional young troops are trained for combat. With certain infections, notably mononucleosis and pertussis (whooping cough), there is a strong shift to the left and intense leukocytosis, resulting in a leukocyte count of 20,000 to 30,000/mm³. This is termed a *leukemoid reaction.* The blood picture is similar to that seen in acute leukemia. Some viral infections do not trigger marked

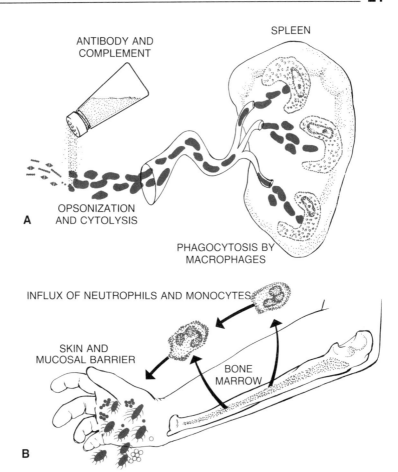

ANTIBODY AND
COMPLEMENT

SPLEEN

OPSONIZATION
A AND CYTOLYSIS

PHAGOCYTOSIS BY
MACROPHAGES

INFLUX OF NEUTROPHILS AND MONOCYTES

SKIN AND
MUCOSAL BARRIER

BONE
MARROW

Figure 2–2. Normal defenses against infection. *(A)* Opsonization and phagocytosis. *(B)* Skin and mucosal barrier.

B

leukocytosis, and other body defenses must be used to combat the illness.

When infection causes leukocytosis, often the neutrophil fraction increases the most. Thus, with common infections caused by staphylococci, pneumococci, and coliforms, the term *neutrophil leukocytosis* (neutrophilia) is often used.

It should be recognized that other conditions besides infection can cause leukocytosis. Inflammatory reactions, tissue necrosis, and neoplastic disease are all associated with an elevated leukocyte count.

Inflammatory Response

Any injury to tissue, including that caused by infection, results in an inflammatory response (see Chapter 3). The consequences of this response may be helpful to the host defense system. For example, the fluid exudate formed during an inflammatory response contains antibodies and other substances that suppress infection. The *cellular exudate,* which contains granulocytes and monocytes, aids in the phagocytosis of bacteria and cellular debris. In addition, *opsonins* and *fibrin,* components of the cellular exudate, aid in the phagocytic process. Opsonins coat bacteria to render them more easily engulfed, and fibrin threads trap bacteria for easier phagocytosis. Finally, endogenous *pyrogen* and *lysozymes* are released from leukocytes in the cellular exudate. These aid in body defense against infection, as previously discussed.

Specific Antibody Formation

In many cases, infection triggers the formation of antibodies specific for an antigen from the invading organism. These antibodies are specific for that particular strain of organism but generally not for anything else. Interaction between antigen and antibody results in inactivation of the antigen. For example, as previously mentioned, infection with hemolytic streptococci causes hemolysis of erythrocytes as a result of the release of the streptococcal antigen, streptolysin O. The infected individual then forms an antibody, antistreptolysin O, that neutralizes the antigen. For a more complete discussion of antigen-antibody interaction, see Chapter 4.

TYPES OF PATHOGENIC ORGANISMS

Although all infections may be considered parasitic because the organism lives off the host, some are specifically called parasitic diseases. These include infections caused by plasmodia (e.g., malaria), helminths (e.g., pinworm infection), trichomonads, (e.g., vaginal infection) and amebae (e.g., intestinal infection) as well as many others. The reader is referred to the many excellent texts on parasitic diseases for further information. This discussion will consider only common infections caused by bacteria, rickettsiae, fungi, and viruses.

Bacteria

Bacteria are single-celled organisms that are plantlike but lack chlorophyll. When treated with Gram's stain (crystal violet, then iodine, then alcohol), some bacteria retain the color of the dye after alcohol treatment and are designated *gram positive*. Those in which alcohol washes out the color are called *gram negative*. This color designation is important, since structural and behavioral properties of organisms often seem to separate on the basis of staining. Among the bacteria of importance to humans are gram-positive and gram-negative cocci, gram-negative rods, mycobacteria, and spirochetes. Rickettsiae, although technically a form of bacteria, will be considered as a separate group.

Cocci

Cocci are round bacteria that usually exist in multiple forms:

1. *Staphylococci* are gram-positive and grow in clusters like grapes (Fig. 2–3). Most strains of staphylococci produce hemolysins and coagulase as well as other compounds. Many strains, notably *S. aureus,* also produce penicillinase. Strains that are generally nonpathogenic, such as *S. epidermidis,* are usually nonhemolytic and do not produce coagulase or penicillinase. Staphylococcal infection causes local skin lesions (boils, impetigo) as well as many respiratory infections (pneumonia) and gastroenteritis.

2. *Streptococci* are gram-positive and exist in chain form. They produce a variety of toxins and enzymes, including streptokinase, hyaluronidase, and hemolysin. A common human pathogen is beta-hemolytic streptococcus group A, which forms streptolysin O and triggers body production of antistreptolysin O. This organism is the causative factor in most cases of impetigo, glomerulonephritis, and rheumatic fever. Normal residents, such as *S. viridans,* do not produce hemolysins or other compounds and are therefore of limited pathogenicity except in unusual circumstances.

3. *Pneumococci* are gram-positive and exist in double form (diplococci), often arranged in chains. They do not produce toxins

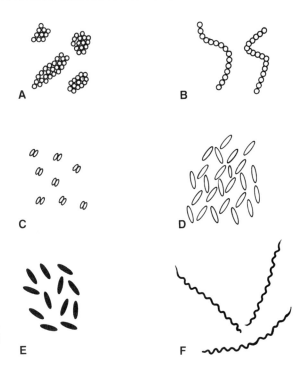

Figure 2–3. Different types of bacteria. *(A)* Staphylococci. *(B)* Streptococci. *(C)* Diplococci. *(D)* Rods. *(E)* Mycobacteria. *(F)* Spirochetes.

or enzymes of importance but cause a tissue reaction in which a large quantity of fibrinous fluid is produced at the site of infection (see the previous discussion of consolidation). Human disease often results from lowered resistance and invasion of pneumococci that are already in the vicinity. Pneumococci cause about 30 varieties of pneumonia as well as ear and sinus infections.

4. *Neisseriae* are gram-negative diplococci. A few forms are normal residents of the respiratory tract and are generally of little importance. Two forms cause important human diseases: *Neisseria gonorrhoeae* is the causative agent in gonorrhea, and *N. meningitidis* causes meningitis.

Gram-Negative Rods

Rod-shaped, gram-negative bacteria form an important group of pathogenic organisms (Fig. 2–3). Most strains are found in the intestinal tract as residents (coliforms). They become pathogenic when they leave their usual surroundings and enter other body areas. Most produce endotoxin and some produce antibiotic substances that kill or inhibit neighboring bacteria (bacteriocins).

Escherichia coli, for instance, causes urinary tract infection, meningitis, and sepsis in debilitated patients. Pathogenic strains of *E. coli* exist that cause intestinal infection, even though other strains are normal intestinal residents. *Enterobacter aerogenes* causes urinary tract infection and, occasionally, systemic sepsis. *Proteus vulgaris* is a common urinary tract pathogen ("vulgaris" means common). It exists in many forms, many of which are quite drug-resistant. *Pseudomonas aeruginosa* is a well-known pathogen that causes urinary tract infection and meningitis. As with many other gram-negative rods, sepsis with Pseudomonas occurs in debilitated patients, in the young, or in the elderly.

Salmonella and *Shigella* are not among the usual coliforms.

Some individuals, however, may harbor these gram-negative rods in the intestinal tract. Often they do not become ill themselves because they develop a resistance to the organisms. They can, though, spread the bacteria to other people, especially if they work in the food industry ("Typhoid Mary"). *Salmonella enteritidis* causes gastroenteritis, and other salmonellae cause typhoid fever and sepsis. *Shigella dysenteriae* causes severe gastroenteritis (dysentery) but only rarely causes sepsis.

Mycobacteria

Bacteria that exhibit some properties of fungi are termed *mycobacteria* (Fig. 2–3). They are rod-shaped and do not stain easily, but once stained, they are resistant to decolorization using acid-alcohol solution (Ziehl-Neelsen technique). Thus, they are called *acid-fast*. Acid-fastness is largely due to the presence of a protective cell wall that contains lipids, waxes, polysaccharides, and proteins. This prevents penetration by stain. However, once a stain succeeds in entering the cell, it is removed only with difficulty. The same protective wall makes penetration with drugs or body chemicals poor, and treatment of mycobacterial infections is often long and difficult. Most mycobacterial strains elicit a granulation reaction that further surrounds the infectious lesion with a body tissue barrier (see Chapter 3). The most important mycobacteria are *Mycobacterium tuberculosis* (tuberculosis) and *M. leprae* (leprosy).

Atypical forms of mycobacteria also exist. These cause several different types of human disease. Atypical mycobacteria have many similarities to the organisms that cause tuberculosis and leprosy, but they often infect in different ways. They have somewhat different properties and growth requirements when cultured. Infections are acquired from soil or animal sources but not by human-to-human contact, as with tuberculosis. An example is *M. scrofulaceum*, which causes lymph node infections in the neck area (cervical adenitis). Because many strains are resistant to standard antituberculous drugs, surgical excision of the infected tissue is often the treatment of choice.

Spirochetes

Spirochetes are slender, spiral-shaped organisms that do not stain easily with Gram's stain (Fig. 2–3). They are virtually transparent and must be specially treated to be visible. One technique for visualization is to angle the light from the microscope lamp indirectly through the preparation, allowing the organisms to contrast more with the surrounding medium. This is called *darkfield illumination*. There are now techniques in which spirochetes can be made to fluoresce that greatly improve visibility. Spirochetes may provoke an immune response, in which small numbers of organisms cause a severe tissue reaction, leading to damage. The most important spirochete in human disease is *Treponema pallidum*, the causative agent for syphilis. Other spirochetes also cause leptospirosis and Vincent's angina (trenchmouth).

Rickettsiae

Rickettsiae were once thought closely related to viruses, but they are now considered a form of small bacterium. They produce toxins and multiply within small blood vessels, leading to vascular thrombosis and tissue necrosis. Most rickettsiae require an insect *vector* for transmission to humans. Therefore, the transmission is either from infected animal to vector to human or, occasionally, from infected human to vector to human. Two well-known human rickettsial diseases are Rocky Mountain spotted fever, caused by *Rickettsia rickettsii* and transmitted by ticks, and louse-borne typhus, cause by *R. prowazekii.*

Fungi   Although some fungal organisms perform useful functions in the environment, such as aiding in the production of bread and cheese, about 100 species are pathogenic for humans. These are divided into two general categories: the *superficial fungi,* which cause surface infection, and the *deep fungi,* which cause infection of the lungs and other body organs. Fungi generally do not produce toxins but cause a granulation reaction in the host, leading to tissue damage (note the similarity to mycobacteria).

Many common superficial infections in humans are caused by fungi. Athlete's foot (tinea pedis) and ringworm of the scalp (tinea capitis) are caused by fungi called *dermatophytes.* These organisms digest the keratin tissue of skin, hair, or fingernails. Systemic therapy of these conditions requires the use of griseofulvin (Fulvicin), a unique drug that penetrates into keratin tissue. Infection with *Candida albicans* (candidiasis, moniliasis) is another common fungal condition occurring on the surface mucosa of the oral cavity, intestinal tract, or vagina.

Deep mycotic infections involve body organs and deeper tissues, such as bones or, rarely, the central nervous system. Examples are histoplasmosis, caused by *Histoplasma capsulatum* and coccidioidomycosis, caused by *Coccidioides immitis.* Both infections start in the lung, but may occasionally spread to involve other body organs. For a discussion of deep mycotic infections, see Chapter 9.

Viruses   Among the most peculiar of the microorganisms that infect humans are the viruses. These consist of only a protein structure containing ribonucleic acid (RNA) or deoxyribonucleic acid (DNA) and have no cell machinery for energy production or self-contained reproduction. There is debate as to whether viruses are truly alive. They attach to cells of the host and inject RNA or DNA, which takes control of the host cell (Fig. 2–4). In this way they reproduce by directing the host cell to synthesize new viral protein and nucleic

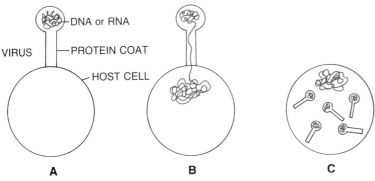

Figure 2–4. Viral infection of host cells. *(A)* Attachment. *(B)* Injection. *(C)* Control.

acid. Viruses cannot reproduce if there is no host cell to use. Since viruses grow only in living cells, culture is often difficult and special tissue culture techniques are required.

Viruses cause a variety of human diseases—probably even more than are currently recognized. Chickenpox, measles, and mumps are examples of common childhood viral diseases. The common cold is caused by a wide variety of *rhinoviruses* and *adenoviruses*. This wide variety of viruses and the short-term immunity developed after illness with these has made the development of a cold vaccine extremely difficult. *Arboviruses* are transmitted by a vector (mosquito, tick, or fly) in a manner similar to that of the rickettsiae. Yellow fever, transmitted by mosquitoes, is an example. Other serious human viral diseases include hepatitis, caused by *hepatitis virus A* and *B*, and rabies, caused by a *rhabdovirus* that infects the nerve tissue of animals and is spread through the saliva. *Herpesvirus* causes shingles (zoster) and various external lesions on the skin or mucous membranes. Genital herpes infection is currently of serious concern, since it can cause birth defects if the mother is infected during pregnancy. There is also evidence that it increases the risk of cervical cancer.

Viruses that have an extremely long incubation period and that can withstand heat, formaldehyde, and irradiation treatment are now recognized. These *slow viruses* may cause several progressive neurologic disorders formerly thought to be degenerative illnesses.

Drug therapy of viral infections has been limited, since most drugs that would kill the virus particles also kill the host cells. However, drugs are now available that block stages in the viral takeover of the host cell and thus do not damage the host cells. Two widely used antiviral drugs are amantadine (Symmetrel), for the treatment of *influenza A* (Asian "flu"), and idoxuridine (Stoxil), for herpes-induced conjunctivitis.

SUMMARY

We live in a world filled with microorganisms. With some we establish a balance that may be mutually beneficial. Others are pathogenic because of special abilities they have to harm the host. The host, likewise, is equipped with a myriad of defense mechanisms to ensure survival. Specific drug therapy is one of the most useful weapons we have.

Questions

1. Using sterile techniques, scientists in a few laboratories can raise animals that have virtually no resident bacteria. What might happen if these animals were exposed to a typical bacterial environment?
2. The immunosuppressive drug azathioprine (Imuran) is used to treat an inflammatory disease called *lupus erythematosus.* What might be a common problem associated with treatment with this type of drug?
3. Do you think that organisms are developing new mechanisms of pathogenicity? How can the host respond to these new weapons, if formed?

Additional Reading

Body defenses. Pharmacy Times, May 1978, p. 55.

Rahal, J. J., and Simberkoff, M. S.: Antibiotics and how to use them. Postgrad. Med., 62(3) to 64(2), 1977 to 1978.

Ross, S., et al.: Staphylococcal susceptibility to penicillin G: The changing pattern among community strains. J.A.M.A., 229:1075, 1974.

CHAPTER 3

INFLAMMATION

Throughout life the human organism is exposed to a variety of harmful influences. From the shock of birth itself to the terminal illness, life is a series of body reactions to external or internal trauma. As previously discussed, factors such as radiation or exposure to irritating chemicals challenge the body's well-being and cause a tissue response. Internal, poorly understood chemical processes also trigger tissue response in conditions such as rheumatoid arthritis. Interestingly, the tissue responses are often similar or identical, regardless of the inciting traumatic event. An infection with hemolytic streptococci causes a tissue reaction in the joints identical to that caused by rheumatoid arthritis, a condition not associated with streptococcal infection. Tissue irradiation causes changes similar to those induced by ischemia or mechanical injury. It appears that the body is "designed" to meet a variety of challenges with a uniform package of defenses.

Inflammation can be defined as the tissue reaction to nonlethal injury. Basically, it consists of blood vessel dilation associated with increased vessel permeability to plasma and leukocytes. Under special conditions, correction of this acute condition does not occur and chronic inflammation results.

Acute inflammation is usually considered to be a helpful body response, since it tends to localize the area of injury and allow the body to resist further injury and clear away cellular debris. In some situations, however, the tissue reaction causes more harm than the initial event itself. In one case, a woman inhaled a bee, which flew down her throat. The bee encountered the woman's vocal cords, which were exploding apart violently as she tried to cough up the bee. The bee promptly stung her on one vocal cord, eliciting an acute inflammatory reaction with its venom. The cord became greatly swollen and caused severe breathing difficulty (dyspnea) and ghastly noises as she tried to breathe (laryngeal stridor). Quick treatment by an ear, nose, and throat specialist, using an anti-inflammatory drug and an antihistamine, avoided the necessity for a tracheotomy.

ACUTE INFLAMMATION

It was recognized as early as the first century A.D. that nonspecific changes occur in the tissues in response to inflammatory stimuli. Celsus described *rubor, tumor, calor,* and *dolor* as the four leading findings in inflammation (Table 3–1). Much later, Hunter maintained that inflammation is a nonspecific response with a helpful effect on the host. This was at the end of the 18th century, but the idea was not accepted at that time. We now know that the tissue alterations occurring in inflammation are usually nonspecific and helpful to the host. Without them, most harmful stimuli would be allowed to spread out more and cause greater tissue destruction than is normally the case.

27

Table 3–1. FEATURES OF ACUTE INFLAMMATION

Celsus's Original Term	Modern Term
Rubor	Erythema
Tumor	Edema
Calor	Warmth
Dolor	Pain
—	Loss of Function

Symptoms and Signs

The terminology of acute inflammation has changed since Celsus's early description, but the meaning is the same. Rubor described the erythema or redness occurring during inflammation; tumor, the edema or swelling; calor, the warmth felt; and dolor, the pain accompanying inflammatory changes in the tissues. A fifth feature, *loss of function of the affected body area,* has been added since Celsus's time. For example, an inflamed joint is kept from flexing or is "favored" to avoid pain and discomfort. The suffix *-itis* denotes inflammation but does not specify a cause for it. The term *arthritis,* therefore, refers to inflammation of the joints, *laryngitis,* inflammation of the larynx, and so forth. Some inflammatory diseases are incorrectly named. Lupus erythematosus and scleroderma are inflammatory disorders but lack the *-itis* ending. This probably reflects the lack of understanding of the etiology and pathogenesis of these disorders when the names were assigned.

Causes

Acute inflammation can result from a variety of causes (Table 3–2):

1. *Physical agents* are frequent causes. These include cuts, scrapes, crush injuries, and the effects of extreme heat, cold, or radiation exposure. Tissue damage is due to physical trauma, and a nonspecific inflammatory response occurs.

2. *Chemical agents* can also initiate inflammation. Most foreign chemicals introduced into body tissues have this effect. A good example is iodine solution, which is used as an antiseptic. Considerable tissue damage often results from application of iodine solution to cuts or scratches. In addition, a number of normal body compounds can cause inflammation when released into the tissues. Examples of these include *kinins,* such as bradykinin, *prostaglandins,* and *histamine.* The exact role of these in inflammatory diseases is not clear at present, but there is evidence that these may be etiologic agents for certain diseases. Histamine, the best known of these compounds, is closely associated with allergic reactions involving the skin and upper respiratory tract. In these cases, release of histamine results in an acute inflammatory reaction.

3. *Impaired circulation* often results in acute inflammation. Thus, *ischemia* or *infarction* of tissue gives the typical nonspecific

Table 3–2. COMMON CAUSES OF ACUTE INFLAMMATION

Physical agents
Chemical agents
Impaired circulation
Infection
Immune reactions

results. In myocardial infarction, inflammation of the infarcted area occurs. This partly resolves if circulation to the area improves as a result of increased collateral blood supply. Likewise, ischemia of the leg caused by arterial blockage results in pain, redness, swelling, and the other typical inflammatory changes.

4. *Infection* results in tissue damage and inflammation. A good example is a *furuncle* or boil. Bacterial infection damages the skin and underlying tissue and inflammatory changes result.

5. *Immune reactions* often cause inflammation. In some cases, antibodies cause the tissue to be vulnerable to damage caused by antigens and damage results. This leads to inflammation. In other cases, a complex of the antigen and antibody is formed and the complex triggers an inflammatory response. (See Chapter 4 on immune response for further information.)

Cellular Changes   In general, acute inflammation consists of hyperemia, decreased rate of blood circulation through the area, formation of a fluid exudate and formation of a cellular exudate. The process takes place as follows.

Hyperemia results from the opening of small arterioles and capillaries, which diverts blood that normally would pass through the area. Blood is retained in these vessels and redness and warmth result.

Next, the *rate of blood circulation through the area* decreases, also because of vasodilation, and stagnation of circulation (stasis) results. In addition, blood vessel permeability increases and plasma and cells are allowed to escape through the vessel wall. Since the loss of plasma is greater initially than that of cells, the blood left in the blood vessel becomes more viscous. Leukocytes begin to stick to the vessel wall as a consequence of increased blood viscosity and reduced flow rate. This is called *pavementation of the endothelium.* This action is likened to that of a stagnant stream, in which debris accumulates along the bank where movement is the slowest. This process may continue to the extent that small vessels are completely occluded with leukocytes.

The third event in the development of acute inflammation is the formation of a *fluid exudate* (Fig. 3–1). This occurs primarily as a result of leakage of water and protein from the plasma through the blood vessel wall. As plasma proteins move outside the vessel, they create an osmotic effect that pulls additional water out of the blood vessel. This increases the fluid tension in the surrounding tissues and contributes to edema and pain. The fluid exudate contains a number of substances that help the body to deal with the cause of the inflammation. Specific *antibacterial compounds* and *antibodies* help to suppress or prevent infection. *Fibrinogen* contained in the fluid exudate is converted to *fibrin,* the matrix of blood clots. Fibrin connects damaged tissue and forms a protective barrier over cuts to prevent bacterial invasion. In addition, it increases phagocytic action in the area to help remove bacteria or cellular fragments.

The fourth event consists of the formation of a *cellular exudate* (Fig. 3–2). This process is facilitated by the heavy layer of leukocytes that have accumulated on the inner walls of the blood vessels. Leukocytes—mostly granulocytes—move through the vessel wall

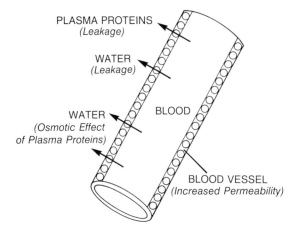

Figure 3–1. Formation of fluid exudate.

and appear outside in the area of inflammation. This is called *emigration of leukocytes*. Some lymphocytes and monocytes, along with an occasional erythrocyte, also frequently leak through. It is thought that the emigration of leukocytes is aided by attraction to certain chemical compounds produced by the body at the site of inflammation. The effect is like that of a magnet pulling iron fillings toward it and is called *chemotaxis*. Compounds produced by lymphocytes, called *lymphokines*, are thought responsible for this phenomenon.

The cellular exudate has several important functions in inflammation. The rich concentration of leukocytes in the area promotes phagocytosis of bacteria or other particles. Phagocytosis is enhanced by the presence of opsonins in the tissues (see Chapter 2). In addition, granulocytic leukocytes contain *pyrogen*, which causes a fever response (see Chapter 2), and *lysozymes*, which help to destroy dead tissue and facilitate a clean-up operation by the body. Cleanup is aided by the action of monocytes that become macrophages when they ingest cellular materials.

Consequences of Acute Inflammation

In most acute inflammations, body responses permit a complete return to normal. The tissues become as they were before the inflammatory event took place. This process, called *resolution*, is the

Resolution desired consequence of an inflammatory reaction and may be has-

Figure 3–2. Formation of cellular exudate.

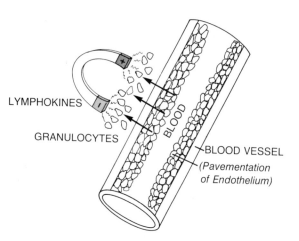

tened by the use of anti-inflammatory drugs. These agents generally block reactions that cause inflammation and thus allow the body to catch up on its clean-up procedures. Macrophages move in to remove battlefield debris, and fluid exudate is reabsorbed via the circulatory and lymphatic systems.

Organization   If resolution does not take place soon enough, there may be other consequences to acute inflammation. If the cellular and fluid exudates are not removed quickly enough, fibrous tissue will invade the area, leading to scar tissue formation. This is *organization.* Examples include the residual scarring of the lungs after pneumococcal pneumonia and the formation of adhesions after abdominal surgery. If necrosis occurs to the extent that resolution is impossible, a cavity containing dead tissue and granulocytes may form. The liquid within the cavity is called *pus* and consists of living and dead microorganisms, necrotic tissue, exudate material, and granulocytes (pus cells). The cavity is called an *abscess.* Abscesses occur occasionally with unresolved streptococcal or staphylococcal pneumonia, and this is terminal *empyema.* Treatment involves antibiotic therapy and, occasionally, drainage of the area to facilitate resolution. Failure to resolve any abscess may lead to a thickening of its contents as a result of reabsorption of water (inspissation) and, eventually, to *calcification* of the area. If the cause of acute inflammation is not removed, the processes of tissue injury and repair continue simultaneously. This leads to *chronic inflammation,* often referred to as "frustrated healing."

CHRONIC   Several situations can lead to a chronic inflammatory response.
INFLAMMATION   Inhalation of *insoluble particles* can lead to chronic lung irritation. The particles are difficult to remove by ciliary action of the bronchial
Causes   mucosa or by expectoration. Asbestos miners and quarry workers are especially prone to chronic lung inflammation (asbestosis, silicosis). Asbestosis may eventually result in malignant tumors of the lung or pleural membrane (mesothelioma).

Infections caused by organisms that evoke a weak body response may persist and cause chronic inflammation. Tuberculosis and syphilis are examples of chronic inflammatory diseases perpetuated by a poor body response. The organisms are not promptly eradicated by body defenses and cause a *chronic granulation reaction* in the tissues. Body response in these cases is one of *hypersensitivity* to the organism or its component(s). Thus, tuberculosis and syphilis result in the formation of inflammatory lesions out of proportion to the number of organisms actually present. In rheumatic fever, the complex formed between streptococcal antigen and tissue antibody causes chronic inflammation of the heart lining (endocarditis).

Another situation in which hypersensitivity evokes chronic inflammation is in the so-called "autoimmune" disorders. In these conditions, for poorly understood reasons, the body apparently produces antibodies against its own tissues. Lupus erythematosus and rheumatoid arthritis are good examples of this phenoneum. Sometimes the antibodies can be detected in the bloodstream and may aid in diagnosis of the condition. *Rheumatoid factor,* an antibody, is found in the blood stream of many people suffering from rheumatoid arthritis.

Types of Chronic Conditions

Chronic Granulomatous Inflammation

As previously mentioned, certain chronic infections to which the body responds with a weak defense result in chronic inflammation. In these cases, which include tuberculosis and syphilis, the body attempts to repair the damage by forming a *granuloma*. The process is *chronic granulomatous inflammation*. Granulomas consist of macrophages that have accumulated in the area combined with *granulation tissue*. Granulation tissue is made up of *endothelial cells*, which form blood and lymph vessels; *fibroblasts*, which form collagen tissue; and *plasma cells*, which secrete immunoglobulins. Sometimes the older terms *tuberculoma* and *syphiloma* are used to describe these particular granulomas.

Chronic Suppurative Inflammation

In this other major type of chronic inflammation, an abscess is created as a result of a persistent infection. "Suppurative" refers to the formation of pus. *Osteomyelitis* is a condition representing this process. Infection within the bone marrow, often with staphylococci, results in formation of an abscess within the relatively inaccessible bone interior. Blood supply is limited and, therefore, body defenses are poor. Chronic suppurative inflammation is easily established. Surgical drainage and the use of specific antibiotics may result in cure.

Consequences of Chronic Inflammation

Some chronic inflammations show evidence of *regeneration*. The body partially repairs the tissue damage by bringing fibroblasts to the inflamed area. These form collagen tissue, which results in *fibrosis* or scarring of the area. This process is somewhat beneficial, but may result in destruction of small blood vessels. As a result, scar tissue, containing no functional blood vessels, remains. Later, the scar may contract (contracture) and cause functional or cosmetic changes in the tissues. We're all aware of the disfigurement caused by a burned, scarred area on the skin. Similar scarring occurs in internal body areas as a result of chronic inflammation and may lead to loss of function. For example, rheumatoid arthritis may lead to scarring of joint surfaces and loss of joint motility. The same process leads to heart valve damage and loss of valve function in rheumatic fever.

Occasionally, regeneration may portend serious disease. Dentists and dental hygienists are well aware of the chronic inflammation of the mucosa of the palate caused by pipe or cigar smoking. The same changes can also occur in the buccal (cheek) area as a result of chewing tobacco or dipping snuff. Whitish patches of cells grow in the inflamed area to replace the damaged cells, and the condition is known as *leukoplakia*. The danger of leukoplakia is that if the inflammatory stimulus is not removed, it may progress to oral cancer. If the stimulus *is* removed, the tissues eventually revert to normal.

SUMMARY

Although there are many causes for acute inflammation, the body responds in much the same way to all. Erythema, edema, warmth, pain, and loss of function are the usual results. Acute inflammation is associated with hyperemia, increased blood vessel permeability, and the formation of fluid and cellular exudates. Acute inflammation that does not resolve may progress to organization, suppuration, or chronic inflammation. Although the inflammatory response is generally a protective and beneficial one, certain consequences may be harmful to the host.

Questions

1. Except for its role in gastric acid production, histamine primarily causes unpleasant allergic reactions. Of what possible benefit to the body is histamine?
2. Simple organisms, such as amebae, lack the capability of an inflammatory response. How do they deal with threatening outside influences, such as bacteria or particulate matter they encounter?
3. Ulcerative colitis, a chronic inflammatory disease of the colon, carries an increased risk of cancer of the colon. How is this condition similar to leukoplakia of the oral cavity?

Additional Reading

Ryan, G., and Majno, G.: Acute inflammation, a review. Am. J. Pathol., 86:185, 1977.

Zarro, V. J.: New nonsteroidal anti-inflammatory drugs. Am. Fam. Physician, 14:142, 1976.

Zigmond, S. H.: Chemotaxis by polymorphonuclear leukocytes. J. Cell Biol., 77:269, 1978.

CHAPTER 4

IMMUNE RESPONSE

Immunity is defined as the state of being resistant to injury, particularly by poisons, foreign proteins, and parasites. If we ignore poisons, which often are rendered less harmful by the use of specific drug products (antidotes), there remain foreign proteins and parasites as agents of potential injury to the body. The body response to most parasitic infections (bacterial, viral, or other) includes the formation of compounds having specific harmful effects on the invading organism. Likewise, the entry of foreign proteins into the body evokes a somewhat similar response. In both situations, the body is taking steps to rid itself of an unwanted visitor. The extent to which the body can inactivate the effects of infiltration by "foreign invaders" is the degree of immunity developed.

SELF VERSUS NONSELF

An amazing feature of humans and other higher animal forms is the ability to distinguish their own cells and other components from those foreign to the body (Fig. 4–1). This requires a surveillance mechanism of some sort that appears to develop during embryonic life. For example, if the wrong type of blood is accidentally transfused, a reaction leading to hemolysis of the transfused erythrocytes may occur. The body not only is aware of what its own cells are but also recognizes the transfused cells as being foreign and engages immunologic machinery to destroy the .foreign cells. The same process applies to infection with bacteria or to allergic responses. An outside agent causes the body to respond in a defensive manner.

The ability to distinguish *self* from *nonself* is not present immediately after fertilization of the egg but develops some time later (Fig. 4–2). Experiments with mouse embryos have shown that if cells from another mouse or even another animal species are

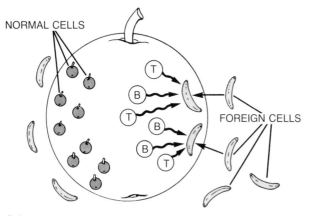

NORMAL CELLS

FOREIGN CELLS

Figure 4–1. Recognition of self versus nonself. Invasion of foreign cells into mature organism causes immediate formation of B and T lymphocytes that destroy or inactivate cells.

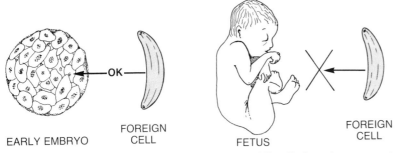

Figure 4–2. Development of self- versus non–self-ability. Early embryos accept foreign cells as their own and convert them to body cells. Later, the fetus rejects foreign cells as shown in Figure 4–1.

EARLY EMBRYO   FOREIGN CELL   FETUS   FOREIGN CELL

injected into the embryo very early in its development, the mouse develops normally. The embryo somehow converts the foreign cells to mouse embryonic cells and they become part of the development scheme. If the same experiment is performed with more developed fetal mice, the cells are rejected. The fetus recognizes that these cells are foreign and destroys them.

ANTIGENS   Substances that cause an immune response are referred to as *antigens*. These are usually proteins (occasionally polysaccharides), having a molecular weight of between 10,000 and 100,000. Generally, substances of less than 10,000 molecular weight are nonantigenic and the antigenicity increases with increasing molecular weight. Antigenicity is partly determined by the number and type of specific antigenic sites on the molecule. These are called *determinant sites* or *epitopes*. The body recognizes not only the *size* of the antigen but also the *shape,* which includes the contributions of epitopes. It is possible for a molecule to have several epitopes, and it is also possible to remove epitopes and thus destroy the antigenicity of a molecule. Removal requires delicate biochemical techniques.

There are three steps in the immune response process:

1. First, the antigen must be *recognized* as being foreign. This requires an immunologically competent cell—one capable of such surveillance—usually a small lymphocyte.

2. Next, the antigen must be *processed.* Its epitopes must be "read" in such a way that a specific compound can be formed to neutralize it. This function is usually the responsibility of macrophages.

3. Finally, a specific compound is *produced* to neutralize the antigen. This is also a protein substance, designed using the antigen as a pattern, and is termed an *antibody.* In addition to antibodies, specially modified lymphocytes are also released into the area of immune response. These aid in neutralization of the antigen and are called *immune lymphocytes.*

HAPTENS   Some proteins are too small to evoke an antigenic response, but they contain determinant factors (antigenic determinants) like those of antigens. These compounds, called *haptens,* can combine with a larger molecule called a *carrier* and form an antigenic compound. For example, contact between a nickel watchband or

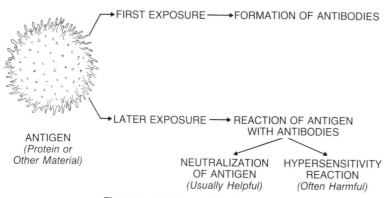

FIRST EXPOSURE ──────→ FORMATION OF ANTIBODIES

LATER EXPOSURE ──────→ REACTION OF ANTIGEN
                          WITH ANTIBODIES

ANTIGEN
*(Protein or
Other Material)*

NEUTRALIZATION   HYPERSENSITIVITY
OF ANTIGEN   REACTION
(Usually Helpful)   *(Often Harmful)*

Figure 4–3. Antigen-antibody response.

earring and skin often causes formation of an antigen. Nickel is the hapten, and a protein in skin is the carrier compound. The body reacts to the hapten carrier (antigen) and forms an antibody to it. Later contact with nickel forms additional antigen and evokes an immune response, leading to skin inflammation. An area of redness and edema develops under the watchband or in the area of contact of the earring. Iodine can also react with tissue proteins to form antigens. Inflammatory responses to iodine applied to the skin are quite common.

**ANTIBODY
RESPONSE**

As previously mentioned, contact with an antigen causes formation of antibodies and gives the body some protection against further antigenic effects. Subsequent contact with the same antigen causes an interaction between antigen and antibody (Fig. 4–3). This generally results in neutralization of the antigen, a helpful outcome. Sometimes the body reacts in a harmful way to the antigen-antibody complex and inflammation results. This is termed a *hypersensitivity reaction*. Examples of this include skin reactions, as in the case of nickel or iodine, or respiratory conditions, such as bronchial asthma. The term *allergy* is often used in place of hypersensitivity reaction. Allergic reactions will be discussed in greater detail later in this chapter.

**IMMUNOACTIVE
LYMPHOCYTES**

Lymphocytes are the cornerstone of the immune response. They are found in the blood stream as well as in lymph nodes, bone marrow, and in specialized lymphoid tissues such as the thymus gland and tonsils.

There are two types of lymphocytes involved in the immune response:

1. The *T lymphocytes* begin in the bone marrow as stem cells and migrate to the thymus gland, where maturation takes place. The mature cells then circulate through the lymphatic system and blood stream, spending part of the time in peripheral lymph nodes. T lymphocytes have a relatively long life span, perhaps 100 to 200 days, and can become sensitized by antigens. When sensitized, they interact with the sensitizing antigen and neutralize it (Fig. 4–4). In addition, there is evidence that they enhance or retard the immune response of other lymphocytes to allow an appropriate body response to occur. These particular T lymphocytes are designed *T-helper* or *T-suppressor cells*.

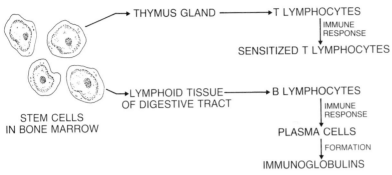

Figure 4–4. Types of lymphocytes and their formation.

2. The *B lymphocytes* also begin as stem cells in the bone marrow but migrate to lymphoid tissue in the colon, small intestine, and appendix for maturation. Mature B lymphocytes populate the peripheral lymph nodes, as do the T lymphocytes, but tend to stay localized and have a shorter life span. The ratio of B to T lymphocytes in the peripheral circulation is about 30:70.

The names of the lymphocytes indicate the area to which they migrate for maturation. For T lymphocytes, it is the thymus gland, as previously mentioned. In birds, B lymphocytes migrate to a structure known as the *bursa of Fabricius*. Although humans do not have an identical structure, it is thought that we have equivalent lymphoid tissue in the intestinal tract. Therefore, the terminology is retained. Upon antigenic stimulation, B lymphocytes are converted to *plasma cells*, which secrete *immunoglobulins*, the source of antibody protection.

Types of Immunoglobulins

Immunoglobulins are complex, high molecular weight proteins that can be separated by their patterns of migration across a charged plate (electrophoresis). Five categories have been identified:

1. *IgA* (immunoglobulin A) appears primarily in secretions from the skin and the respiratory, urinary, and gastrointestinal tracts. It appears to function in destroying bacteria that attempt body invasion from the outside.

2. *IgD* is present in very small quantities in the blood stream. It seems to aid the B lymphocytes in attaching to antigens.

3. *IgE* is intimately concerned with allergic reactions and is found attached to mast cells and basophils, as well as in small amounts in the blood stream. Mast cell rupture caused by IgE-antigen interaction forms the basis for allergic reactions.

4. *IgG* comprises about 80 per cent of the immunoglobulins. It functions to protect against infection with bacterial and viral organisms that have penetrated the body's outer defenses. Because it crosses the placental barrier and enters the fetal circulation, it is present at birth and gives immunity during the first few weeks of life. (Some immunoglobulins also appear in breast milk, giving extra antibody protection to the infant who is nursed). Among the antibodies making up IgG are hemolysins, precipitins, and hemagglutinins.

5. *IgM* appears first after an infectious challenge to the body. It aids IgG in body defenses, especially by means of its ability to cause cell lysis.

Immunoglobulin Response

Initial contact with an infectious agent causes a slowly developing level (titer) in the blood stream of primarily IgM. IgM titer reaches a peak after several weeks and then gradually decreases over several months to a low value. This is called the *primary response*. If another contact is made with the same agent, a faster, stronger response occurs and the titer shoots up higher than before. This is the *secondary response* and is associated mostly with formation of IgG. It appears that the body "remembered" the first encounter and that this memory facilitated a faster response the second time. This phenomenon is known as *immunologic memory* and may be aided by production of special lymphocytes called *memory cells* during first contact.

Immunologic memory is the basis for *booster shots,* which quickly bolster body defenses against infectious diseases. For example, in a person already immunized against tetanus (primary response), a booster injection will quickly build up IgG and protect against infection. This is the rationale for using a tetanus booster in a child who steps on a rusty nail. Since the child is already immunized against tetanus, immunologic memory is retained and the booster will quickly cause buildup of a titer of antitetanus antibodies. The relatively long incubation period of the tetanus organism gives time for this to happen. (This is not the case with infections in which the incubation period is very short).

It appears that the body remembers better for some infections than for others. Common childhood diseases such as chickenpox and mumps are rarely contracted more than once, since the memory for these is excellent and IgG titer is quickly raised upon a second exposure. On the other hand, syphilis and gonorrhea, unfortunately, are often acquired more than once by the same person. In these cases the body "forgets" as soon as the disease is cured and the individual again becomes vulnerable.

IMMUNIZATION

The process of rendering a person immune to an infectious agent is termed *immunization*. This consists of bolstering the body's defenses, primarily by increasing immunoglobulin formation. If the body is stimulated to produce its own immunoglobulins, *active immunity* results (Table 4–1). If immunoglobulin is applied to the host, *passive immunity* is developed. Both types of immunity can also be natural or artificial. *Natural immunity* develops from actual infection with a specific agent (active, natural) or by receiving immunoglobulin from the mother through the placenta before birth

Table 4–1. TYPES OF IMMUNITY

Type	Characteristics
Active	Results from contact with antigen; organism produces its own antibodies
Natural	Results from active infection
Artificial	Results from administration of a vaccine or toxoid
Passive	Results from "borrowing" antibodies from another human or animal
Natural	Results from transfer of antibodies via placenta or nursing
Artificial	Results from administration of antitoxin or antiserum

or via nursing after birth (passive, natural). *Artificial immunity* comes from the injection of antigenic material into the host (active, artificial) or by the use of immunoglobulin preparations (passive, artificial).

Active, Artificial Immunity

The most frequently used products for inducing active, artificial immunity are *vaccines* and *toxoids*.

Vaccine

Vaccines are suspensions of living, attenuated, or killed bacteria, rickettsia, or viruses. The choice of whether to use live, attenuated, or killed organisms depends upon the virulence and growth characteristics of the organism in question. Some organisms will infect and cause clinical disease if used in live form. In these cases, the organisms can be attenuated by growing them on poorly supportive media or by treating them with toxic agents to weaken them. For extremely invasive organisms, such as *Salmonella typhosa* (cause of typhoid fever), killed organisms are used. They still retain antigenicity, however, and will produce an immune response in the host. Common examples of vaccines are poliomyelitis (polio) vaccine and rubella (German measles) vaccine.

Toxoid

Toxoids are made from *toxins* produced by pathogenic bacteria ("toxoid" means "toxinlike"). These products are relatively pure, since the other bacterial components have been removed by filtration. The toxin thus obtained is treated with formaldehyde to weaken it but still retains antigenicity. Toxoids for tetanus and diphtheria are routinely used in childhood immunization. A few toxins are also available, primarily as diagnostic agents. Tiny amounts of these will react with the skin to cause inflammation if insufficient antibody is present in the host. Skin reaction, therefore, signifies susceptibility to the disease. An example is the *Schick test,* which uses diphtheria toxin to determine the antibody protection against diphtheria. It should be noted that this type of test merely measures the degree of protection and neither increases nor decreases the immunity for the disease itself.

Passive, Artificial Immunity

Two types of preparations are commonly used to produce passive, artificial immunity: *antitoxins* and *antisera*.

Antitoxin

Antitoxins are formed when toxins, or more often toxoids, are injected into animals. Horses are usually preferred because of their large size and generous blood volume. After the antitoxin titer is high enough, the animal is bled (not a lethal amount) and the blood is fractionated to obtain the portion containing the antitoxin. The purified fraction is an antitoxin, relatively free of other proteins, and is specific for a particular disease.

Tetanus antitoxin is a good example. These products provide a temporary "loan" of antibodies to the recipient and are used if exposure to the organism has already occurred and symptoms of disease are imminent or actually present. With tetanus, the toxoid would be used as a booster injection if exposure were suspected and if the time elapsed since the suspected exposure permitted adequate IgG titer to develop. If time did not permit the use of the toxoid booster, especially if symptoms were already developing, the anti-toxin would be the most helpful. The situation is likened to a quick trip to the finance company (antitoxin) as compared to a long-term bank account (toxoid immunization).

Antiserum

Antisera represent serum fractions containing antibodies. These contain antitoxins or other antibodies produced in response to immunization or infection. In the days before penicillin, antisera were prepared against the different types of pneumococcal pneumonia. The individual receiving the antiserum thus borrowed antibodies from someone who had recovered from infection with that particular strain of pneumococcal organism. The principle here is the same as with antitoxin preparations. The difference between antisera and antitoxins is that antisera contain other serum elements besides antitoxin. Some elements, such as hemolysins and hemagglutinins, may also contribute to defense against infection. Others, such as plasma elements, are primarily impurities.

Gamma globulin, obtained from pooled human blood, is an example of an antiserum. It contains a variety of antibodies and can be used as a "shotgun" treatment to increase body defenses against many infections. It is especially useful in certain viral infections for which vaccines and antitoxins do not exist. More specific antisera, such as that for mumps (mumps immune globulin), will give selective protection against a particular disease.

A problem that exists with antitoxins and with antisera obtained from animal blood is that these products may contain traces of animal serum proteins. Even relatively pure antitoxin preparations may contain small amounts of these "foreign proteins." In people who are highly sensitive to these, they may cause an allergic reaction, sometimes a life-threatening one. Often, a small test dose of the product is injected under the skin of the recipient before the recommended amount is given. If no reaction occurs with the test dose, a larger amount may be tried. The method is not foolproof, however, since the small test dose occasionally causes sensitization (but no reaction) itself, and a reaction then follows administration of the larger amount.

Suppressed Immune Response

Many drug products can depress the immune response and increase the likelihood of infection or the severity of an existing infection. *Corticosteroids,* used to treat a variety of inflammatory disorders, suppress the inflammatory response and thus reduce the symptoms and signs of inflammation. They can promote infection because they prevent lymphocyte responses necessary for organism control. An example is the spread of tuberculosis infection from its primary site in the lung to multiple sites (miliary spread) in patients given high-dose corticosteroid therapy. *Anticancer drugs,* which kill or prevent formation of malignant cells, have the same actions on lymphocytes, granulocytes, and other cells important to body defenses. Cancer patients taking these drugs develop a wide variety of infections not commonly seen in normal individuals.

Congenital deficiency in the ability to produce B lymphocytes, T lymphocytes, or both renders the individual susceptible to an assortment of infections that normally would be resisted by body defenses. Unfortunately, there is, at present, no way to correct the problem and the individual suffers from repeated infections. If the deficiency is slight, the person survives with the help of good medical care. In combined deficiency disease, the life span may be only a matter of months.

Acquired immune deficiency disease (AIDS) is becoming a recognized problem. The disorder is most often seen in homosexuals, Haitian refugees, and those receiving intravenous drugs. The cause of AIDS is not known at present, but the syndrome is thought to have an infectious etiology.

AUTOIMMUNITY   The immune response is quite complex, if we consider all the known steps involved in recognition of the antigen, processing, and formation of immunoglobulins and specialized lymphocytes. Occasionally, it appears that the body makes a mistake and targets the normal tissue or other component as a foreign invader. Why this happens is not known. Perhaps there is a defect in the surveillance system, so that a normal body component is misread as being an antigen. Normal tissue could also be marked in some way through minor chemical alteration, so that it *is* slightly different from normal. In this case, the surveillance system would be functioning correctly, although its purpose would be misdirected. In any event, the immune response is then directed against the target tissue and a disease state results. Diseases of this type are called *autoimmune diseases* ("auto" means "self"), since the body is, in effect, reacting against itself.

The number of disorders thought to be associated with autoimmune reactions is increasing almost daily. *Rheumatoid arthritis* is the best known of these. It consists of inflammatory reactions in the joints and other tissues that closely resemble the arthritic changes seen with rheumatic fever (see discussion of chronic inflammation in Chapter 3). Other less common disorders include *lupus erythematosus* (a systemic connective tissue disorder), *dermatomyositis*, and *scleroderma*. Dermatomyositis primarily affects the skin and muscular system; scleroderma is associated with inflammation of skin and most internal organs. *Myasthenia gravis*, a disease formerly thought to be caused by failure to manufacture adequate acetylcholine at the junction of somatic nerve ending and skeletal muscle (myoneural junction), is now thought due to an autoimmune reaction that damages the receptors for acetylcholine. Muscle weakness then occurs because the nerve message, carried by acetylcholine, produces too weak a response on the limited number of receptors remaining in the muscle. Rheumatic fever is discussed more fully in Chapter 10, and rheumatoid arthritis and lupus erythematosus are covered further in Chapter 17.

Causes of Immune   Several situations seem to initiate an autoimmune reaction:
Reactions   1. In some cases, it appears that antigen has been stored within tissue and is inaccessible to the surveillance system. Injury to the tissue causes release of the antigen and the body then recognizes it as foreign. An immune response results. The best example of this is in Hashimoto's thyroiditis, in which thyroglobulin leaks out of the thyroid tissue and causes formation of antithyroid antibodies. Inflammation of the thyroid gland then results.

2. If the tissue is damaged, as in burns or chemical destruction of the skin, the body senses the tissue alteration and forms antibodies against the "antigen" tissue. Skin inflammation and sloughing result.

3. If a hapten comes in contact with normal body protein, an antigen can be formed. The body then reacts to the new antigen and inflammation results. This is not completely autoimmune, since part of the antigen comes from outside.

4. If the body fails to recognize a normal component, antibodies may be directed against it. This seems to occur in hemolytic anemia associated with chronic lymphocytic leukemia. The body misreads the normal erythrocyte and produces an autohemolysin, which destroys normal erythrocytes, leading to anemia.

It should be pointed out that the etiology and pathogenesis of some disorders considered to have an autoimmune basis cannot be explained using these mechanisms and additional processes may be operating.

Organ-Specific and Non–Organ-Specific Responses

Antibodies formed during autoimmune reactions are of two types (Fig. 4–5). Some antibodies are specific for a particular tissue or organ and are called *organ-specific*. In Hashimoto's thyroiditis, mentioned previously, only the thyroid gland is affected. Other antibodies are *non-organ-specific* and attack several different body organs or tissues. Rheumatoid factor, an antibody found in the blood stream of some people suffering from rheumatoid arthritis, appears to be non-organ-specific. Besides joint inflammation, immune responses affecting the subcutaneous tissues, sclera of the eye and vascular system are often seen in rheumatoid arthritis. Systemic lupus erythematosus also seems to be caused by non-organ-specific antibodies acting on a variety of body components.

ALLERGY

Whereas autoimmune disorders are characterized by formation of antibodies against body tissues, allergic reactions result from contact with an external antigen, termed an *allergen*. In allergy, as in autoimmunity, the body appears to consider as foreign or threatening something that is relatively harmless. An immune reaction results, the symptoms of which are troublesome or even threatening to the host. Again, the body's mistake leads to an unnecessary immune response.

Allergens are usually proteins. Occasionally, however, other large molecules, such as polysaccharides, can cause allergic reactions. Although these are not really "self," they are not perceived as

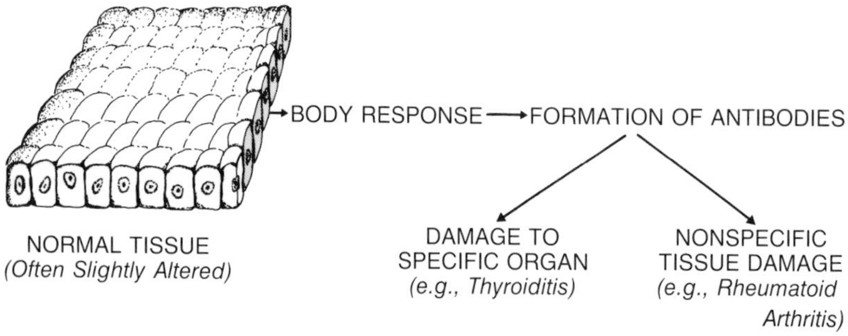

NORMAL TISSUE
(Often Slightly Altered)

→BODY RESPONSE──→FORMATION OF ANTIBODIES

DAMAGE TO SPECIFIC ORGAN *(e.g., Thyroiditis)*

NONSPECIFIC TISSUE DAMAGE *(e.g., Rheumatoid Arthritis)*

Figure 4–5. Autoimmune reaction.

"nonself" by the normal individual. The allergic person, however, reacts to these, presumably in an attempt to remove them from the body or to localize their effects, and inflammation results.

Types of Allergens

Common allergens include *inhalants,* such as pollen, dust, mold, and tobacco smoke; *contact materials,* including poison ivy exudate, ingredients in cosmetics, and certain drugs applied to the skin; and *foods,* such as eggs, chocolate, or strawberries. These are among the most common of the allergens, but virtually anything can cause allergic response in the right (or wrong!) person. Careful testing is often required to identify the particular offenders in a given case. Small amounts of extracts of the common allergens are applied to the skin or injected between the layers of skin (intradermally). If allergy is present, the skin will form redness and edema (wheal) at the site of injection after a few minutes. Serum tests are now available for some allergens and elimination tests are used for many food items.

Types of Allergic Disorders

The incidence of allergy is estimated to be 10 to 20 per cent in the general population, making it extremely common. There is often a family tendency toward it, suggesting a hereditary defect in the immune system passed through family generations. Within the same family, though, the exact manifestations of allergy may be different. One family member may have *hay fever* (allergic rhinitis), in which sneezing, nasal congestion, and discharge are the major symptoms. Another may have attacks of *bronchial asthma,* characterized by bronchoconstriction and wheezing. A third member may react to substances placed on the skin with the formation of *hives* (urticaria). A fourth may develop indigestion and diarrhea upon ingesting certain foods. The principle is the same in all these cases, but the *target tissue* (tissue affected by the reaction) differs with each person.

Antibody Response

Allergic Process

The steps in an allergic reaction are parallel with, but not identical to, those of a response to an infectious organism. Initial contact with an allergen causes an increased titer of IgE to develop (Fig. 4–6). This is similar to the primary response seen with infection. In this case, though, most of the IgE attaches to *mast cells,* which

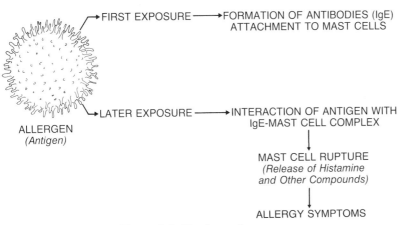

ALLERGEN
(Antigen)

FIRST EXPOSURE ⟶ FORMATION OF ANTIBODIES (IgE)
ATTACHMENT TO MAST CELLS

LATER EXPOSURE ⟶ INTERACTION OF ANTIGEN WITH
IgE-MAST CELL COMPLEX
↓
MAST CELL RUPTURE
*(Release of Histamine
and Other Compounds)*
↓
ALLERGY SYMPTOMS

Figure 4–6. Allergic reaction.

are located mainly in the respiratory tract, digestive tract, and skin. The mast cell–IgE complex is "cocked for firing," so to speak, since it can then interact with additional amounts of the same allergen entering the body.

Subsequent contact with the same allergen results in mast cell rupture and release of its contents, which include *histamine* and other inflammatory compounds. These compounds cause an inflammatory response primarily in the area in which mast cell rupture takes place. If the nasal mucosa is affected, allergic rhinitis results. Mast cell rupture in the bronchi causes an attack of bronchial asthma. If the skin is the target tissue, urticaria results. Gastrointestinal mast cell rupture causes symptoms of indigestion and diarrhea.

It is possible that allergy is an asset to the body that has changed into a liability. Most areas in which allergic reactions are seen are on the "outside" of the body (skin, respiratory and gastrointestinal mucosa). Perhaps the "intention" of the body is good—to rid itself of a harmful substance by sneezing, local skin reaction, diarrhea, or bronchial secretion—but the process becomes misdirected against substances that are of no threat to the human organism.

Severe Allergic Reaction

Occasionally, allergic reactions are more than just troublesome to the afflicted individual. Severe drop in blood pressure (shock), laryngeal edema, and intense bronchoconstriction combine to form a life-threatening combination. The individual loses consciousness and becomes pale from lack of circulation. This severe reaction is called *anaphylactic shock* and is caused by massive release of histamine and other compounds from mast cells. It may follow bee or wasp stings or administration of certain drugs, such as penicillin. Reaction to animal proteins in blood derivatives, such as antitoxins and antisera, is another important cause of this condition. Almost always, the person has had at least one prior exposure to the allergen, after which a massive buildup of IgE occurred. Sometimes, the reaction is initially mild but worsens with each subsequent exposure to the agent. Thus, a mild skin reaction later leads to mild bronchoconstriction and finally to anaphylactic shock.

Treatment for anaphylactic shock consists of administration of antihistamines, epinephrine (which helps to reverse the bronchoconstriction and low blood pressure), corticosteroids, oxygen, and fluids to increase the blood volume. Persons known to be allergic to drugs or insect stings should wear a bracelet or carry a card informing others of their allergy, so that they may be helped immediately if a reaction occurs.

Types of Hypersensitivity

Allergic reactions, including anaphylactic shock, are representative of a general type of hypersensitivity reaction known as *type I hypersensitivity*. This type is characterized by IgE formation and mast cell rupture, as previously mentioned.

Type II is uncommon and is associated with the formation of antibodies to normal cells. The penicillin derivative methacillin (Staphcillin), used for staphylococcal infections, can cause the formation of such antibodies. Red cell lysis then occurs, and the condition is termed **hemolytic anemia**.

Type III results from the formation of immune complexes between antigen and antibody. As a result of this interaction, skin rash, fever, and other symptoms occur. Probably the reaction is due to release of compounds such as *lysozymes* from granulocytes caught up in the antigen-antibody interaction. Reactions to drugs like aspirin or sulfonamides seem to be of this type.

In *type IV* (cell-mediated hypersensitivity), sensitized T lymphocytes are formed. These trigger immune attack on invading organisms, as in the primary response to tuberculosis infection.

Treatment for Allergies

Avoiding the Allergen

Allergic people obtain relief from symptoms when they avoid the offending allergen. This is easy if only one or a few uncommon foods are involved but becomes almost impossible if common foods such as eggs or wheat are allergens, since they are present in many different food products. Contact allergens can usually be avoided, but inhalants may be difficult to avoid.

Antihistamines

Air conditioning and static precipitators work well indoors to purify the air, but outdoor air is still contaminated. In these cases, good relief is often obtained through the use of antihistamines, which block the cellular sites (receptors) to which histamine attaches when it is released through mast cell rupture. Antihistamines work especially well for skin allergies and allergic rhinitis, but they are much less effective for bronchial asthma and most food allergies affecting the gastrointestinal tract.

Hyposensitization

An alternative form of treatment to those previously mentioned is hyposensitization, by which the allergic response is attenuated by repeated exposure to tiny amounts of the offending allergens. The person is first given skin tests (or occasionally serum or food restriction tests) to determine which substances are troublesome. Extracts of these are prepared and minute amounts are injected below the skin (subcutaneously) at weekly or twice-weekly intervals. The doses of the extracts are gradually increased over a period of months, ideally well in advance of the time when protection is most needed (e.g., the onset of hay fever season). This causes formation of IgG, instead of the IgE formed upon heavier exposure (as during normal contact with the allergen), and a serum titer of IgG is established. IgG does not attach to mast cells; it remains in the blood stream and intercepts an allergen that enters the body. The mental picture formed here is of the "good guys heading the bad guys off at the pass." Intercepted allergen fails to reach the IgE-mast cell complex, and mast cell rupture does not take place.

In practice, some reaction often occurs (not all allergen is intercepted) but it is a milder one. This method of treatment is theoretically better than the other ways of treating allergy, since it actually alters the immune response itself, rather than blocking histamine receptors or merely controlling the symptoms of the attack. The benefit of hyposensitization must be weighed against the cost and discomfort to the patient in each case to see if it is worthwhile.

SUMMARY

Early in fetal development, the human organism learns to recognize its own cells and to identify those that are different. Out of this "self versus nonself" ability comes the immune response, which helps the body to eliminate nonself material. The immune response protects us from invading organisms and is an important part of the defense against infection. Two different types of lymphocytes make separate contributions to the immune response.

Alteration of the normal immune mechanism gives rise to autoimmunity and allergy. In autoimmunity, the body's immune system is directed against its own tissue components and clinical disease results. In allergy, the reaction is to outside agents and characteristic clinical states occur upon exposure to the agents.

Questions

1. Why is there rarely, if ever, an immune response to sugar molecules?
2. What would happen to the immune response if all thymus gland tissue were removed at birth?
3. Which type of immunoglobulin (IgA, IgD, IgE, IgG, or IgM) could we *least* afford to do without, with respect to body defenses?
4. Do the same "memory cells" that "remember" previous contact with infectious organisms persist throughout life? How else might lifetime immunity be maintained?
5. What might be the harmful outcome of using long-term, high-dose corticosteroid treatment to control a chronic inflammatory disorder such as rheumatoid arthritis? What if the patient also had a tubercular granuloma in the lung?

Additional Reading

Craddock, C. G., Longmire, R., and McMillan, R.: Lymphocytes and the immune response. N. Engl. J. Med., 285:324, 1971.

DiPalma, J. R.: Pharmacology of myasthenia gravis. Am. Fam. Physician, 22:158, 1980.

Passero, M. A., and Dees, S. C.: Allergy to stings from winged things. Am. Fam. Physician, 7:74, 1973. (*This is a valuable discussion of hyposensitization.*)

Rapaport, H. G.: Disarming insect stings. Drug Ther., May 1975. (*This article provides important information on the treatment of anaphylactic shock.*)

Speer, F.: Food allergy: The 10 common offenders, Am. Fam. Physician, 13:106, 1976.

Spiegelberg, H. L.: Biological activities of immunoglobulins of different classes and subclasses. Adv. Immunol., 19:259, 1974.

CHAPTER **5** WOUND HEALING

One of the truly remarkable features of multicellular organisms is their ability to make tissue repairs necessitated by disease or injury. We are accustomed to the regrowth of plants following pruning or trimming, but do not consider that the animal kingdom is also endowed with similar abilities. Crabs and lobsters often lose a claw or leg in battle and are able to grow another. Certain amphibians, such as salamanders, can also regrow lost limbs. This is amazing when we consider that several different kinds of specialized tissue must be formed simultaneously in these cases.

HOW DO WE HEAL?

The ability to regrow limbs, unfortunately, does not extend to the higher animals, including humans. Perhaps this reflects adaptation of lower species to harsher conditions than are experienced by higher forms of animal life. Nevertheless, higher animal species retain considerable ability to repair damaged tissue and, in some cases, to replace lost tissue with an identical substitute. Were it not for this ability, survival of the higher animal world would be impossible.

Primary Mechanisms of Healing

Repair

If lost or damaged tissue is replaced by scar tissue, the process is called *repair*. This tissue is no longer functional, but it is structurally sound. For example, scar tissue formation in the lung leads to loss of alveolar or bronchial function in that area, but it does hold the other tissues together.

Regeneration

If the damaged tissue is replaced with tissue that is similar to, but not identical to, the original tissue, *regeneration* takes place. Although the regenerated tissue may be functional, it is often different in appearance from the parent tissue. *Leukoplakia* is a good example of this. The whitish patches of cells that replace damaged tissue in the oral cavity are easily distinguished from normal oral mucosa. Regeneration of the colonic mucosa in ulcerative colitis leads to pseudopolyp formation. Here, the regenerated tissue is irregular and obviously different from the normal mucosa. In both leukoplakia and ulcerative colitis, the regenerated tissue is prone to malignancy, indicating that there are other differences besides just gross appearance.

Reconstitution

With certain tissues, complete replacement of the damaged tissue with identical new tissue occurs. This process is known as *reconstitution*. It is commonplace among lower animal forms, but humans have the capability for it with only a few tissues. Damage to the cornea of the eye, the skin, or the liver may result in reconstitution of the affected tissues in humans. Corneal abrasions usually heal by complete replacement of damaged tissue with new corneal tissue. Many skin wounds heal by reconstitution. Removal of a portion of the liver usually leads to its regrowth to former dimensions. In laboratory rats, a common practice is to remove two thirds of the liver in the process of testing certain anticancer drugs. Within a few weeks, the liver is back to normal.

Other Considerations

Some tissues are not easily replaced in higher animals. Nerve tissue, in general, is not reconstituted and may not even regenerate. (It depends upon the type of injury—damaged axons often are reconstituted, but damaged nerve cell bodies usually die or fail to regenerate.) Nerve damage in the brain or spinal cord is almost always permanent.

Damage to long nerve fibers in the limbs can sometimes be repaired with extremely skillful surgery. The advent of successful reattachment of severed arms, hands, and fingers attests to this fact.

Heart muscle heals only by repair. Therefore, nonfunctional scar tissue fills in areas of damage. If the area of damage is large, the heart is definitely weakened by this loss of functional myocardium.

Smooth muscle, likewise, fails to reconstitute and heals by scar formation (repair). Voluntary muscle, in contrast, often can reconstitute and become functional again after injury. Suturing of severed limb muscles often results in restored muscle function.

The stimulus for wound healing is unknown. It is possible that local substances are released at the site of injury and trigger the healing process. Evidence for the existence of these *trephones* is scanty.

Another theory is that tissues normally form chemical compounds that prevent regrowth of cells. When damage occurs and inhibition by these *chalones* ceases, repair begins. Again, evidence is lacking. An understanding of the action of chalones, if they do exist, might help to explain the means of control of cell growth. This might unravel the mystery of tumor growth.

STEPS IN WOUND HEALING

Wound Contraction

When a wound occurs, the severed tissues move toward each other during the first few days after injury. This is called *wound contraction*. This movement reduces the size of the injured area, making it easier for repairs to take place. If good contraction occurs, the resulting scar is smaller than if little contraction has been possible. The exact process of wound contraction is not completely understood but seems to depend upon the formation of *granulation tissue* around the edges of the wound. If granulation tissue is prevented from forming, contraction will be poor and significant scarring will result. The use of corticosteroid drugs or radiation treatment, both of which interfere with the formation of granulation tissue, inhibits wound contraction.

Formation of Granulation Tissue

Granulation tissue forms a temporary covering over damaged tissue and prevents infection until permanent tissue can be developed by the body. Once granulation tissue covers the damaged area, action of newly formed fibroblasts called *myofibroblasts* causes the wound edges to pull closer together. The other elements of granulation tissue also exert benefit to promote healing. *Endothelial cells*

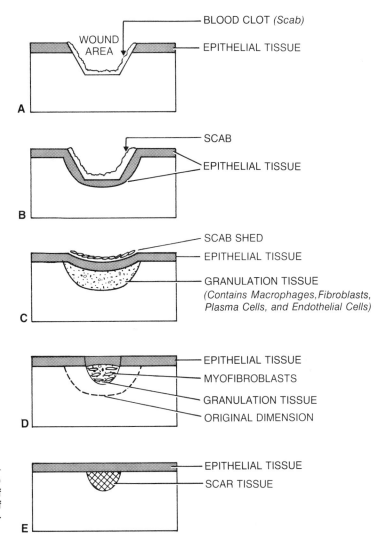

Figure 5–1. Process of wound healing, starting with injury to tissue. *(A)* Formation of scab. *(B)* Formation of epithelial tissue. *(C)* Formation of granulation tissue. *(D)* Wound contraction. *(E)* Healing complete.

form new blood and lymph vessels in the area, *plasma cells* release immunoglobulin to prevent infection, and *macrophages* engulf bacteria or cellular debris in the vicinity of the injury. Older fibroblasts lay down collagen tissue, which binds the wound together and forms a scar (Fig. 5–1).

Additional Factors Affecting Healing

In order for optimal healing to take place, a number of conditions must be met (Table 5–1). Most important is an *adequate blood supply* to the injured area. Without suitable circulation, most steps in the repair process fail to take place. This problem is often seen clinically when extensive disease or prior surgery has damaged the blood supply to an area. The *normal immune system* must be operating to protect the injured area so that healing can occur. This situation is like that of military troops protecting a battle area so that a bridge can be built. *Optimal nutrition* is also a requirement. Deficiency of vitamin C, zinc, or protein cause impaired collagen formation and delayed or incomplete healing.

Old age tends to slow the healing process, possibly through reduced circulation or a slowdown in body processes in general.

Table 5-1. FACTORS AFFECTING WOUND HEALING

Factors promoting healing
Adequate blood supply
Normal immune system
Optimal nutrition

Factors hindering healing
Old age
Foreign materials in wound
Infection

(Old age itself is not a deterrent to most types of surgery, however.) *Foreign materials* (e.g., talcum powder) left in a wound delay or prevent healing. *Infection* slows the repair process and may cause additional tissue damage. Conversely, attempts to prevent infection by the use of harsh antiseptics like iodine solution may also cause tissue damage and delay healing.

HEALING BY PRIMARY INTENTION
When a wound is closed by means of sutures or clips, the edges are brought together and healing is greatly facilitated. The amount of wound contraction required is minimal, and there is a much smaller area to be covered with granulation tissue. Ultimately, the scar is smaller and less noticeable. This is desired in surgery, and great pains are taken to make a neat, clean incision and to close it carefully. Interestingly, this result was also desired in certain primitive tribes, who used large ants to grip the edges of the wound with their jaws. The heads of the ants were removed and left along the suture line, much as clips are now used. Since the first intent in all of these cases is to obtain good healing with only a small scar, the process is called *healing by primary intention*.

A day or so after bleeding and clotting occur in the area of injury, epithelial tissue grows beneath the clot (which by this time has formed a scab) and begins to force the clot (scab) toward the surface (Fig. 5-2).

Approximately 2 days later, *granulation tissue* forms under the epithelial tissue, followed by infiltration of *collagen fibers* between the edges of the incised tissue. Collagen forms the basis of the *scar* and provides strength to the healed incision. The scar is usually only 70 to 80 per cent as strong as the original tissue, but this is normally quite adequate.

Finally, the scab is shed and the avascular scar remains. Scar tissue becomes white when it loses its vascular tissue and fails to tan, since it lacks the *melanin pigment* necessary for darkening of the skin. Scars are, therefore, more noticeable when the rest of the skin is tanned.

HEALING BY SECONDARY INTENTION
Wounds in which the tissue is not (or cannot be) brought together undergo *healing by secondary intention* (Fig. 5-3). In this case, a larger area is left to be filled with epithelial and granulation tissue. This occurs when an injury large enough to require sutures is not sutured or if excessive tissue damage occurs during the injury. A large defect is left, and a larger clot forms than if the wound is closed. The steps in healing are the same as in healing by primary intention. After clotting, the injured area contracts and the processes of epithelial growth and formation of granulation tissue begin, as

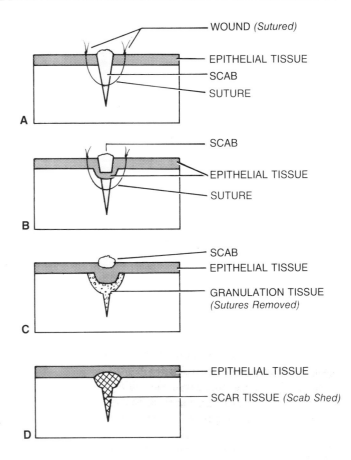

WOUND *(Sutured)*
EPITHELIAL TISSUE
SCAB
SUTURE

A

SCAB
EPITHELIAL TISSUE
SUTURE

B

SCAB
EPITHELIAL TISSUE
GRANULATION TISSUE
(Sutures Removed)

C

EPITHELIAL TISSUE
SCAR TISSUE *(Scab Shed)*

D

Figure 5–2. *(A–D)* Wound healing by primary intention.

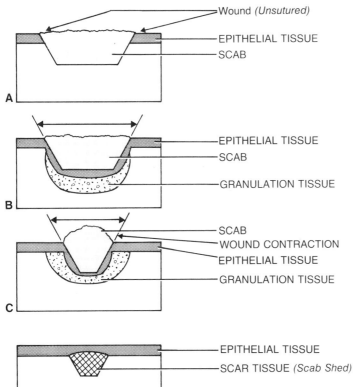

Wound *(Unsutured)*
EPITHELIAL TISSUE
SCAB

A

EPITHELIAL TISSUE
SCAB
GRANULATION TISSUE

B

SCAB
WOUND CONTRACTION
EPITHELIAL TISSUE
GRANULATION TISSUE

C

EPITHELIAL TISSUE
SCAR TISSUE *(Scab Shed)*

D

Figure 5–3. *(A–D)* Wound healing by secondary intention.

Table 5–2. **COMPLICATIONS TO WOUND HEALING**

· Herniation of scar
· Dehiscence of scar
· Infection of injured area
· Contracture of scar
· Keloid formation

previously described. A base of granulation tissue also forms at the bottom of the wound and moves upward toward the surface.

Finally, the scab is shed and the epidermis (outer layer of skin) is replaced. The end result is not as good as if healing by primary intention had taken place, however. The scar is larger and is more prone to contracture. On the surface of the body this causes mostly cosmetic problems, but within deeper body structures it can result in impaired organ function. (See the discussion on pyloric stenosis as a complication of chronic ulcer in Chapter 12.)

Healing by secondary intention renders the individual more susceptible to complications than does healing by primary intention, although the same complications occur in both situations (Table 5–2). The wound may bulge (herniation) or burst (dehiscence), since the scar is larger, and therefore the tissue is weaker. Infection is more likely because the protective epithelial covering is more precarious. Healing takes longer, since a greater amount of tissue must be restored. Contracture is more likely because the scar is larger. Because of the large amount of collagen tissue present, *keloids* form more readily. These are tumorlike masses of scar tissue and represent, essentially, overgrowth of the healed area. Black people and pregnant females of all races are more prone to keloid formation than are other groups. If keloids are removed, they often grow back larger than before.

SUMMARY

One of the great mysteries of life is the process of wound healing and tissue repair. Lower animals are better equipped for organ or even limb regeneration than are higher animals, including humans. We are able, though, to repair injury to the skin and other surface tissues quite well and to reconstitute liver tissue if damaged or lost. Generally, neural tissue of the central nervous system and heart muscle tissue do not regenerate or become reconstituted, although repair, by means of scar tissue formation, takes place.

Injury to the skin is followed by a predictable series of events that usually lead to good repair, regeneration, or reconstitution of the tissue. Certain factors are required for optimal wound healing, including adequate circulation, a normal immune system, accessory substances such as vitamin C and zinc, and adequate protein intake.

Questions 1. Diabetics often have delayed wound healing and are prone to complications to wounds, especially in the legs and feet. Discuss factors that might be operating in the diabetic to cause this. (Refer to the discussion of diabetes mellitus, if needed.)

2. Would you expect repair, regeneration, or reconstitution to occur if the oral mucosa is damaged by biting down on the edge of a sharp potato chip? Which process would likely operate if a tendon were accidentally severed but were expertly sutured back together?
3. Would you expect healing to be faster or slower than normal in a skin wound that was constantly exposed to cold temperature, as in outdoor winter exposure? Why?

Additional Reading

Majno, G.: *The Healing Hand*. Cambridge, Mass., Harvard University Press, 1975.

Neldmar, K. H., and Hambridge, K. M.: Zinc therapy. N. Engl. J. Med., 17:289, 1975.

Peacock, E., and Van Winkle, W.: *Wound Repair,* 2nd ed. Philadelphia, W. B. Saunders Company, 1976.

Ross, R.: Wound healing. Scientific American, 220:40, 1969.

CHAPTER 6

TUMORS

Many disease states are characterized by the abnormal growth of cells. Although the term *tumor* suggests abnormal cell growth to most people, it actually means swelling or edema. (Remember that *tumor* was one of Celsus's signs of inflammation.) Because most conditions of abnormal cell growth do produce a swelling, the term usually applies, but there are exceptions to this. Leukemia, for example, is caused by abnormal proliferation of leukocytes but is not associated directly with swelling or edema. In earlier times, names were often applied on the basis of physical appearance of disease rather than with an understanding of the disease process involved. Swellings caused by abnormal cell growth, inflammation or infection were often called tumors. *Neoplasia* (see Terms in Pathophysiology earlier in this book) is perhaps a better term to describe abnormal cell growth. Neoplasia means "new growth" and applies to conditions in which cell proliferation is the major feature. Even this term is not without confusion, however, since it can refer to both malignant and nonmalignant cell growth.

Tumors are generally named using the ending *-oma*. Although this system is usually accurate, there are several diseases ending with -oma that are not associated with cell proliferation. *Glaucoma,* for example, is associated with increased intraocular pressure and retinal damage, leading to loss of visual field. A *hematoma* is caused by accumulation of blood at the site of an injury. Lesions associated with infection are often also misnamed as tumors. For example, *tuberculoma* refers to an inflammatory lesion caused by infection with tuberculosis. Likewise, a *syphiloma* is an inflammatory lesion formed in response to infection with syphilis. *Granuloma* is a more general term that includes syphilomas and tuberculomas as well as strictly inflammatory lesions.

Tumors are generally classified on the basis of the tissue of origin and whether *benign* or *malignant* (Table 6–1). Benign tumors are named with the ending -oma following the tissue of origin (e.g., lipoma = benign tumor of fatty tissue). Malignant tumors are named with the tissue of origin plus the ending *-sarcoma* or *carcinoma* (e.g., liposarcoma = malignant tumor of fatty tissue). Sarcomas develop from connective tissue, blood vessels, or lymphatic vessels (mesenchyma); carcinomas develop from surface tissue or the lining of vessels or cavities (epithelium). Some tumors fall in between benign and malignant categories in terms of behavioral properties and are designated *intermediate.* These may be named as malignant tumors (e.g., basal cell carcinoma) or the problem of naming may be avoided by using other terminology (e.g., giant cell tumor).

This chapter deals with the common types of tumors and their behavioral characteristics and considers tumor formation as a disease process. Diseases caused by tumors or associated with them are

Table 6–1. TERMINOLOGY OF TUMORS

Parent Tissue	Classification		
	Benign	*Intermediate*	*Malignant*
Connective tissue			
Cartilage	Chondroma		Chondrosarcoma
Bone	Osteoma	Giant cell tumor	Osteosarcoma
Adipose	Lipoma		Liposarcoma
Fibrous	Fibroma		Fibrosarcoma
Smooth muscle	Leiomyoma		Leiomyosarcoma
Skeletal muscle	Rhabdomyoma		Rhabdomyosarcoma
Nerve sheath	Neurofibroma		Neurofibrosarcoma
Epithelial tissue			
Surface	Papilloma	Basal cell carcinoma	Carcinoma
Gland	Adenoma		Adenocarcinoma
Embryonic tissue			
Kidney			Nephroblastoma
Retina			Retinoblastoma
Nerve			Neuroblastoma
Compound	Benign teratoma		Malignant teratoma

considered elsewhere. Chapter 21 deals exclusively with malignant disorders and includes causes and treatment of common forms of malignancy. Benign tumors that cause clinical disease are discussed with the appropriate disease. For example, approximately 0.5 per cent of the cases of hypertension are caused by a *pheochromocytoma,* a tumor (usually benign) of the adrenal medulla. Pheochromocytomas are discussed in Chapter 10, Cardiovascular Disorders.

BENIGN TUMORS

Tumors that tend to remain localized and in which the cells show cohesiveness (tend to stick together) are termed *benign* (Table 6–2). The tendency of benign tumor cells to stick together causes formation of a discrete mass of cells that offers a good possibility for surgical removal.

Pressure Atrophy

As a benign tumor grows, it causes pressure on adjacent tissues and compresses their blood vessels, causing ischemia and death of surrounding tissue. This is called *pressure atrophy*. As a result of this, tissue requiring good circulation for survival undergoes necrosis, leaving only the tough connective tissue that is not as dependent upon a good blood supply. The remaining connective tissue forms a *capsule* around the tumor mass. The encapsulated tumor is therefore further contained in shape and is even more easily removable than before. If rigid structures prevent expansion of the tumor, increased

Table 6–2. PROPERTIES OF BENIGN AND MALIGNANT TUMORS

Benign	Malignant
Remain localized	Spread by metastasis
Have good cell cohesiveness	Have poor cell cohesiveness
Are easy to remove surgically	Are difficult to remove surgically
Often cause pressure atrophy	Usually penetrate surrounding area
Usually are encapsulated	Usually are not encapsulated
Cause local obstruction	Cause local obstruction
Are well differentiated	Are poorly differentiated
Ulceration and bleeding are uncommon	Ulceration and bleeding are common

local damage occurs. A good example of this is a benign brain tumor that causes headaches and brain damage if not removed.

Obstruction

Benign tumors do not spread into distant sites in the body, but they can cause *local obstruction* of body areas. A bronchial adenoma (benign tumor of bronchial lining) causes blockage of the bronchial lumen and leads to wheezing and cough. Since there is impairment of the normal ciliary action that removes bacteria from the lung, infection often results. Benign tumors in the intestinal tract cause obstruction, pain, and constipation.

Deranged Hormone Production and Tissue Changes

Another pathogenic effect of benign tumors is that they destroy normal tissue in the area they invade. For example, benign ovarian tumors largely replace the affected ovary with tumor tissue and therefore destroy its function in secreting estrogen and progesterone. Conversely, some tumors cause increased secretion of hormones and clinical disease results from this hypersecretion. An example is an adrenal medullary tumor (pheochromocytoma) that secretes epinephrine and norepinephrine and raises the blood pressure by the constant influx of these compounds into the blood stream. Other examples of secreting benign tumors include tumors of the islet cells of the pancreas (islet cell adenomas), which cause overproduction of insulin and a severe drop in blood glucose (hypoglycemia), and adrenal *cortical* tumors that overproduce cortisone-type compounds, leading to the clinical condition *Cushing's syndrome*. In Cushing's syndrome, there is edema, atrophy of muscle, and hypertrophy of fatty tissue, plus a wide assortment of other metabolic disturbances. Figure 6–1 show some representative tumors.

Benign tumors are more often associated with hypersecretion of a hormone than are malignant tumors. The reason is that benign tumors tend to resemble the tissue of origin very closely and are said to be *well differentiated*. Therefore, if the parent tissue is differentiated to form an adrenal cortex, a tumor in the adrenal cortex may also have a similar function and will produce cortisonelike compounds. If the parent tissue is specialized as thyroid tissue, the tumor also will produce thyroid hormones. When the amount of hormone produced by the tumor is added to that produced by the remainder of the gland, the total is greater than the normal amount. Sometimes tumor cells resemble the parent tissue so closely that it is hard to tell where they stop and the normal tissue begins, especially if a good capsule has not been developed. This is often the case with benign smooth muscle tumors (leiomyomas).

Stroma Formation

In addition to the capsule that develops around the tumor, a network of connective and vascular tissue develops within the tumor to provide structural integrity and nutrition for it. This is the *stroma.* The stroma is not actually a part of the neoplastic growth but serves to support it. Capillary growth within the stroma seems to be dependent upon a compound called *tumor angiogenesis factor* (TAF) released by the tumor. Since the stromal blood supply is often poor with benign tumors, the rate of growth may be limited and complete surgical removal very likely possible.

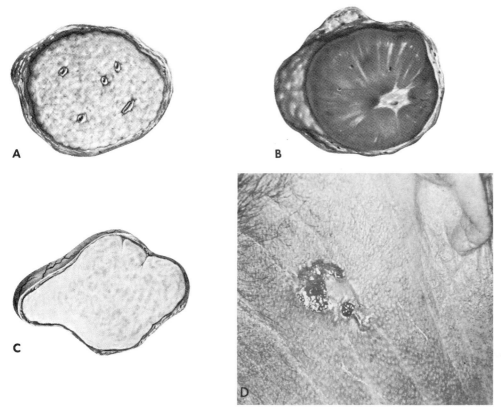

Figure 6–1. Representative tumors. *(A)* Cortical adenoma, a benign tumor of the adrenal cortex, causes Cushing's syndrome. *(B)* Pheochromocytoma, a benign tumor of the adrenal medulla, causes hypertension. *(C)* "Tuberculoma" is actually an infectious inflammatory lesion of the adrenal gland. *(A-C reproduced by permission of Merck Sharp & Dohme, Division of Merck & Co., Inc.) (D)* Basal cell carcinoma of the skin, classified as intermediate.

Ulceration

Ulceration or bleeding is generally uncommon with benign tumors, since they do not invade surrounding tissue planes of the body. Thus, blood vessels are not eroded to cause oozing of blood and the capsule maintains a smooth surface for the tumor that is not prone to erosion, leading to ulceration. Surface tumors in the bladder and intestine, however, may ulcerate and bleed, since they are relatively unprotected and are directly exposed to body excretory products and to the mechanical trauma of urination or defecation.

MALIGNANT TUMORS

Behavioral and Physiologic Properties

The term *cancer* is applied to malignant tumors because of their behavioral properties. "Cancer" comes from the Latin word for "crab," and this connection is seen in the use of the crab as the symbol for the astrological sign Cancer.

Malignant tumors have crablike tendencies: fingers of tissue growth extend into surrounding tissues like claws; the tumors are tenacious like crabs. This tendency to penetrate surrounding tissues distinguishes malignant from benign tumors and increases their risk to the host (Table 6–2).

Since malignant tumors do not normally have a firm capsule, they are not well circumscribed. Probably the invasive nature of malignant tumors is the reason why they do not develop a capsule. Rather than creating pressure that causes necrosis of surrounding tissue and survival of connective tissue as do benign tumors, they penetrate surrounding tissues and invade them. A capsule is not formed, and the tentacles of the tumor go deeper into the surrounding tissues. If the tumor is removed, parts of the tentacles may remain to regrow in the same area. Therefore, malignant tumors are more difficult to remove than benign tumors and a much wider excision is needed.

Two other factors aid in the crablike spread of malignant tumors. The cells have little or no cohesiveness and thus do not readily form a well-defined mass. Also, they do not exhibit *contact inhibition,* or the tendency for cell growth to stop when the normal boundary for growth is reached. Normal cells grown in a petri dish will stop growing when they form a layer across the dish one cell thick. Malignant cells will pile up on each other without regard for the limiting size of the dish or the physical contact between them. Malignant tumors can cause local obstruction because of their bulk just as benign tumors can.

Malignant tumors invade and destroy normal tissue and cause loss of tissue function, as do some benign tumors. It is much less common, however, for malignant tumors to secrete hormones than for benign tumors to do this. The reason is that malignant cells are more primitive histologically and therefore rarely have specialized functions such as hormone synthesis. They are described as being *poorly differentiated* or as resembling embryonic cells closely. An exception to this is the secretion of antidiuretic hormone (ADH, vasopressin) or adrenocorticotropic hormone (ACTH) by certain malignant lung tumors that, by rights, should not have this capability.

Most malignant tumors are basically growth machines and expand at a rate exceeding that of surrounding tissues. Histologically, this is detected by finding cells with larger nuclei, multiple nuclei, or additional chromosome material. The mitotic cycle is usually shorter than with normal cells or benign tumors and sometimes *two* new cells are formed by mitosis instead of one (triradiate mitosis). Cells having these described histologic characteristics are called *anaplastic.* In general, the more anaplastic a tumor is, the more malignant. Thus, oat cell carcinoma of the lung (also called small cell anaplastic carcinoma) spreads faster than does squamous cell carcinoma of the lung. Certain anaplastic thyroid tumors are so malignant that they are incurable before they are able to be diagnosed.

Ulceration and bleeding occur often with malignant tumors, since they are not usually encapsulated. Bleeding occurs because the tumor does not respect tissue boundaries and invades surrounding blood vessels. Ulceration occurs because of the irregular, loosely cohesive surface of the tumor. Some malignant tumors grow so rapidly that they "outrun their blood supply"; i.e., the vascular system does not increase at the same rate as the tumor mass. These tumors become ischemic, then necrotic, and ulceration is very likely.

Local Spread   Although benign tumors can cause local tissue destruction and pressure atrophy or obstruction, they do not leave the primary site and are thus usually completely removable. Malignant tumors also cause local tissue destruction and obstruction, but they have a greater tendency to penetrate surrounding tissues without regard for tissue type. This is called *direct spread.* A gastric tumor may penetrate the wall of the stomach and invade the pancreas. Some tumors enter the lymph channels and form a long string of cells, moving down the channel as in a single-file march. This phenomenon, *lymphatic permeation,* is different from the cells being seeded into the lymph fluid and transported to distant sites in the body. Local spread to vascular tissue may cause formation of thrombi, which block small blood vessels locally.

Metastatic Spread   The process whereby malignant cells are transported to distant sites and then form new growth colonies is called *metastasis.* This is different from local spread, since there is no chain of malignant cells leading from the primary site to the new site but a stretch of normal tissue in between. In lung cancer, for example, metastatic lesions frequently appear in the brain, and it can be shown histologically that these were derived from the original lung lesion. They therefore had to have traveled from the original site to the new site in the brain. Likewise, breast tumors often metastasize to bones—traveling from the original site to the new site.

Three major pathways for metastasis seem to exist: the blood stream, the lymphatic system, and fluid exudates.

Some malignant cells are carried by the *blood stream* to new body areas. Presumably, the tumor penetrates blood vessels and deposits cells within them. The cells are carried in the circulation to the new sites. The site chosen depends upon the vascular supply to it (how accessible it is to circulation) and the "climate" of the tissue. It appears that some tissues have a favorable climate for metastatic growth, while others do not. Lung, liver, brain, and bone are common sites for metastasis, whereas heart and skeletal muscle are uncommon sites—even though the latter two receive excellent circulation.

Other malignant cells travel through the *lymphatic system* in the lymph fluid. When they encounter a lymph node, they multiply and cause the node to enlarge (lymphadenopathy). The enlarged node restricts the flow of lymph fluid and slows the spread of tumor cells. Usually, however, the cells eventually pass the node and move farther to the next node. In surgery for malignant tumors, nodes in the vicinity of a tumor are often removed and examined histologically for tumor cells. The finding of "positive" nodes means that cells have already reached them and may have gone farther. "Negative" nodes in the immediate surroundings of the tumor indicate that malignant cells have not yet reached them and are a good indication that complete removal of the tumor may be possible. Since lymph fluid drains into the blood stream after passage through the tissues there is often a mixture of the two types of spread with advanced tumors.

A third route of metastasis is by production of a fluid exudate containing malignant cells. Areas reached by this exudate can be seeded with malignant cells. This is called *transcelomic spread.* Thus, pancreatic tumors seed into the peritoneal cavity and cause widespread metastasis. Lung tumors cause seeding of the pleural cavity with cells contained in the inflammatory exudate from tissue surrounding the tumor (pleural effusion). Exudate fluid can be aspirated from the chest or abdominal cavity and such malignant cells can be detected histologically.

Types of Malignant Tumors

Malignant tumors are usually named on the basis of tissue of origin plus the ending -*sarcoma* or *carcinoma*, as previously mentioned (Table 6–1). For example, an *osteosarcoma* is a malignant tumor of bone. Sarcomas involve, in addition to bone, other *mesenchymal tissues,* such as cartilage, fibrous or adipose (fatty) tissue. Tumors of these tissues are called, respectively, *chondrosarcomas* (cartilage), *fibrosarcomas* (fibrous tissue), and *liposarcomas* (fatty tissue). If the parent tissue is of *epithelial* origin, such as skin, mucous membrane, or glands, the ending *carcinoma* is used. Examples are squamous cell carcinoma of the skin and adenocarcinoma (adeno = gland) of the thyroid gland.

OTHER TUMORS

Some tumors show both benign and malignant tendencies. They may be locally invasive, yet may fail to metastasize or metastasize very slowly. These are designated *intermediate tumors*. Basal cell carcinoma of the skin is a good example. Although the name suggests malignancy, the tumor does not metastasize; it spreads by local invasion of tissue. Progression of the lesion is slow, and there is plenty of time for diagnosis and treatment with surgery or topical anticancer drugs. *Carcinoid tumors* of the intestinal tract are also considered intermediate. They usually secrete hormones such as serotonin or histamine and cause flushing of the face and abdominal cramps. *Carcinoid* means "carcinomalike" and points up the similarity to malignant tumors. The fact that carcinoid tumors secrete hormones suggests that they are well differentiated and therefore resemble benign tumors.

Teratomas are tumors containing several types of well-differentiated tissue. These bizarre tumors usually grow in the ovary, are benign, and contain teeth, hair, skin, bone, and specialized organ tissue. They resemble a fetus that failed to develop normally, but instead grew within the ovary from a fertilized egg. The origin of these is unclear.

Choriocarcinomas (chorion = placenta) contain placental tissue and occur in both males and females. Embryonic tumors such as *nephroblastomas* (blast = primitive cell) form from differentiating cells—in this case, the kidney. Embryonic tumors are most common in children, who are closer to the period of embryonic development than are adults.

Tumors involving the lymphatic system are called *lymphomas* and develop in the lymph nodes, bone marrow, or organs such as the spleen. These conditions do not result from lymphatic spread of primary tumors (as do metastases from lung cancer, for example) but represent distinct disease entities. *Hodgkin's disease,* the most common lymphoma, will be discussed in detail in Chapter 21.

SUMMARY

Abnormal cell growth is always a cause for investigation. Tumors, or areas of abnormal cell growth, may be benign, intermediate, or malignant, depending upon their histologic and behavioral characteristics. Although some terminology is faulty, tumor nomenclature generally indicates the tissue of origin and whether the tumor is benign or malignant. The expected behavior of a tumor may often be predicted by knowing the type and location of it. Malignant tumors spread to distant sites or metastasize, whereas benign tumors cause local invasion and damage but do not metastasize. Some tumors show characteristics of both benign and malignant lesions and are thus called intermediate. Others arise from a mixture of tissues and are designated teratomas.

Questions
1. Spontaneous remission occurs occasionally with malignant tumors. Discuss ways in which the body might cause a tumor to shrink or disappear without surgery, radiation treatment, or drug therapy.
2. An elderly female with inoperable breast cancer breaks a leg after a trivial bump against a chair. Describe the events leading to this "pathologic fracture," including those related to the underlying disease process and to the effects of advanced age.
3. Tumor cells injected into volunteers usually fail to "take" and are destroyed by the body. What defense process is likely operating here?
4. What might be a very obvious effect of a benign tumor in the anterior pituitary? In the posterior pituitary?

Additional Reading
Foulds, L.: *Neoplastic Development.* New York, Academic Press, 1969.

Gerald, P. S.: Origin of teratomas. N. Engl. J. Med., 292:103, 1975.

Kessler, I. I., and Clark, J. P.: Saccharin, cyclamate, and human bladder cancer: No evidence of an association. J.A.M.A., 240:349, 1978.

Pitot, H. C.: The natural history of neoplasia. Am. J. Pathol., 89:402, 1977.

CHAPTER 7

FLUID AND ELECTROLYTE DISTURBANCES

A fundamental property of mammals is their ability to maintain physiologic parameters within narrow limits by means of internal controls. This process, *homeostasis,* is less well developed in non-mammals, such as fish or reptiles. These "cold-blooded" animals are adapted for survival under a wide variety of environmental conditions, but they lack the sophistication of mammals in controlling their internal environment.

Nowhere is the homeostatic process more evident than in control of water and electrolyte balance in humans. Deviation from a narrow range of normal values causes illness or death, and a complex set of physiologic mechanisms is employed to keep these parameters within the norm. Since humans are less well adapted than lower animals for survival under adverse conditions, internal stability must be closely maintained for life to be possible.

FACTORS CONTROLLING WATER AND ELECTROLYTE BALANCE

Water balance is maintained through the combined action of *ingestion* and *excretion* processes. Ingestion is in the form of liquid intake and water contained in foods. The total is approximately 2.5 liters per day. In addition, 0.3 liter per day is formed as a metabolic by-product of chemical reactions within the body. Excretion must equal ingestion over the long run, or dehydration or overhydration will result. Of the 2.8 or so liters per day lost by the body, 1.5 liters appear as urine, 0.2 liter is lost as fecal water, 0.7 liter is exhaled as water vapor, and 0.4 liter evaporates from the skin.

Fortunately for us, we do not have to consciously regulate water intake. (If so, we would be in the position of the centipede that tried to figure out which foot to move first!) Water intake is controlled through the action of *osmoreceptors* located in the hypothalamus. These receptors sense the osmolality of circulating blood and determine whether more or less water is needed to maintain the correct osmolality. If more is needed (if the blood is too concentrated), a feeling of thirst is generated and we drink until it is satisfied. If less water is needed (if the blood is too dilute), thirst is suppressed until sufficient water is excreted to reach the correct osmotic level.

The hypothalamus, by means of osmoreceptor activity, also controls the release of antidiuretic hormone (ADH, vasopressin) from the posterior pituitary gland. ADH increases the pore size in the renal collecting duct and allows water already filtered out by the glomerulus to leak out of the duct and become reabsorbed (Fig. 7–1). Thus, release of ADH leads to water reabsorption. In severe

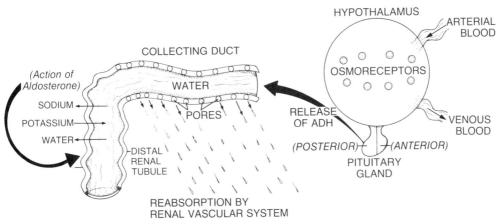

Figure 7–1. Renal action of antidiuretic hormone (ADH) and aldosterone. ADH acts on the collecting duct to increase pore size and promote leakage of water from duct and reabsorption into the blood stream.

dehydration, ADH release is maximal and the body conserves as much water as possible. Conversely, if the individual is overhydrated, ADH release is suppressed and a larger volume of water appears as urine. This is the major way by which the body adjusts for variations in water intake and in the rate of evaporation, fecal excretion or exhalation of water vapor. Individuals with *diabetes insipidus* (diabetes = siphon; insipidus = dilute) lack ADH or, in rare cases, are insensitive to normal quantities of it. Accordingly, they fail to reabsorb the normal quantity of water under ADH control and excrete a very large volume (up to 20 liters/day) of dilute urine. Forms of ADH (lypressin, Pitressin) administered to these individuals are usually of benefit.

Aldosterone, a hormone from the adrenal cortex, has a somewhat less important action on water balance than does ADH. Aldosterone causes an exchange of potassium for sodium in the distal renal tubule and also promotes water reabsorption through the osmotic effect of the retained sodium (Fig. 7–1). Insufficient production of aldosterone causes a major portion of the clinical condition known as *Addison's disease,* in which reduced blood volume (hypovolemia), reduced sodium content of the plasma (hyponatremia), and increased plasma potassium level (hyperkalemia) are important features. Conversely, excessive aldosterone production or the administration of drugs having a similar effect causes reduced plasma potassium level (hypokalemia), increased sodium level (hypernatremia), and increased extracellular fluid volume, leading to *edema.*

Water is maintained at a constant level in the various body areas through the action of electrolytes, proteins, and other osmotically active compounds. Active transport of these from one area to another causes shifts of water and equilibrium is then re-established. In plasma, the force of blood pressure, which tends to squeeze water through the capillary walls (hydrostatic pressure), is counterbalanced by the osmotic effect of plasma proteins (oncotic pressure), which tends to keep water within the capillaries.

Electrolyte balance is also the result of the interaction of ingestion and excretion processes. Intake varies with the type and

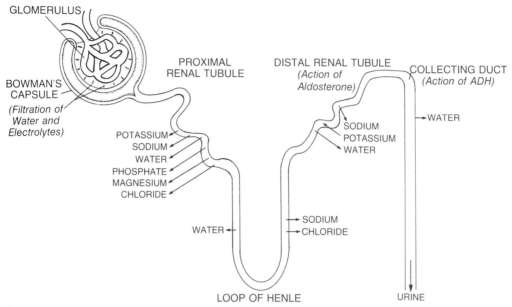

Figure 7–2. Renal influence on water and electrolyte balance. Movement out of the tubule or loop of Henle (reabsorption) and movement into the tubule or loop of Henle (secretion) are shown.

quantity of food and drink ingested. As with water, the body must adjust excretion to maintain electrolyte values within normal limits. A minor portion of body electrolytes is excreted in sweat, feces, tears, and milk, but the major part is removed through action of the kidneys. It is estimated, for example, that most Americans ingest ten to a hundred times the required amount of sodium per day. The kidneys remove the excess by excretion. In reality, the excretion of sodium is largely caused by failure to reabsorb sodium that has already been filtered by the glomeruli and is in the tubular system (Fig. 7–2). Likewise, with potassium and other electrolytes, a complex combination of filtration, reabsorption and secretion is employed by the kidneys to maintain physiologic values for electrolytes in the face of variable intake and changing conditions in the internal and external body environment. Renal failure has devastating effects on electrolyte and water balance (see Chapter 11). Typically, the urine is dilute and there is retention of potassium and calcium with depletion of sodium, since the renal mechanisms for maintaining physiologic values for these are impaired.

NORMAL COMPOSITION OF WATER AND ELECTROLYTES

Approximately 60 per cent of body weight is water. Water exists as two major pools in the body: *intracellular water* (water contained within the cells—40 per cent) and *extracellular water* (water contained outside the cells—20 per cent). Extracellular water consists of *interstitial water* (between the cells—15 per cent) and *plasma water* (contained in blood plasma—5 per cent), making a total of three distinct areas, or compartments, for water. Water is generally free to move among these compartments; however, because some time is required for movement, a temporary deficiency or excess can occur in one compartment until equilibrium has been re-established. Thus, the patient with severe blood loss has a temporary shortage of plasma water, but not necessarily a shortage of intracellular or

Table 7–1. NORMAL PLASMA VALUES FOR COMMON ELECTROLYTES

Electrolyte (Ion)	Range (mEq/L)
Sodium	136–145
Potassium	3.5–5.5
Calcium	4.5–5.7
Magnesium	1.5–2.5
Phosphate	1.2–2.3
Chloride	96–106

interstitial water until equilibration takes place. Administration of sufficient intravenous fluid (as 5 per cent dextrose in water, for example) replenishes the depleted plasma water.

In edema states, there is an excess of interstitial water, usually accompanied by retained sodium. Actually, retention of sodium is the most common *cause* of edema, since it attracts water into the interstitial area by osmosis. Generalized edema is called *anasarca* and is especially characteristic of congestive heart failure (see Chapter 10.) Abdominal edema is referred to as *ascites* and most often develops as a result of cirrhosis of the liver (see Chapter 13).

The normal values for common electrolytes (ions) are shown in Table 7–1. These are measured as plasma concentrations (plasma is blood with the cells removed). Values are usually expressed as milliequivalents of electrolyte per liter (mEq/L) rather than as equivalents per liter because of the small quantities represented in plasma. A milliequivalent is the molecular (or atomic) weight of an electrolyte (ion) divided by its valence and expressed in milligrams. Thus, for calcium, which has a molecular (ionic) weight of 40 and a valence of 2, a milliequivalent is 20 mg. For sodium, with a molecular (ionic) weight of 23 and a valence of 1, a milliequivalent is 23 mg. To convert milliequivalents to equivalents, divide by 1000.

Sodium is contained primarily in the extracellular fluid and is in low concentration within the cells. Plasma sodium concentration, therefore, gives an accurate representation of the bulk of sodium in the body. Potassium, on the other hand, is contained mainly within the cell and plasma levels reflect only a small part of the total body content. Low plasma levels do not always reflect low cellular levels, since sufficient time may not have elapsed for equilibration to have taken place and for the plasma potassium to have been replenished.

FLUID AND ELECTROLYTE IMBALANCES

Water

Dehydration

Depletion of body water can result from a number of causes (Table 7–2). Although the initial water loss is primarily in the interstitial compartment, rapid shifts occur from the other two compartments in the body's attempt to equalize the loss. Thus, the intracellular and plasma water volumes soon begin to be depleted. The mechanism operating here is *osmosis*. As interstitial water is depleted, interstitial fluid becomes hypertonic and attracts water from the other two compartments. Eventually, all compartments become hypertonic and a dangerous situation exists. The skin is flaccid, the eyes are sunken into the sockets, the tongue is swollen and sticky, and pressure on the skin leaves depressions (fingerprinting). Blood pressure is low because of the reduced blood volume, and shock can easily occur. Treatment consists of removing the

Table 7–2. CAUSES OF DEHYDRATION

Vomiting, diarrhea, or gastric suction
Inadequate fluid intake
Hyperventilation or mechanical respiration (loss of water vapor)
Evaporation from normal skin during heavy exercise
Evaporation from burned surfaces
Diuresis (from diuretic drugs or from the diuretic effect of glycosuria in
  diabetes mellitus)
Diabetes insipidus

cause of the dehydration, if possible, and administering oral fluids (water, juices) or intravenous solutions (e.g., 5 per cent dextrose in water). Adequate time must be allowed for re-equilibration of water in all three compartments.

Overhydration   Overhydration results from overadministration of intravenous solutions or by exceeding the excretory capacity in a patient with reduced renal function by the use of enemas or excessive oral intake of fluids. Occasionally, self-ingestion is the cause of overhydration in a psychotic individual who compulsively drinks 1 liter per hour or more of liquid. Usually, such individuals are obsessed with the idea of cleansing themselves internally by means of the excessive water ingestion. All water compartments become overhydrated, and the plasma volume increases, leading to an increased cardiac workload. In a person predisposed to *congestive heart failure,* this extra volume load can precipitate an attack of failure. *Edema* results from increased extracellular water volume. Increased intracellular water volume causes cells to swell. This is especially noted in the central nervous system, where delirium, convulsions, or coma may result from swollen nerve cells (water intoxication).

Sodium   Lowered levels of plasma sodium (<136 mEq/L) result from a variety of causes (Table 7–3). Since sodium is found primarily in the *Hyponatremia* extracellular water, depletion occurs mainly from this fraction and affects plasma and interstitial water. Chloride levels usually parallel sodium levels and will also be depleted in this case (<96 mEq/L), since most sodium exists in the form of sodium chloride. The symptoms of hyponatremia include mental confusion or delirium, muscle weakness, abdominal cramps, and hypotension. Severe hyponatremia can lead to vascular collapse and shock, resulting from low blood volume. Depletion of sodium and water from blood causes increased red blood cell count (hemoconcentration) and increased levels of plasma proteins (hyperproteinemia), since these blood elements remain when water is lost from the blood.

Table 7–3. CAUSES OF HYPONATREMIA

Vomiting, diarrhea, or gastric suction
Excessive sweating without sodium replacement
Loss of sodium from burned surfaces
Certain renal conditions ("salt-losing" nephritis)
Excessive use of diuretics
Cystic fibrosis (excessive loss of sodium in sweat)
Addison's disease (insufficient production of corticosteroids, causing
  reduced reabsorption of sodium by kidney)

Treatment of hyponatremia consists of fluid restriction with increased intake of sodium chloride (salt) or, in more severe cases, the use of intravenous hypertonic saline solution.

Hypernatremia   Overloading with sodium (plasma level >145 mEq/L) occurs when an excess of sodium is ingested or normal saline solution is infused too vigorously in a hospitalized patient. Impaired renal function may also lead to accumulation of sodium, even with normal sodium intake. As previously mentioned, the "normal" sodium intake of most Americans is greatly in excess of body needs and hypernatremia easily occurs with renal impairment. The practice of eating salt tablets to replace sodium lost through sweating is usually unnecessary and further increases the burden of sodium to be removed by the kidneys. All that is usually needed is for the person to use some salt on food after the period of excessive sweating. Plasma chloride level is usually greater than 106 mEq/L in hypernatremia, since, as previously mentioned, most sodium is in the form of sodium chloride.

Hypernatremia is occasionally seen in individuals who have been forced to drink sea water for survival. Since approximately 1.25 liters of body water are required to excrete the sodium in 1 liter of sea water, ingestion of sea water leads to hypernatremia and dehydration. Humans cannot concentrate the urine enough to effectively use sea water for water replacement. Certain animals, such as the desert rat, adapted for extremely arid conditions, can excrete a much more concentrated urine and could use sea water to advantage.

The symptoms of hypernatremia include fever, thirst, dry, sticky mucous membranes, and edema (since most of the sodium enters the interstitial compartment). Hypernatremia can be treated by restricting salt intake, increasing the intake of sodium-free fluids, or administering an intravenous solution of 5 per cent dextrose in water.

Potassium   Low potassium levels (<3.5 mEq/L) result from a great variety of clinical states (Table 7–4). Among the common causes are the *Hypokalemia*   administration of most diuretics, such as furosemide (Lasix), hydrochlorothiazide (Hydrodiuril), or ethacrynic acid (Edecrin), vomiting or diarrhea, and removal through gastric suction. As previously stated, plasma potassium levels do not accurately measure *intracellular* potassium, the major fraction found in the body. In hypokalemia, potassium shifts from intracellular pools into the blood stream, but before equilibration occurs, complications of hypokalemia can develop.

Table 7–4. CAUSES OF HYPOKALEMIA

Inadequate potassium intake
Malabsorption by intestinal tract
Vomiting, diarrhea, or gastric suction
Loss of potassium from burned surfaces
Use of "potassium-losing" diuretics
Certain renal conditions (renal tubular defects)
Cushing's syndrome (excessive production or overingestion of
   corticosteroids, causing reduced reabsorption of potassium by kidney)

Potassium is required for normal function of nerve and muscle tissue, as well as for many metabolic processes. Hypokalemia can cause muscle weakness, cardiac arrhythmias, irritability, and slowed gastric motility. A particular problem occurs in persons taking digitalis products for the treatment of congestive heart failure along with diuretics that cause potassium loss. Hypokalemia that is induced by the diuretic causes increased digitalis effect (potentiation) because of the intracellular loss of potassium, and toxicity may result. It is necessary for those taking digitalis and most diuretics concurrently to use potassium supplements (e.g., Kaon) or to eat foods with a high potassium content (apples, bananas, oranges).

Two diuretics cause potassium *retention* instead of *depletion*. These drugs, called *potassium-sparing diuretics,* are spironolactone (Aldactone) and triamterene (Dyrenium). They can be used with digitalis to prevent hypokalemia and digitalis toxicity.

Hypokalemia is treated by correcting its cause, if possible, and by the administration of oral potassium supplements (Kaon) or intravenous potassium solutions (e.g., potassium chloride solution). Intravenous potassium should be given carefully, since it is easy to overtreat and cause *hyperkalemia*. Repeated plasma potassium determinations should be made to determine the rate of infusion necessary to replenish potassium in the intracellular compartment.

Hyperkalemia

Hyperkalemia (>5.5 mEq/L) is less common than hypokalemia, but it is equally hazardous. Common causes (Table 7–5) include renal disease, overadministration of potassium orally or by infusion, and overuse of potassium-sparing diuretics. Severe crushing injury to tissues causes release of potassium from damaged cells and elevates the plasma potassium level. Symptoms include increased intestinal activity leading to diarrhea and colic, sedation, muscle cramps, and cardiac slowing, leading eventually to cardiac arrest. Many individuals with abnormally high potassium levels feel quite well, although they are in danger of cardiac toxicity.

Treatment of hyperkalemia involves restriction of oral intake or discontinuation of parenteral potassium solutions. In more severe cases, an ion exchange agent (Kayexalate) is used orally or by enema. Kayexalate attaches to potassium in the intestinal tract and removes it, facilitating further secretion into gastric and intestinal fluid and removal of potassium from body water compartments.

Calcium

Calcium levels in the body are controlled by a complex set of factors. Vitamin D promotes calcium absorption from the digestive tract. Two hormones influence plasma calcium levels. *Parathormone,* secreted by the parathyroid gland, raises the plasma level, and

Hypocalcemia

Table 7–5. CAUSES OF HYPERKALEMIA

Excessive potassium intake
Overuse of "potassium-sparing" diuretics
Renal failure
"Crush" injury to muscle or other tissue (potassium is released into blood stream from damaged cells)
Addison's disease (insufficient production of corticosteroids, causing reduced secretion of potassium by kidney)

Table 7–6. CAUSES OF HYPOCALCEMIA

Inadequate calcium intake
Inadequate vitamin D intake (reduced absorption of calcium)
Renal failure (failure to reabsorb calcium)
Hypoparathyroidism
Inadvertent removal of parathyroid tissue

calcitonin, produced by modified thyroid tissue, lowers the plasma level. Only about 1 per cent of the total body calcium appears in body fluids. Most is in the bone tissue and teeth, with bone tissue serving as a pool for calcium storage and release as needed.

Calcium has important functions in nerve and muscle activity, in enzyme activity, and in blood coagulation. The importance of calcium was appreciated by early surgeons who inadvertently removed the parathyroid glands during thyroid removal (thyroidectomy). A day or two after sugery, their patients developed signs of hypocalcemia. Other causes of hypocalcemia include disease of the parathyroid gland and overadministration of calcium-free solutions or citrated blood (which has the calcium removed to prevent clotting) (Table 7–6).

Low levels of calcium (<4.5 mEq/L) cause malfunction of nerve tissue, leading to numbness or tingling of the extremities and muscle hyperactivity, resulting in hyperreflexia, muscle cramps, and eventually *tetany* (locking of muscles in the flexed position). In extreme cases, laryngeal tetany occurs, causing stridor (noisy breathing) and dyspnea (difficulty in breathing). Treatment is with oral calcium salts (e.g., calcium lactate) or, in severe cases, with calcium gluconate by intravenous infusion.

Hypercalcemia   Hypercalcemia (>5.7 mEq/L) often results from overingestion of calcium-containing antacids and milk in the treatment of ulcer (milk-alkali syndrome), from hyperparathyroidism or as a result of metastatic cancer that causes bone deterioration and release of calcium into the blood stream (Table 7–7). Symptoms include muscle weakness, vomiting, constipation (because of reduced gastrointestinal motility), and sedation. In severe cases, coma and death can occur as a result of impaired nerve and muscle function. Renal damage often occurs, because of precipitation of calcium compounds from the urine into kidney tissue. Most calcium compounds have limited solubility in urine, and high plasma levels encourage crystallization in the kidney (crystalluria).

Mild cases of hypercalcemia respond to restriction of oral intake of calcium (especially in the form of dairy products) and hydration (2 liters or more of water per day, which helps to lower plasma and urine levels of calcium). In extreme cases, especially where bone

Table 7–7. CAUSES OF HYPERCALCEMIA

Excessive calcium intake (milk-alkali syndrome)
Excessive vitamin D intake (excessive absorption of calcium)
Hyperparathyroidism
Metastatic cancer involving bone tissue (release of calcium from bone
  breakdown)

metastases are involved, mithramycin (Mithracin) can be given orally. Mithramycin is an anticancer drug, but in lower doses decreases the plasma calcium level.

OTHER ELECTROLYTE IMBALANCES

Magnesium, phosphate, and chloride ions are also important electrolytes; however, disturbances in balance of these ions are less commonly causes of clinical disease states than are those of sodium, potassium and calcium.

Magnesium

Hypomagnesemia

Low magnesium levels (<1.5 mEq/L) are associated with severe vomiting, diarrhea, or prolonged gastric suction, or as a result of impaired absorption. The chief consequence of hypomagnesemia is hyperreflexia, sometimes leading to convulsions or tetany. Intravenous or intramuscular magnesium solution corrects the problem.

Hypermagnesemia

Elevated magnesium levels (>2.5 mEq/L) nearly always occur as a result of impaired renal function and reduced excretion. Symptoms include muscle weakness, sedation, and mental confusion. Treatment is directed toward improving renal function or involves the use of hemodialysis to clear magnesium from the body.

Phosphate

Hypophosphatemia

Low phosphate levels (<1.2 mEq/L) occur as a result of reduced intake or decreased absorption, increased renal loss, or hyperparathyroidism. Bone pain, fracture, muscle pain, and loss of appetite are common results of prolonged low plasma phosphate levels. Treatment is with oral phosphate salts (K-Phos; Neutraphos) along with adequate vitamin D to ensure optimum absorption.

Hyperphosphatemia

High phosphate levels (>2.3 mEq/L), although uncommon, result from reduced renal excretion of phosphate (seen in renal failure), hypoparathyroidism, or excess intake of vitamin D (hypervitaminosis D). Treatment is directed toward the underlying cause, occasionally with the use of hemodialysis to remove excess phosphate ion from the blood stream.

Chloride

Hypochloremia

Reduced levels of plasma chloride (<96 mEq/L) occur with severe vomiting or diarrhea, sodium depletion, or the excessive use of diuretics (which also cause sodium depletion). As previously mentioned, chloride ion tends to follow sodium ion, since most body sodium is in the form of sodium chloride. Replacement of chloride with ingested sodium chloride or the intravenous administration of 0.9 per cent sodium chloride solution (normal saline) is effective.

Hyperchloremia

Increased chloride levels (>106 mEq/L) occur with excessive salt intake, dehydration, or renal insufficiency. Restriction of salt intake is usually adequate for treatment.

SUMMARY

A constant internal environment is necessary for human survival. Disruption by disease processes or alterations in intake of water and electrolytes is met with body adjustments directed at the maintenance of homeostasis. If body adjustments are not adequate to restore the water or electrolyte value to within the normal range, clinical disease results. The advent of accurate assay techniques for plasma electrolytes and specific treatments for electrolyte abnormalities has vastly improved recovery from water and electrolyte disturbances.

Questions

1. Spironolactone (Aldactone) is a diuretic that blocks the action of aldosterone at the distal tubule. What are the effects of spironolactone on extracellular water, plasma sodium level, and plasma potassium level?
2. What is the milliequivalent weight of potassium (molecular weight = 39; valence = 1) and magnesium (molecular weight = 24; valence = 2)?
3. Would intravenous administration of fluid (for example, 5 per cent dextrose in water) *immediately* correct severe dehydration? Explain.
4. If we reduced our salt intake to 10 per cent of its present quantity, would we become hyponatremic? Explain.

Additional Reading

Deftos, L. J., and Neer, R.: Medical management of the hypercalcemia of malignancy. Ann. Rev. Med., 25:323, 1974.

Fitzgerald, F.: Clinical hypophosphatemia. Ann. Rev. Med., 29:177, 1978.

Iseri, L. T., Freed, J., and Bures, A. R.: Magnesium deficiency and cardiac disorders. Am. J. Med., 58:837, 1975.

Moses, A. M., and Miller, M.: Drug-induced hyponatremia. N. Engl. J. Med., 291:1234, 1974.

Nardone, D. A. *et al.*: Mechanisms in hypokalemia: Clinical correlation. Medicine, 57:435, 1978.

Schrier, R. W. (ed.): *Renal and Electrolyte Disorders.* Boston, Little, Brown & Company, 1976.

CHAPTER 8

ACID-BASE DISTURBANCES

The ability to maintain acid-base balance within narrow limits is a feature of higher animals and a necessity for their survival. Even lower organisms must operate within a relatively constant acid-base environment to survive or thrive. As the phylogenetic scale is ascended toward humans, the degree of sophistication of balance mechanisms increases and the dependence upon these for survival also escalates. Thus, the same tight control is required for acid-base balance that is required for water and electrolyte balance.

The concept of *pH,* familiar to most college students, helps us to understand the regulatory processes for acid-base balance. pH is defined as the negative logarithm of the hydrogen ion concentration ([H$^+$]) and is expressed by the following equation:

$$[H^+] \times [OH^-] = 10^{-14}.$$

The product of hydrogen and hydroxyl ion concentrations equals 10^{-14}. If [H$^+$] = 10^{-7} and [OH$^-$] = 10^{-7}, the pH is 7. If [H$^+$] = 10^{-3} and [OH$^-$] = 10^{-11}, the pH is 3. If [H$^+$] = 10^{-9} and [OH$^-$] = 10^{-5}, the pH is 9.

A pH of 7 is *neutral,* lower than 7 is *acidic,* and between 7 and 14 is *basic* (alkaline). The normal pH of blood is slightly alkaline (7.35 to 7.45), and imbalance conditions occur if it is outside the normal range. The absolute limits for survival are approximately 6.8 to 8.0. Urine pH varies from 4.8 to 8.5 (average = 6), but changes in response to diet variations, disease conditions, and other factors to keep blood pH within normal limits.

Body metabolism causes a constant production of acidic compounds, including carbonic acid (H_2CO_3), lactic acid, sulfuric acid, and phosphoric acid. Without acid-base control mechanisms, body pH would gradually shift further and further below 7.35 until death occurred. Likewise, the ingestion of acidic or basic foods, drinks, or drug products would cause lethal variations in blood pH, were it not for the body's ability to maintain a physiologic pH range.

BODY BUFFER SYSTEMS

Several chemical systems designed to resist changes in blood pH exist in the body. *Hemoglobin* in red blood cells has the following relationship with hydrogen ion:

$$H\text{-Hemoglobin} \rightleftarrows H^+ + \text{Hemoglobin}^-.$$

Thus, extra H$^+$ added (more acidity) results in the formation of more H-Hemoglobin and in the "using up" of the excess H$^+$.

Similarly, *plasma proteins* can buffer additional H^+ in the following manner:

$$H\text{-Protein} \rightleftharpoons H^+ + \text{Protein}^-.$$

Phosphate ion also buffers added H^+ as expressed in the equation:

$$H_2PO_4 \rightleftharpoons H^+ + HPO_4^-.$$

This is referred to as the *phosphate buffer system.*

In all three systems, the ability to buffer acid is limited by the quantity of buffer compound in the body (hemoglobin, protein, or phosphate ion). Thus, with extended influx of excess H^+, the buffering capacity is finally exhausted and blood pH begins to fall. However, the body has additional ways of dealing with excess H^+.

The *carbonic acid–bicarbonate buffer system* is represented by the equation:

$$H_2CO_3 \rightleftharpoons H^+ + HCO_3^-.$$

As with the other buffer systems, additional H^+ causes formation of more un-ionized compound (H_2CO_3). In this case, though, H_2CO_3 can dissociate to form carbon dioxide (CO_2) and water (H_2O). Water is excreted in the urine, and CO_2 is exhaled in the air. The body can form more HCO_3^- (bicarbonate ion) by the reactions:

$$H_2O + CO_2 \xrightarrow{\boxed{\text{carbonic anhydrase}}} H_2CO_3$$
$$H_2CO_3 \rightleftharpoons H^+ + HCO_3^-.$$

The normal serum level of bicarbonate ion (HCO_3^-) is 25 to 30 mEq/L. Carbonic anhydrase, an enzyme found in the red blood cell, lung, kidney, and other body areas, catalyzes the combination of H_2O and CO_2 and greatly speeds up the formation of H_2CO_3 (which hydrolyzes to form $H^+ + HCO_3^-$). In the kidney, carbonic anhydrase functions in the manner described to cause formation of H_2CO_3 from H_2O and CO_2. Hydrolysis of H_2CO_3 then causes formation of $H^+ + HCO_3^-$. H^+ is then exchanged for sodium at the distal tubule (one molecule of H^+ is secreted for each molecule of sodium reabsorbed). In this way, the kidney removes excess H^+ and helps to correct the imbalance. Urine pH is more strongly acidic in this case (< 6.0), because of the larger amount of H^+ being secreted. It should be noted that reduced H^+ intake or formation by the body shifts the buffer equations to the right (in favor of increased H^+ formation by ionization) and helps to maintain optimum blood pH.

Short-term changes in blood pH primarily affect the respiratory system, which responds to decreased serum pH (more acidity) by increasing activity. This favors the removal of more CO_2 in the exhaled air. Carbon dioxide is considered to be "potential acid," since it forms H_2CO_3 when dissolved in water. Thus, CO_2 removal depletes H_2CO_3 from the serum and helps to shift the pH back to normal. Increased serum pH (more alkaline) results in suppression of respiratory activity, causing accumulation of CO_2 (less removed

Table 8–1. CAUSES OF RESPIRATORY ACIDOSIS

Respiratory depression from barbiturates, narcotics, alcohol or other
   drugs
Reduced alveolar oxygen uptake (bronchial asthma, emphysema)
Foreign material in air passage
Laryngeal edema
Insufficient ventilation with respirator
Carbon dioxide poisoning

in the expired air). This causes formation of more H_2CO_3 and lowers the pH to normal. Respiratory adjustments to changes in serum pH occur within seconds to minutes.

Longer-term changes in blood pH, which cannot be completely resolved by respiratory adjustments, result in compensatory changes in the chemical buffer systems previously described, especially the carbonic acid-bicarbonate system. Hours to days are required for these changes. Therefore, long-term excess H^+ production or intake results in a lowering of serum HCO_3^- level (but not its complete depletion) and the body starts forming more HCO_3^-. Insufficient H^+ results in increased levels of HCO_3^-, and production of HCO_3^- is decreased by the body.

Although it is often possible for the body to adjust to severe changes in serum pH, a certain amount of time is required for the adjustment to take place. Temporarily, the serum pH will remain at an abnormal level. If the level is below 7.35, the term *acidosis* is used to describe the clinical state. *Alkalosis* represents a level above 7.45. In these cases, body processes are operating to correct the condition but have not yet done so.

Conditions that result in accumulation of CO_2 cause *respiratory acidosis,* and increased respiratory action is the primary adjustment that takes place. Clinical states causing depletion of CO_2 result in *respiratory alkalosis,* and depression of respiration is the result. Conditions resulting in depleted HCO_3^- lead to *metabolic acidosis* and those resulting in accumulation of HCO_3^- cause *metabolic alkalosis.* In general, it is helpful to think of respiratory acidosis or alkalosis as short-term problems and metabolic acidosis or alkalosis as long-term problems, since there is a considerable difference in the time needed for body response in the two situations.

ACID-BASE IMBALANCES

Respiratory Acidosis

Respiratory acidosis results from a variety of causes (Table 8–1). The common denominator of the causes is interference with gas exchange in the lung, either by impaired alveolar action, as in emphysema, or by decreased respiration, as with barbiturate poisoning. As a result, CO_2 accumulates (normal partial pressure in serum [PCO_2] is 35 to 45 mm Hg of mercury) and the serum pH shifts below 7.35 (Table 8–2). Urine pH decreases as H^+ is secreted to

Table 8–2. LABORATORY FINDINGS IN RESPIRATORY ACIDOSIS

Serum pH	Below 7.35
Urine pH	Below 6.0
PCO_2	Above 45 mm Hg (cause of acidosis)
HCO_3^-	30–35 mEq/L

Table 8–3. CAUSES OF RESPIRATORY ALKALOSIS

Hyperventilation (from anxiety or intentional overbreathing)
Lack of oxygen (high altitude or partial asphyxia)
Fever
Overventilation with respirator

compensate for the acidosis. Serum bicarbonate level is slightly elevated as a result of formation of H_2CO_3 from the retained CO_2, which hydrolyzes to form H^+ and HCO_3^-, but long-term adjustments in HCO_3^- have not yet taken place. Symptoms include weakness, disorientation, and central nervous system depression, leading, in severe cases, to coma.

Treatment   Treatment is directed toward increasing the respiratory rate and/or the rate of gas exchange in the alveoli. Respiratory rate can be increased by removal of depressant drugs from the blood stream with hemodialysis or by the use of specific antidotes for them (e.g., naloxone [Narcan], a specific narcotic antagonist). Respiratory assistance by means of a mechanical respirator or the use of respiratory stimulant drugs (e.g., doxapram [Dopram]) increases respiratory function and removal of CO_2. Treatment of conditions such as emphysema (see Chapter 14), in which alveolar gas exchange is depressed, results in increased CO_2 removal. Bronchial asthma is treated with drugs that dilate the bronchi and provide more opportunity for alveolar gas exchange (see Chapter 14). This causes removal of more CO_2 and the respiratory acidosis is corrected.

Respiratory Alkalosis   In this condition, deficiency of CO_2 results in an upward shift in serum pH (>7.45). Although there are many causes of respiratory alkalosis (Table 8–3), they have in common that respiratory rate and/or depth are increased, resulting in excessive removal of CO_2 in the expired air ("blowing off" of CO_2). Since CO_2 is considered to be potential acid, its removal raises serum pH (Table 8–4). Serum bicarbonate level is slightly lower than normal, since less CO_2 is available for formation of H_2CO_3 and, therefore, HCO_3^-. However, long-term adjustments utilizing the carbonic acid-bicarbonate system have not yet occurred. Renal adjustment in respiratory alkalosis consists of restricting H^+ secretion to counteract the alkalosis condition.

Since the central nervous system is stimulated by alkalosis, the chief symptoms are nervousness, anxiety, tremors, and, in severe cases, convulsions. Ironically, some anxious individuals begin a vicious cycle of *hyperventilation,* caused by their anxiety, which leads to respiratory alkalosis, increased anxiety, and further hyperventilation.

Table 8–4. LABORATORY FINDINGS IN RESPIRATORY ALKALOSIS

Serum pH	Above 7.45
Urine pH	Above 7.0
P_{CO_2}	Below 35 mm Hg (cause of alkalosis)
HCO_3^-	20–25 mEq/L

Treatment   Treatment involves breathing into a paper bag (which causes rebreathing of expired CO_2 and increased uptake of CO_2 into the serum). This is generally quite effective in breaking the cycle of anxiety-hyperventilation. Hyperventilation caused by fever will disappear when the fever is lowered or when infection is brought under control. *Hypoxia,* another common cause of respiratory alkalosis, improves with treatment of the underlying lung condition or with the administration of oxygen. In all cases of respiratory alkalosis, increased CO_2 retention reverses the alkalosis condition.

Metabolic Acidosis   A wide variety of clinical states cause metabolic acidosis (Table 8–5). Some common causes include:

1. Severe diabetes mellitus that is not adequately controlled.
2. Starvation.
3. The use of a high-fat (ketogenic) diet for weight control.

In all three cases, the body begins metabolizing fats (either body or dietary fat) for energy in place of carbohydrate. In severe diabetes mellitus, body fat is utilized to provide energy unavailable from glucose metabolism (see Chapter 16). Long-chain fatty acids are broken down into two-carbon (acetate) fragments, leaving only the ends of the fatty acid chains *(ketone bodies)* These can be likened to the core of the apple that must be discarded. Accumulation of ketone bodies (consisting of acetone, beta-hydroxybutyric acid, and acetoacetic acid) causes *ketosis* and results in metabolic acidosis, called in this case *ketoacidosis* or *diabetic acidosis.* Acidosis develops partly because two of the ketone bodies are acids and affect pH when retained by the body, and partly because the body excretes sodium and potassium ions in order to eliminate the acids as salts. Loss of sodium and potassium (so-called "fixed bases") results in systemic acidosis. A similar situation occurs in starvation, in which the body breaks down its own fats for energy, and with the use of a high-fat diet.

Lactic acidosis, a form of metabolic acidosis, is caused by accumulation of lactic acid as a result of reduced tissue perfusion (causing tissue hypoxia) and dependence upon anaerobic metabolism for energy. It is seen in shock or if cardiac pumping action is severely impaired, as in congestive heart failure or in temporary arrest following a myocardial infarction. Certain drugs can also cause lactic acidosis, the most notable being the oral antidiabetic drug phenformin (DBI), which was removed from the market several years ago as a result of this adverse effect.

Metabolic acidosis develops more slowly than respiratory acidosis and involves more extensive compensation by the body. Laboratory findings (Table 8–6) include:

1. Low serum pH (<7.35).

Table 8–5. CAUSES OF METABOLIC ACIDOSIS

Starvation or severe weight loss
Ketogenic diet
Uncontrolled severe diabetes mellitus
Renal disease (reduced tubular H^+ secretion)
Drug ingestion (acids or drugs having acidic metabolic
  products)

Table 8–6. LABORATORY FINDINGS IN METABOLIC ACIDOSIS

Serum pH	Below 7.35
Urine pH	Below 6.0
P_{CO_2}	Below 35 mm Hg (compensation for acidosis by hyperventilation)
HCO_3^-	Below 20 mEq/L

2. Urine pH below 6.0, since H^+ is secreted to compensate for the acidosis.

3. HCO_3^- level lowered, since HCO_3^- is used up to buffer the excess acid.

Symptoms of metabolic acidosis include weakness; central nervous system depression, leading to sedation and coma; and hyperventilation. Hyperventilation (called "air hunger" in this situation) is a compensatory mechanism that removes CO_2 and creates a respiratory alkalosis, which counteracts the metabolic acidosis. It is of interest that the central nervous system depression caused by acidosis renders the individual less susceptible to seizures. In the early days of epilepsy treatment, before effective drugs were discovered, ketogenic diets were employed to reduce seizure activity. Even today, carbonic anhydrase inhibitors, such as acetazolamide (Diamox), are used as adjunctive treatment for epilepsy. These drugs, by virtue of their action on renal carbonic anhydrase, prevent H^+ secretion and cause metabolic acidosis.

Treatment   Treatment of metabolic acidosis is directed toward the cause and includes:

1. Control of diabetes mellitus.

2. Discontinuation of drugs that cause severe acidosis.

3. Adjustments in the diet to maintain less dependence upon fat metabolism for energy (usually more carbohydrate added to the diet).

In cardiac arrest, sodium bicarbonate solution is given intravenously to replace the HCO_3^- used to buffer acid. As cardiac function improves and tissues perfusion increases, infusion of sodium bicarbonate becomes unnecessary.

Metabolic Alkalosis   Accumulation of HCO_3^- leads to metabolic alkalosis, which requires some time to develop, in comparison with respiratory alkalosis. Common causes (Table 8–7) include:

1. Vomiting or excessive gastric suction (both of which remove H^+).

2. Excessive administration of sodium bicarbonate.

3. Hypokalemia.

Table 8–7. CAUSES OF METABOLIC ALKALOSIS

Vomiting or excessive gastric suction (loss of H^+)
Excessive intake of sodium bicarbonate
Hypokalemia (inadequate intake of potassium, overuse of potassium-losing diuretics, or excessive corticosteroid activity)

Sodium bicarbonate (baking soda) is often taken orally as an antacid, and its overuse leads to rebound acid production and escalated intake. Since both Na^+ and HCO_3^- are well absorbed from the gastrointestinal tract, excessive use leads to increased levels of both ions in the body. Sodium buildup expands the extracellular fluid volume and leads to edema and increased cardiac workload (see Chapter 7 regarding hypernatremia). Bicarbonate ion accumulation results in metabolic alkalosis.

An interesting connection exists between lowered potassium levels and metabolic alkalosis. Hypokalemia, whether induced by diuretics, deficient intake, or administration of corticosteroids, can cause metabolic alkalosis. If there is insufficient K^+ to exchange for Na^+ at the distal tubule (see Chapter 7 regarding aldosterone activity), H^+ is secreted in exchange for Na^+ in place of K^+. Loss of H^+ and reabsorption of HCO_3^- that would have been lost as sodium bicarbonate leads to metabolic alkalosis.

Laboratory Findings

Laboratory findings in metabolic alkalosis (Table 8–8) include:
1. High serum pH (>7.45).
2. Increased urine pH (>7.0).
3. Increased serum HCO_3^- level.
4. Reduced serum K^+ (if hypokalemia is the cause).

Respiratory depression occurs as a compensation for the alkalosis, leading to accumulation of CO_2.

Symptoms and Signs

In addition to respiratory depression, symptoms include central nervous system stimulation leading to hyperreflexia, increased muscle tone, and, eventually, tetany and convulsions.

Treatment

Metabolic alkalosis is treated by eliminating the underlying cause. Treatment can include:
1. Suppression of vomiting or cessation of gastric suction.
2. Discontinuation of sodium bicarbonate administration.
3. Administration of potassium (if hypokalemia is the cause).

Mixed Acid-Base Disturbance

It is possible, under certain circumstances, to have both acidosis and alkalosis at the same time. If an uncontrolled diabetic (metabolic acidosis) travels quickly to a high altitude or hyperventilates because of anxiety, respiratory alkalosis develops along with the metabolic acidosis. The more severe of the two conditions would prevail and, with time, cancellation of one or both of them would occur.

It is also possible to have respiratory and metabolic acidosis or respiratory and metabolic alkalosis simultaneously. The same uncon-

Table 8–8. LABORATORY FINDINGS IN METABOLIC ALKALOSIS

Serum pH	Above 7.45
Urine pH	Above 7.0
P_{CO_2}	Above 45 mm Hg (compensation for alkalosis by depression of respiration)
HCO_3^-	Above 30 mEq/L
K^+	Below 3.5 mEq/L (in those cases caused by hypokalemia)

trolled diabetic who was overdosed with a barbiturate drug would suffer respiratory depression, leading to respiratory acidosis along with metabolic acidosis caused by the diabetes. The two processes would tend to reinforce each other, increasing the severity of the acidosis.

SUMMARY

Serum pH is maintained relatively constant through the interaction of a complex set of control mechanisms, including the carbonic acid-bicarbonate, phosphate, hemoglobin, and protein buffer systems, CO_2 expiration by the lungs, and H^+ secretion by the kidney. Variations of serum pH below 6.8 or above 8.0 cause death in humans. Values between these extremes and the normal range (7.35 to 7.45) are abnormal and are attended by compensatory body adjustments. Both respiratory acidosis and alkalosis, caused by excess or lack of CO_2 retention, and metabolic acidosis and alkalosis, caused by lack or excess of HCO_3^-, exist.

The causes of acid-base disorders are legion and include disease states, treatment procedures, environmental influences, and variations in diet. Treatment involves alteration of contributing factors to allow the normal body mechanisms to return acid-base values to within physiologic range.

Questions
1. It is known that mixed (respiratory and metabolic) acid-base disturbances can occur, at least temporarily. What combination of disturbances would result from starvation in conjunction with high altitude exposure? From excessive use of potassium-losing diuretics in conjunction with barbiturate overdose? From prolonged vomiting coupled with high fever? From a ketogenic diet along with emphysema?
2. Assuming that all other acid-base control mechanisms remained constant, what would be the effect on serum pH of reduced and increased H^+ secretion by the renal tubule? What would be the effect of reduced and increased rate of CO_2 removal by the lungs?

Additional Reading
Coe, F. L.: Metabolic alkalosis. J.A.M.A., 238:2288, 1977.
Davenport, H. W.: *The ABC of Acid-Base Chemistry*. Chicago, University of Chicago Press, 1974.
Filley, G. F.: *Acid-Base and Blood Gas Regulation*. Philadelphia, Lea & Febiger, 1971.
Ganong, W. F.: *Review of Medical Physiology*. Los Altos, Calif., Lange Medical Publications, 1977. *(Good discussion of acid-base balance.)*
Relman, A. S.: Lactic acidosis and a possible new treatment. N. Engl. J. Med., 298:564, 1978.

CHAPTER 9

INFECTIOUS DISORDERS

Clinical disease in which infection is the major feature accounts for a large number of physician visits and hospitalizations. In the areas of broad medical practice, such as family practice, internal medicine, or pediatrics, infectious diseases may constitute the major type of disorder encountered. The practitioner must be well versed in the diagnosis and treatment of infectious diseases, especially in the selection of appropriate drug therapy. Even in the narrowest of medical specialties, infectious diseases form a significant fraction of the cases. Some subspecialties—for example, tropical medicine—are almost totally concerned with infections, their diagnosis, treatment, and complications.

Infection is a pathophysiologic mechanism and has been discussed in detail in Chapter 2. The disorders covered in this chapter reflect infection as the *major* or as a *significant contributing factor* to disease. It should be appreciated, however, that infection rarely occurs without involving other responses in the body. Intimately intertwined with infection are the processes of inflammation, immune response, and wound healing. It is often difficult to separate the pathologic consequences of these related processes, and the histologic findings suggest a mixture of all three. It is somewhat arbitrary to call bronchitis an infectious disorder, for example, since the name suggests inflammation. However, most cases of acute bronchitis are caused by infection and many cases of chronic bronchitis are associated with infection, either as a cause or as a complication. Likewise, a certain amount of tissue repair occurs in chronic bronchitis as a consequence of damage caused by inflammation and/or infection. Squamous metaplasia is often seen in bronchitis associated with exposure to chronic irritants, such as cigarette smoke. This results in alteration of the bronchial mucosa, as previously mentioned, and may increase the risk of malignancy. Therefore, other disease processes are at work and the total picture is more complicated than one in which organisms merely infect the tissues.

No attempt is made in this chapter to cover all infectious diseases. A number of common infections are discussed in some detail. These are organized into three general areas: respiratory, genitourinary, and central nervous system infections. (Pharyngitis, laryngitis, and sinus infections are covered in Chapter 18 as eye, ear, nose and throat disorders, as is infectious conjunctivitis.)

It should be recognized that the process of infection is often similar in different body areas and that an organism frequently has the same invasive, propagative, and virulent properties in several types of body tissue. For example, *Staphylococcus aureus* causes skin infections (boils, carbuncles), oral infection, and lung infection (pneumonia). In each case, the organism usually forms an abscess, becomes partially walled off from surrounding tissue, and secretes penicillinase. Therefore, the treatment of staphylococcal infection is usually with penicillinase-resistant penicillins or cephalosporins, along with drainage of the abscessed area, if necessary. Many streptococcal infections cause formation of antibodies that can trigger inflammatory kidney disease. Therefore, treatment of streptococcal infections, whether in the form of "strep throat," impetigo (skin infection), or tonsillitis, requires attention to the kidney as a possible victim of the immune response, in addition to treatment of the infection itself with penicillin or ampicillin.

As each individual infection is studied, it is helpful to think about the causative organism and its properties. This will aid in better understanding of the symptoms, required treatment, and complications of the infection.

RESPIRATORY INFECTIONS

BRONCHITIS   Inflammation of the bronchial mucosa can be either acute or chronic and can be related to other lung conditions, such as emphysema or bronchial asthma. *Primary bronchitis* is caused by infection or by the inhalation of irritating materials (smoke, particulate matter, or allergens). *Secondary bronchitis* occurs in conjunction with other respiratory conditions and represents only a part of the total disease process.

Acute Bronchitis   Acute bronchitis is usually caused by infection with one of the 30 or more respiratory viruses and often results from an extension of a cold or flulike illness into the chest ("chest cold"). Adenoviruses and rhinoviruses are among the most common infectious agents. Secondary bacterial infection, especially with pneumococci or *Haemophilus influenzae,* is also common in tissue whose resistance is lowered by viral infection.

Pathogenesis   Following irritation, infection, or allergic reaction, the bronchial mucosa becomes inflamed and edematous and forms a fluid exudate in response to the inflammatory stimulus. The large amount of fluid exudate occupies the intrabronchial space, interfering with inhalation and exhalation. Cough with expectoration of mucus then results.

Symptoms and Signs   Common symptoms and signs of acute bronchitis include malaise, fever, and a brassy cough that produces sputum (productive cough) which often contains pus (purulent). Head cold symptoms of nasal congestion, rhinorrhea (runny nose), sore throat, and headache often coexist with acute bronchitis. Cervical (neck) lymph nodes are enlarged as virus particles are trapped and prevented from circulating through the blood stream.

Laboratory Findings   X-ray films of the chest in acute bronchitis are often unremarkable, since the alveoli are not affected. The only benefit of a chest x-ray exam is to rule out other respiratory conditions (such as pneumonia, emphysema, or lung tumor) that produce definite x-ray changes. If bacterial infection is present, leukocytosis generally is found. However, the white blood cell count is often normal in viral infections.

Diagnosis   Acute bronchitis must be differentiated from pneumonia, emphysema, bronchial asthma, and neoplastic lung disease. Chest x-ray findings, along with a careful history and investigation as to cause, permit accurate diagnosis. In children, acute bronchitis is often the first manifestation of a systemic infectious disease (chickenpox, measles) and a knowledge of current epidemic diseases helps to predict which disease will surface.

Treatment   Uncomplicated acute bronchitis resolves with bed rest, administration of adequate fluids, and cessation of smoking or exposure to other irritants. Excessive coughing can be controlled with codeine or dextromethorphan. Some coughing is desirable, however, to keep the airway clear. This is especially important in those with chronic respiratory diseases such as emphysema, in whom retained mucus causes further respiratory obstruction. Antibiotics are used occasionally if secondary bacterial infection is present or in a debilitated person in whom secondary bacterial infection might be extremely dangerous. Penicillin, ampicillin (Polycillin), or tetracycline (Achromycin) is the drug of choice. Coexisting cold symptoms are treated with aspirin, decongestants (e.g., pseudoephedrine [Sudafed]), and antihistamines (e.g., chlorpheniramine [Chlortrimeton]). These do not change the course of infection but make the patient more comfortable until recovery occurs.

Complications   Healthy adults rarely suffer complications from acute bronchitis. Debilitated individuals may develop pneumonia, and those with chronic respiratory diseases can develop life-threatening respiratory insufficiency. Small children can be in danger of asphyxiation from severe respiratory obstruction in acute bronchitis because of the narrow diameter of respiratory passages. In these cases, oxygen therapy and the use of bronchodilators may be of great benefit.

Chronic Bronchitis   Chronic bronchitis is considered to be present in an individual who has had persistent productive cough for at least 3 months in two or more consecutive years. It is most common in middle-aged men (10 to 25 per cent in city dwellers) and is associated with cigarette smoking and air pollution. Of the two, cigarette smoking is the more important, since it alone will increase the incidence of chronic bronchitis four to ten times that in nonsmokers. Air pollutants, such as nitrogen dioxide and sulfur dioxide along with particulate matter, also increase the risk of chronic bronchitis, especially when coupled with heavy smoking.

Pathogenesis   Chronic irritation of the bronchial mucosa leads to hyperplasia of the mucus-producing glands and increased formation of goblet cells, which secrete mucus. Long-term exposure to irritants, particularly cigarette smoke, also destroys ciliary action and causes squamous metaplasia. These changes reduce the self-cleaning ability of the lung and may cause a cycle of further irritation from inhaled materials.

Infection frequently accompanies inflammation in chronic bronchitis. Although infection is less important than inflammation in the development of the condition, it probably helps to maintain it and accounts for periodic exacerbations of symptoms. Pneumococci and *H. influenzae* are often found in sputum cultures in chronic bronchitis and probably invade tissues already made less resistant by chronic inflammation. Smoking seems to facilitate infection, possibly by interfering with ciliary and macrophage activity needed to remove bacteria from the respiratory tract. Certainly, infection further burdens the already poorly functioning bronchial system by causing edema and partial obstruction of small bronchi.

Symptoms and Signs

Productive cough is the chief symptom of chronic bronchitis. Bloody or foul-smelling sputum suggests infection or lung tumor. In long-standing cases, expansion of the chest and hypertrophy of the respiratory musculature may occur because of the extra effort required for breathing. The term "pink puffer" is sometimes applied, since the victim tends to hyperventilate and may overoxygenate the blood with excessive respiratory effort.

Laboratory Findings

Physical examination often reveals breathing noises (bronchial rales), presumably caused by air passing over inflamed and swollen tissue. Unless infection is present, the leukocyte count is generally normal. The erythrocyte sedimentation rate (ESR), which is usually elevated in inflammatory states, is commonly normal in this case. Sputum culture is often positive for pneumococcus or *H. influenzae* (opportunistic infection).

Diagnosis

Chronic bronchitis must be differentiated from tuberculosis or fungal infection of the lung, conditions caused by inhalation of specific particles (silicosis, asbestosis), neoplastic respiratory disease, or foreign bodies in the respiratory tract. Tuberculosis or fungal infection can be identified by chest x-ray examination in conjunction with organism identification in the sputum and skin tests to determine immune response to the causative organism. History of occupational exposure to silica or asbestos is of major benefit in differential diagnosis. Lung tumors usually appear on x-ray films or are observable using bronchoscopy (visualization of the bronchi with a lighted tube inserted through the mouth and throat).

Foreign bodies remaining in the respiratory tract for a long time can cause chronic cough. In one case, a man was smoking a pipe while standing next to a factory. The factory exploded and, in reaction to it, the man bit off part of the stem of his pipe and inhaled it. For the next 25 years or so, he was troubled with a chronic cough. Finally, one day he coughed up the piece of pipe stem and his problem disappeared!

Treatment

Cessation of smoking is the single most important factor in the treatment of chronic bronchitis. Change of location out of heavily populated areas will also improve symptoms dramatically. Steam inhalation serves to soothe inflamed bronchial tissue and reduce cough. Expectorant drugs, such as ammonium chloride or glyceryl guaiacolate, aid in mucus removal. Excessive coughing can be suppressed with small doses of codeine or dextromethorphan. For coexisting infection, ampicillin (Polycillin) or tetracycline (Achromycin) is a useful agent. These should be used only during the acute infectious episode.

Prognosis

Chronic bronchitis usually improves if the treatment program described is implemented. Progressive obliteration of small bronchioles occurs in severe, untreated cases, causing increasing respiratory difficulty. The development of squamous metaplasia may be a forerunner of bronchial tumors.

PNEUMONIA

Inflammation of the lung parenchyma (outer portion) is usually caused by infection, but it may be caused by inhalation of irritating chemicals or by aspiration of gastric contents. The latter situation is most common during surgery in a patient who has not fasted. Anesthesia both suppresses the cough reflex and increases the tendency toward vomiting. These effects increase the risk of gastric aspiration. This discussion will be limited to infectious pneumonia, and will emphasize the most common type caused by pneumococcal infection.

As discussed in Chapter 2, the upper respiratory tract harbors organisms that are kept from proliferating in the lower respiratory tract by normal body resistance. Factors that lower body resistance favor the development of pneumonia. These include alcoholism, debilitating diseases, malnutrition, and overdose of respiratory depressants, such as barbiturates. The predilection of pneumonia for the very young and the very old and infirm earned it the nickname "friend of the old and enemy of the young," since it was a tragedy for a young person to die of it but a relatively painless death for a nursing home resident. Although pneumonia is much more effectively treated today than in earlier times, it is still the fifth leading cause of death in the United States. In many cases, resistance has been severely reduced by debility, old age, alcoholism, or treatments such as anticancer therapy.

Pathogenesis

Two major types of pneumonia are recognized: *bronchopneumonia* and *lobar pneumonia*. In bronchopneumonia, infiltration occurs from the bronchi into the immediate surrounding lung parenchyma (Fig. 9–1). Inflammation occurs and a large amount of exudate is formed with a patchy distribution. Lobar pneumonia affects a large section of a lobe or an entire lobe. A key feature in both types is *consolidation*, or the formation of a semisolid mass of exudate containing fibrin. The affected area of the lung is virtually nonfunctional until the consolidation liquefies and is removed by blood and lymph circulation and by expectoration. *Pneumonitis* describes minimal alveolar involvement with a less dramatic white blood cell response to infection. This condition is often seen with viral infection and usually produces fewer symptoms than do bacterial pneumonias.

Symptoms and Signs

Cough, chest pain, chills, and high fever are common findings in both bronchopneumonia and lobar pneumonia. Respiration is hindered by exudate formation in the lung, and tachypnea (rapid

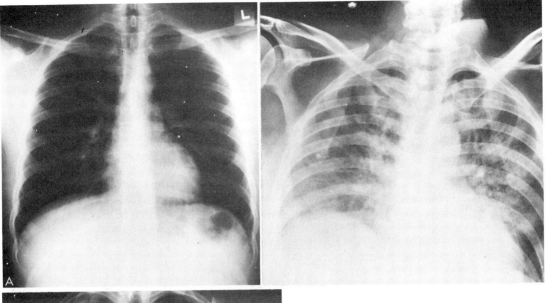

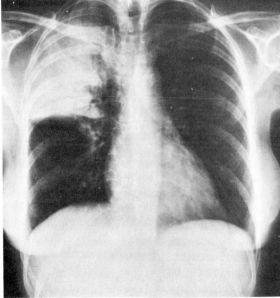

Figure 9–1. Bronchopneumonia versus lobar pneumonia. *(A)* Normal lungs. *(B)* Bronchopneumonia. *(C)* Lobar pneumonia. (From Griffiths, H. J., and Sarno, R. C.: *Contemporary Radiology: An Introduction to Imaging.* Philadelphia, W. B. Saunders Company, 1979.)

breathing) results. Inspiratory rales occur as air passes over the areas of inflammation and exudate in the lung. Rales usually disappear at the peak of consolidation (likened to the silence in the eye of a hurricane) and then reappear as the consolidation is being cleared. Cough, often producing a blood-streaked ("rusty") sputum, is common.

Laboratory Findings   Bacterial pneumonias cause leukocytosis or leukemoid reaction (20,000 to 25,000/mm³), whereas viral pneumonias generally produce little or no white blood cell response. Most causative organisms can be identified by sputum smear or culture (85 per cent of bacterial pneumonias are caused by pneumococci). Although viruses can be cultured, they are usually identified by elimination of bacterial or other causes of pneumonia because culture is difficult. Chest x-ray films show areas of patchy distribution in bronchopneumonia or more well-defined areas in lobar pneumonia.

Diagnosis With a clear picture of laboratory findings, symptoms, and signs, the diagnosis of bacterial pneumonia is not difficult. Pneumonia caused by nonbacterial organisms may be more difficult to identify, since the disease produces less typical findings. Other respiratory conditions, such as acute bronchitis and bronchial asthma, can mimic some of the findings in pneumonia. Chest x-ray and sputum examinations are probably the most helpful laboratory tests in the differential diagnosis.

Treatment Pneumococcal pneumonia nearly always responds to penicillin, usually given intramuscularly or intravenously. Doses are two to ten times the usual oral dose of penicillin to provide the high blood level needed for rapid cure. In individuals allergic to penicillin, erythromycin (Ilotycin), tetracycline (Achromycin), or sulfa drugs are also useful. Often oxygen is required during the acute episode to provide a richer air mixture, since alveolar gas exchange is impaired by the exudate formed. This can be given by nasal catheter, tent, or mask, depending upon the severity of the condition. Fluid replacement is also important, since the combination of high fever and tachypnea removes moisture from the body very rapidly. Table 9–1 lists the various drug therapies for pneumonia.

Complications Pulmonary edema is a common complication to pneumonia. Oxygen administration helps to reduce its severity. Shock (severe drop in blood pressure) is another life-threatening complication and must be treated by the use of blood volume expanders and/or drugs that increase blood pressure, such as methoxamine (Vasoxyl). Delirium often occurs as a result of fever and the toxic effects of infection. This is managed with diazepam (Valium) or phenobarbital (Luminal). Some degree of pulmonary fibrosis is often seen after recovery, but this rarely causes difficulty.

Prognosis Most deaths from pneumonia occur in very young and very old individuals and in those with debilitating illnesses. The overall mortality rate is 5 to 10 per cent with good medical care. For those at high risk of pneumococcal pneumonia, a polyvalent vaccine (which protects against 14 strains of pneumococci) is available for added protection.

Other Gram-Positive Pneumonias Gram-positive pneumonias other than those caused by pneumococci are generally caused by hemolytic streptococci or staphylococci. *Hemolytic streptococcal pneumonia* often develops as a

Table 9–1. DRUG THERAPY OF PNEUMONIAS

Causative Organism	Drug of Choice
Pneumococci	Penicillin, erythromycin, tetracycline, sulfas
Streptococci	Same as for pneumococcal pneumonia
Staphylococci	Nafcillin, methicillin
Klebsiella, Pseudomonas, Proteus, Serratia	Gentamicin, cephalosporins
Legionella	Erythromycin, rifampin
Mixed organisms	Ampicillin, tetracycline
Mycoplasma	Erythromycin, tetracycline
Viruses	No specific drug therapy

complication to viral pneumonia, especially in those with chronic lung disease. Pleural effusion and empyema (collection of pus in the pleural space) are common complications. Treatment is similar to that of pneumococcal pneumonia.

Staphylococcal pneumonia develops under similar circumstances and often appears after antibiotic therapy. In this case, the antibiotic eradicates most organisms except *S. aureus,* which then proliferates in the lungs. Cavitation of the lung (a cavity formed by tissue destruction) is common, and empyema and pneumothorax (lung collapse) are also frequent complications. X-ray films often show the presence of air or fluid in cavitation areas.

Treatment　　Since most staphylococcal strains are penicillin-resistant because they produce penicillinase, special penicillinase-resistant drugs such as nafcillin (Unipen) or methicillin (Staphcillin) are used for treatment. Empyemic areas often require surgical drainage and prolonged antibiotic treatment for cure.

Gram-Negative Pneumonias　　Pneumonias caused by Klebsiella, Pseudomonas, Proteus, and Serratia are relatively common, especially in the hospital environment and in those with contributing factors of alcoholism, malnutrition, or debilitating diseases. Generally, symptoms are severe and massive consolidation occurs, leading to death without drug intervention. Lung abscess and necrosis are extremely common. Diagnosis is similar to that of other pneumonias, primarily using x-ray findings and sputum smears or cultures. Pneumonia caused by Klebsiella responds to gentamicin (Garamycin) or cephalosporins, such as cefazolin (Ancef). Gentamicin is also useful for pneumonias caused by Pseudomonas, Proteus, and Serratia.

Legionnaire's disease is a gram-negative pneumonia caused by *Legionella pneumophila,* which grows in dust or soil. A famous epidemic of it occurred in 1976 at the American Legion Convention in Philadelphia and was traced to contamination in dust from the air-conditioning system of the hotel. The symptoms are similar to those of other pneumonias, but the organism is difficult to recover from sputum, pleural fluid, or blood and requires special medium for growth. Organism identification was originally very difficult, and deaths occurred because the exact treatment was not known (penicillin is ineffective). The cause of death is usually shock, respiratory failure, or renal failure. Erythromycin (Ilotycin) has been found effective, and rifampin (Rifadin) is used as a backup drug for resistant cases.

Mixed Pneumonia　　Infection with a variety of organisms often occurs as a terminal event in severely debilitated individuals. With greatly reduced resistance, organisms are allowed to invade the alveoli and bronchopneumonia develops. Sputum culture or smear shows several organisms to be actively growing in the lung, rather than one prominent organism as with other pneumonias.

Treatment　　Treatment is often ineffective, owing to the underlying condition of the patient. Broad-spectrum antibiotics, such as ampicillin (Polycillin) or tetracycline (Achromycin) are agents of choice, since they inhibit most, if not all, of the infecting organisms.

Primary Atypical Pneumonia

Infection with organisms other than gram-positive and gram-negative bacteria produces a pneumonia that is generally milder in symptomatology and is called primary atypical pneumonia. The common causative agents are adenoviruses, influenza viruses, and *Mycoplasma pneumoniae* (Eaton agent), a bacterialike organism without a cell wall.

Symptoms and Signs

The disease usually starts as an influenzalike upper respiratory illness that spreads to the trachea and bronchi and then involves the alveoli. Sore throat and bullous myringitis (eardrum infection that causes blisters) are frequently associated with the respiratory infection.

Laboratory Findings

Laboratory findings are usually nonspecific, with patchy infiltration seen on chest x-ray exam. The white blood cell count is normal or slightly depressed, and sputum culture is negative for growth with standard media. Both viruses and mycoplasma can be grown under special conditions, but culture is more difficult than with common pathogens.

Diagnosis

Diagnosis rests primarily on the findings of a pneumonialike illness in a person with a history of upper respiratory tract infection but without the typical laboratory findings of bacterial pneumonia. Infection with mycobacteria or fungi can cause a similar-appearing condition, but the organism can usually be identified with skin tests or recovery of the organism from the sputum. (See the discussion of tuberculosis and fungal respiratory infections later in this chapter.)

Treatment

No treatment, other than bed rest and fluid replacement, is needed for mild cases of primary atypical pneumonia. Aspirin helps to relieve pain and lower temperature. More severe cases of mycoplasmal pneumonia respond to erythromycin (Ilotycin) or tetracycline (Achromycin). There is no specific drug therapy for viral pneumonias.

TUBERCULOSIS

Infection with *Mycobacterium tuberculosis,* once a major cause of death in the United States (200 per 100,000 population in 1900), is now an uncommon cause of death (2 per 100,000 population), although it is still a scourge in many areas of the world. Most cases in the United States occur in slums, where overcrowding and lack of sanitation prevail. Alcoholism, malnutrition, and chronic disease also predispose to tuberculosis, as does the use of agents that suppress the immune response (anticancer drugs, corticosteroids). Some natural resistance to tuberculosis exists and Caucasians seem to have more innate resistance than do blacks or Eskimos.

Most cases of tuberculosis seen in the United States are lung infections because they are diagnosed at a relatively early stage. In other countries (as was the case in the United States at the turn of the century), tuberculosis infection in the kidney, larynx, or central nervous system is common and produces different presenting symptoms and signs than does pulmonary tuberculosis. "Tuberculosis" comes from the word tubercule (small potato), which describes the appearance of the infectious lesions.

Pathogenesis   Tuberculosis is spread in droplets coughed into the air by an infected person and inhaled by the victim. Spread via contaminated surfaces or articles handled by an infected person is a very minor source of infection. *M. tuberculosis,* an acid-fast bacillus, enters the lung and sets up a *primary* infection.

In most persons, body resistance is great enough to limit the infection to a small area of the lung, often in the periphery. Organisms migrate to the nearby hilar lymph nodes (Fig. 9–2) and become trapped. A granulation reaction occurs and necrosis develops in the infected tissue, forming a caseous (cheesy) center to the lesion. Eventually, the lesion becomes fibrotic and calcifies, but it can contain viable organisms for an extended period of time. The calcified lesion is called a *Ghon tubercle.* It, plus the enlarged hilar lymph nodes, represents the *Ghon complex,* usually visible by x-ray exam.

Most individuals with this type of infection develop a positive skin test for tuberculosis but have no symptoms and do not develop further infection. The mild exposure confers lifetime immunity to tuberculosis for most people. Only if immunity is severely suppressed does active lung infection develop at this point.

Secondary tuberculosis occurs from reactivation of the primary infection as organisms previously trapped within calcified lesions are released. Occasionally, very heavy exposure to an infected person occurs and the immunity developed from the primary infection is overwhelmed. In these cases, hypersensitivity developed on prior exposure leads to significant lung damage.

The secondary lesion is granular and is almost always located in the lung apex (top portion) where oxygen supply is greatest (Fig. 9–3). Caseation necrosis again occurs, and the lung tissue may cavitate or form fibrosis and calcification. Eventually, collagen tissue

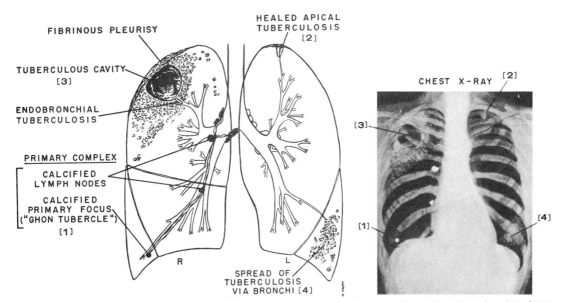

Figure 9–2. Primary infection in tuberculosis. (From *Introduction to Lung Disease,* 6th ed. New York, American Lung Association, 1975. Used by permission.)

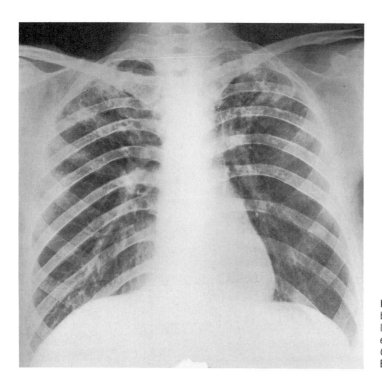

Figure 9–3. Secondary infection in tuberculosis. (From Squire, L. F., Colaiace, W. M., and Strutynsky, N.: *Exercises in Diagnostic Radiology: The Chest,* vol. 1, 2nd ed. Philadelphia, W. B. Saunders Company, 1981.)

may completely wall off the lesion and prevent its spread (but also restrict the penetration of drugs into the area).

The causes of secondary tuberculosis are variable. Often, primary infection occurs in childhood, but secondary infection surfaces in adulthood. This is especially likely if contributing factors such as alcoholism or debilitating disease are present. Actual reinfection is quite uncommon. The greatest danger is from reactivation of quiescent primary lesions.

Symptoms and Signs

Cough, chest pain, weakness, and loss of weight are common symptoms with tuberculosis, although mild cases may be asymptomatic. Mild fever is often present. Fever worsens in the afternoon and breaks at night, causing *night sweats*. Wheezing, rales, and expectoration of blood occur in more advanced cases.

Laboratory Findings

Tuberculosis can be identified by the use of a combination of chest x-ray exam, skin tests, and sputum exam.

X-ray Exam. Chest x-ray films demonstrate the Ghon complex and secondary lesions, along with any cavitation present in the lung. Often, multiple x-ray exposures are required to visualize lesions hidden by ribs or other structures.

Skin Tests. These measure the hypersensitivity developed to antigenic bacterial proteins and show prior exposure to the organism. The *tine test* uses small prongs coated with tuberculin antigen that puncture the skin. It is a commonly used screening test, especially in children. The *Mantoux test* utilizes the same principle, but the antigen is injected intradermally (between the layers of skin). It is considered more sensitive for the diagnosis of tuberculosis. The degree of reaction is determined by the size of the area of induration (raised, hardened tissue). Induration of 10 mm or more with the Mantoux test is considered positive (prior exposure to *M. tuberculosis*).

Sputum Test. Sputum examination for acid-fast organisms also aids in diagnosis. (See the discussion of Ziehl-Neelsen technique in Chapter 2.) Smears provide rapid identification of the causative organism. Culture requires a special growth medium and often takes 1 to 2 months for definite growth to occur. However, culture is recommended as a definitive test, even though treatment is usually started before culture results are obtained. Since organisms are often coughed up and swallowed, the stomach may yield mycobacteria upon *gastric washing*. If accessible lymph nodes are infected (as in the neck area), lymph node biopsy and culture can be performed to aid in diagnosis.

Diagnosis   Many respiratory conditions can mimic the profile of pulmonary tuberculosis. Atypical mycobacteria (see Chapter 2) produce tuberculosislike infection and may even give a positive skin test for tuberculosis. They often require special drug therapy or surgical excision of the infected lesion for cure. Fungal infections (to be discussed) resemble tuberculosis in many ways but require different treatment. Lung tumors can produce many of the symptoms of tuberculosis, including cough, fever, weight loss, and expectoration of blood. Although x-ray findings are often confusing when comparing the various conditions, sputum examination and skin tests help to pinpoint tuberculosis as the culprit.

Treatment   Prevention of spread of tuberculosis can be accomplished by the use of face masks and covering of the mouth while coughing. After 2 or 3 weeks on medication, most patients are noncontagious. Close contacts of the infected individual should be examined (by skin test and chest x-ray) for tuberculosis. These contacts could be either the source or the result of infection in the patient, but they would need to be identified and treated in either case.

Bacille Calmette-Guérin (BCG) vaccine is used as a preventive measure in high-risk people (especially those working with tuberculosis patients) and is used as a routine immunization in some high-risk areas of the world. The vaccine will give increased (but not absolute) protection against tuberculosis, but it has the disadvantage of causing a permanently positive skin test. This deprives the individual of an important clue to recent exposure (conversion to positive in a previously negative person). For this reason, it is not considered desirable as a routine immunization in the United States, a low-risk area for tuberculosis. Those who have recent conversion to a positive skin test but who show no evidence of active disease (negative x-ray and sputum findings) are treated with isoniazid (INH) for 12 to 18 months to prevent active infection.

For secondary tuberculosis infection, a variety of drugs are also available. Combinations are recommended for clinical tuberculosis because the organism develops resistance to single drugs fairly easily. Also, with combination therapy, a lower dose of each drug can be used, thus reducing the incidence of toxicity and side effects.

Currently used combinations include isoniazid plus rifampin (Rifadin) and isoniazid plus ethambutol (Myambutol). Streptomycin is added as a third drug in more extensive cavitary tuberculosis or if other organs are involved.

Current practice emphasizes careful compliance to treatment programs for a period of 9 to 18 months. The cure rate is currently over 95 per cent.

Other treatment measures, such as special diets or climate changes, are of little importance. Surgery has limited application in tuberculosis, primarily in the removal of severely caseated lung areas or areas that might harbor tumors within the granulation area.

Complications   Severe cough is harmful in tuberculosis and should be partially suppressed with codeine or dextromethorphan. Normal productive cough should be encouraged because it clears the lungs and helps to prevent secondary infection with other organisms.

Hemorrhage causes the danger of shock, but mainly it spreads the infection by aspiration of blood. Cough suppressants help to reduce the severe coughing that encourages bleeding. If bleeding is extensive, vasopressin (Pitressin) can be used intravenously to constrict pulmonary blood vessels and reduce oozing of blood into the bronchioles.

The use of high doses of corticosteroids in persons with arrested tuberculosis encourages breakdown of inflammatory tissue that serves to localize infection. Consequently, seeds of infected material spread from the previously walled-off area and cause widespread lung infection (Fig. 9–4). This is called *miliary spread* because of the likeness of the new lesions to millet seeds, and it may result in overwhelming infection and death. Therefore, corticosteroid use should be discouraged in tuberculosis patients, except in unusual circumstances.

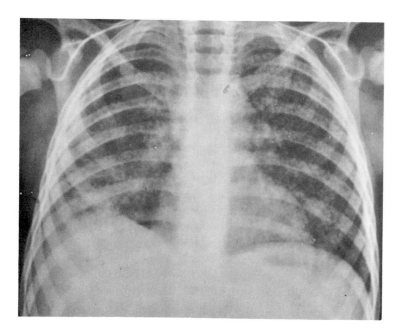

Figure 9–4. Miliary spread of tuberculosis. (From Griffiths, H. J., and Sarno, R. C.: *Contemporary Radiology: An Introduction to Imaging.* Philadelphia, W. B. Saunders Company, 1979.)

FUNGAL RESPIRATORY INFECTIONS

Deep mycotic infections begin as lung infections as a result of inhalation of organisms from the environment. The similarity of fungi and mycobacteria is noted in their growth patterns and in the body response to infection. Likewise, the pathogenesis of these diseases parallels that of tuberculosis in an uncanny way. There is a *primary infection,* often with hilar lymphadenopathy, as in the Ghon complex. The disease may remain at the primary stage and then heal or it may produce *secondary infection* at a later time. Widespread involvement of body organs and central nervous system occasionally occurs in poorly resistant individuals. Miliary spread can occur, giving an x-ray pattern identical to that of miliary tuberculosis.

Fungal respiratory infections begin as flulike illnesses with productive cough, fever, arthralgia (joint pain), chest pain, and lymphadenitis (inflamed lymph nodes) as early symptoms. They are often misdiagnosed as viral infections early in their course. Later, they may be mistaken for tuberculosis as characteristic x-ray changes develop. Even in advanced stages, they may be confused with tuberculosis, since the two disease courses run parallel to each other. Since the common fungal respiratory infections are quite similar, their pathophysiology and treatment will be discussed together.

The pulmonary lesion seen in fungal infection is a granuloma, virtually identical to that of tuberculosis. Fibrosis, calcification, and cavitation can occur, as with tuberculosis. In severe cases, involvement of the liver, spleen, bones, and central nervous system is seen.

Coccidioidomycosis

Infection with *Coccidioides immitis* is called *desert fever* or *valley fever* (because of the high incidence in the San Joaquin Valley of California.) It affects about 80 per cent of the residents of the San Joaquin Valley and is common in the southwestern United States. Contact is made by inhaling organisms or spores in dust. The disease is generally mild and only rarely causes cavitation or spread to other body organs.

Laboratory Findings

Leukocytosis and increased ESR are present.

Diagnosis

X-ray findings closely resemble those of tuberculosis. A skin test that measures antibody response to coccidioidin antigen is available. Serum antibodies can also be titrated to aid in diagnosis.

Symptoms and Signs

Coccidioidomycosis is usually a self-limited condition and rarely progresses beyond the primary stage. Often, symptoms are minimal or absent.

Treatment

No treatment is required in these cases except bed rest and symptomatic drug therapy (aspirin, cough suppressants). Treatment of severe cases is discussed under North American blastomycosis.

Histoplasmosis

Lung infection with *Histoplasma capsulatum* produces an infection similar to coccidioidomycosis. It is contracted by inhaling organisms or spores in dust from bird droppings. Infection is especially prevalent in the Midwest and southeastern United States. In a documented case occurring in an acquaintance from Louisiana, the individual had been clearing land that was a blackbird roosting area. Pigeons, chickens, and turkeys are also common carriers of the disease. The initial illness is similar to coccidioidomycosis, but there is somewhat greater tendency for spread of infection to occur. Infiltration of the liver and spleen is fairly common, associated with enlargement of these organs (hepatosplenomegaly).

Symptoms and Signs   In addition to the usual symptoms of fungal respiratory infection, ulceration of the throat, diarrhea, and anemia are common findings.

Laboratory Findings   Laboratory tests show decreased red and white blood cell counts, increased ESR, and typical x-ray findings.

Diagnosis   Skin test for histoplasmin is usually positive, which is a major help in diagnosis.

Treatment   Mild cases require no treatment and heal by calcification, producing permanent x-ray changes in the lung. More severe cases are treated with drug therapy, as is the case with coccidioidomycosis and North American blastomycosis.

North American Blastomycosis   Infection with *Blastomyces dermatitidis* is seen almost entirely in North America, especially on the East Coast and in the Mississippi and Ohio River valleys. It is the least common and most severe of the three fungal respiratory infections discussed.

Blastomycosis is thought to be contracted from organisms that reside in soil, probably by the inhalation of contaminated dust. The primary lung infection is similar to that of the other mycotic infections, but the primary focus often spreads within the lung to cause extensive infection and then invades other body areas. The skin is involved about 25 per cent of the time (hence the name *dermatitidis*). Less frequently involved are bones, organs such as the liver, and the central nervous system.

Symptoms and Signs   Symptoms may be mild and resemble those of other fungal lung infections but often become more severe, with loss of weight and the expectoration of bloody or purulent sputum as prominent features.

Laboratory Findings   Leukocytosis, anemia, increased ESR, and an x-ray pattern resembling that of tuberculosis are present.

Diagnosis   Skin tests are not reliable, but diagnosis can often be made by culture of the organism, especially from skin lesions.

Treatment   In those cases of North American blastomycosis requiring drug therapy, amphotericin B (Fungizone) is the drug of choice; it is also used for more severe cases of coccidioidomycosis and histoplasmosis. It is given intravenously by slow drip, dissolved in a large volume of 5 per cent dextrose solution. Small doses should be tried at first, since the drug is toxic to the kidney and bone marrow and causes vein irritation (phlebitis) when administered. Cure of the fungal infection often requires treatment for 1 to 2 months.

GENITOURINARY INFECTIONS

URINARY TRACT INFECTIONS

Acute Urinary Tract Infection

Short-term infection of any portion of the urinary tract is called acute urinary tract infection (acute UTI). In most cases, the bladder is the focus of infection and the condition is known as *cystitis*. In more extensive infection, the kidney itself is infected, especially in the pelvic area in which urine collection occurs (*pyelonephritis*). Pyelonephritis will be discussed in detail in Chapter 11.

A number of factors predispose to urinary tract infection. *Congenital deformities* of the urinary tract are common and include twisted or constricted ureter, bladder deformities causing reflux of urine, and bladder neck obstruction.

Males are more prone to congenital deformities than females and thus have a higher incidence of acute UTI as newborns or infants. In older males, prostatic obstruction accounts for a large percentage of urinary tract infections. Prostatic hypertrophy prevents complete voiding and encourages longer retention of urine, which fosters bacterial growth in the urinary tract. Prostatic carcinoma, also common in elderly males, has the same effect.

The shorter urethra of females makes them more vulnerable to external entry of bacteria than males, and in the age range between infancy and old age, females have the higher incidence of acute UTI. Entry of bacteria into the bladder via fecal contamination (wiping fecal organisms into the urethral opening), sexual activity, catheterization, or instrumentation of the urinary tract is thus much more likely in females than in males.

Other factors of importance are *reduced fluid intake,* which results in a concentrated urine and decreased flushing action on urinary bacteria, and *pregnancy,* which encourages infection by causing pressure of the expanding uterus on the bladder. Occasionally, a localized abscess in the kidney is the source of widespread acute UTI.

Pathogenesis

Two theories are proposed to explain the development of acute UTI:

1. *Hematogenous infection.* According to this theory, organisms are carried in the blood stream and cause infection when they are deposited in the kidney and other structures. Since the kidney and bladder are normally resistant to infection, this occurs primarily if urinary obstruction is present and the flushing and diluting effects of urine are reduced. Serious septic infection, as with staphylococci, would also tend to encourage deposition of bacteria in urinary tract structures. It is also possible that organisms could travel from the colon to the kidney via the blood stream and cause infection.

2. *Ascending infection.* The second theory, more plausible and generally more applicable, is that organisms enter the bladder via the urethra and may then move up the ureter into the kidney. This would apply if fecal contamination of the urethra, sexual activity, catheterization, or instrumentation of the urinary tract were involved. Obstruction of urine outflow would also promote ascending infection, as it would in hematogenous infection.

The vast majority of urinary tract infections are caused by fecal gram-negative, rod-shaped organisms that normally inhabit the colon (coliforms). Among these, the common offenders are *Escherichia coli, Klebsiella, Proteus* and *Pseudomonas* species. Other organisms, such as gram-positive cocci, mycobacteria, and fungi, cause infection much less frequently but must be kept in mind as possible causes.

Although the bladder is normally sterile and in fact may resist infection with substances secreted by its mucosa, the outer third of the urethra houses a normal flora of organisms. These do not cause infection but may cause confusion in the interpretation of urine samples or cultures. (See the discussion of significant bacteriuria later in this chapter.)

Symptoms and Signs Lower abdominal pain, pain or burning upon urination (dysuria), urinary frequency (frequent voiding), and urgency (urge to void often) are common symptoms of cystitis. If the kidneys are also involved, nausea, vomiting, headache, and low back pain often occur. The systemic effects of kidney infection lead to fever, chills, and weakness. Many females, especially school-age girls, maintain chronic urinary tract infection that produces no symptoms and rarely causes complications (asymptomatic bacteriuria). The only laboratory finding is that of bacteria in the urine.

Attempts to eradicate the infection are often unsuccessful, and the condition may run its course with time. The cause is unknown, but factors such as changing hormone levels or personal hygiene may be important, especially in school-age females. Boys are seldom affected. The incidence is 2 per cent for girls but only 0.05 per cent for boys.

The inflammation associated with most urinary tract infections leads to hyperemia of the involved tissue, along with bleeding in some cases. Hematuria is the result. Long-term infection may have little or no consequence or may lead to the typical findings in chronic inflammation: fibrosis and scarring. In some cases, bladder or kidney damage occurs and malfunction may result. The bladder fails to contract normally and the kidney begins to lose function as scar tissue replaces functional kidney tissue.

Laboratory Findings Urine samples from infected individuals show the presence of bacteria, pus (pyuria), and occasional red blood cells. The white blood cell count is normal in cystitis, but if the kidneys are involved, it is often elevated with a shift to the left. Damage to the glomerular membrane caused by kidney infection leads to loss of protein molecules normally kept in the blood stream by the intact membrane (proteinuria).

Since there is a normal bacterial flora in the outer urethra, urine samples contain urethral organisms as contaminants. Voiding washes out normal urethral organisms and they appear in the sample. Catheterization of the urethra prevents sample contamination but increases the risk of bladder infection (1 to 2 per cent of catheterizations), since organisms can be introduced on the catheter.

An alternative is the *voided midstream specimen.* The urethral opening is cleansed and the first portion of the voided specimen is discarded. The middle portion is collected in a sterile container and the last portion is discarded. This procedure washes out urethral bacteria in the first portion and provides an uncontaminated sample at no risk to the patient. In infants, in whom a voided midstream specimen is difficult to obtain, *suprapubic aspiration* (puncture of the abdominal wall and bladder with a sterile needle and withdrawal of urine) is a relatively safe alternative. Only rarely does bladder injury occur.

The presence of contaminating organisms in urine samples can cause misleading results. It has been shown that background contamination resulting from faulty technique or the presence of urethral bacteria is usually below 10,000 organisms per milliliter, while true UTI gives a count of at least 100,000/ml. Consequently, values of less than 10,000/ml are considered normal, whereas values of greater than 100,000 ml signify clinical infection. This is referred to as *significant bacteriuria.* Values between 10,000/ml and 100,000/ml are equivocal. Additional samples should be obtained and the results considered in the light of any symptoms present.

Urine samples can be examined microscopically, using stained or unstained preparations. More than 10 bacteria per field indicates significant bacteriuria. Culture of urine, using traditional techniques or by means of disposable tubes or sticks coated with nutrient medium, is also highly useful. Dipstick tests that utilize chemicals reduced by bacterial action are also very helpful in determining the presence of UTI. The latter are good for screening and can be followed by culture of the organism for confirmation.

Diagnosis   Acute UTI must be differentiated from appendicitis or kidney stone, which can cause abdominal or back pain, and from various gynecologic conditions such as dysmenorrhea or ovarian cyst. A urine sample is the most useful diagnostic aid, since it will show the bacteriuria, pyuria, and hematuria seen in UTI.

Treatment   In a first attack of uncomplicated urinary tract infection, sensitivity tests to determine organism susceptibility to drugs are not needed. Sulfisoxazole (Gantrisin) or co-trimoxazole (Bactrim, Septra) is the drug of choice. Alternative drugs are tetracycline (Achromycin), ampicillin (Polycillin), nitrofurantoin (Macrodantin), or cinoxacin (Cinobac). Penicillin is not generally useful, since it has very limited coverage of gram-negative organisms.

Treatment is continued for 10 to 14 days, after which a recheck for significant bacteriuria should be done. If infection is still present, the drug should be continued for an additional 10 to 14 days or sensitivity tests should be performed for selection of a more appropriate drug. If infection persists or recurs, further investigation as to causes of urinary obstruction or reflux are indicated and careful attention should be paid to other predisposing factors as well. Additional treatment measures include adequate water intake and analgesic drugs to relieve bladder or kidney pain.

Chronic Urinary Tract Infection   Chronic UTI develops in individuals in whom acute UTI is not adequately controlled. Sometimes the appropriate drug has not been chosen or the duration of treatment has been too brief. In other cases, predisposing factors that increase the difficulty of successful treatment exist. Among the most common are urinary tract obstructions and reflux of urine. Males, especially, with chronic UTI should be carefully examined for predisposing factors, since the chance of repeated infection is much less than it is with females. Chronic UTI in males, therefore, more often signifies a contributing underlying condition than is the case with chronic UTI in females.

Symptoms and Signs   Symptoms and signs in chronic UTI are usually less severe than with acute UTI and may be absent in some cases. The danger of this is that the infection will continue without treatment until renal damage results. In long-standing cases, fibrosis and scarring of the kidney occur, associated with loss of renal function and/or hypertension. (See the discussion of renal hypertension in Chapter 10.)

Laboratory Findings   Significant bacteriuria is present in chronic UTI. Culture of the urine may demonstrate typical organisms but often shows atypical, drug-resistant strains (e.g., strains of Proteus resistant to common antibacterial agents). Infections with gram-positive organisms, fungi, and mycobacteria are more common in chronic UTI than in acute UTI and may persist because of incorrect drug therapy. It is imperative not only that the organism be identified but also that sensitivity tests be performed to establish the most effective drug therapy.

In many cases, special tests are performed to demonstrate abnormalities in the urinary tract that encourage infection. A *voiding cystourethrogram* allows observation of the bladder as it empties and checks for the presence of reflux of urine into the ureters. An *intravenous pyelogram* (IVP) measures dye excretion through the renal pelvis, ureters, and bladder. The dye is injected intravenously and x-ray films are taken at intervals as the dye is being excreted through the urinary tract. The result is a clear outline of the urinary tract, so that anatomic abnormalities can be easily noted.

If hypertension develops as a complication of chronic UTI, the individual is at risk for its harmful effects, including stroke, congestive heart failure, and further kidney damage. Renal damage caused by chronic UTI impairs the ability of the kidney to remove waste materials and to concentrate the urine. This is reflected in an increased blood urea nitrogen (BUN) level, an increased serum creatinine level, a decreased creatinine clearance, and a decreased specific gravity of the urine. (See the discussion of chronic renal failure in Chapter 11.)

Diagnosis   Chronic UTI is diagnosed using the results of urinalysis and any findings resulting from complications (e.g., increased blood pressure, increased BUN) as aids. A history of repeated or continuous UTI and/or urinary tract abnormalities is also helpful.

Treatment   Surgical treatment is indicated if urinary tract abnormalities that encourage infection are found. Surgery is primarily directed toward prevention of obstruction or urine reflux.

Drug therapy is continued for a longer time period in chronic UTI than in acute UTI. After determining the appropriate drug to use on the basis of sensitivity tests, the full dose is administered for at least 4 weeks. Repeat checks for bacteriuria after completion of treatment show whether or not the infection has been eradicated. If the infection cannot be cured in this manner, long-term suppressive therapy (6 to 12 months) is indicated. Drugs of choice for this therapy include nitrofurantoin (Macrodantin), methenamine salts (Mandelamine, Hiprex), and cinoxacin (Cinobac).

The urine should be maintained at an acidic pH, perhaps with the use of ammonium chloride or ascorbic acid (vitamin C). This is especially important with the methenamine salts, which require an acidic medium for decomposition into formaldehyde, their active derivative.

VENEREAL INFECTIONS (Sexually Transmitted Diseases)

The term *venereal* derives from Venus, the goddess of love, and refers to infections transmitted by sexual contact. Among the common venereal infections are gonorrhea, syphilis, chlamydial infection, and herpes infection. Often, multiple infections result from the same contact.

CHLAMYDIAL INFECTION

Chlamydial infection is a cause of *nongonococcal urethritis* (NGU), an infection that produces symptoms similar to those of gonorrhea. Tetracycline (Achromycin) or erythromycin (Erythrocin) is the drug of choice for treatment and is given for 2 weeks.

HERPES

Herpes genitalis, caused by infection with herpesvirus type II, is currently a major venereal infection. Local genital pain, fever, and dysuria are common symptoms in males and females. Males are not known to suffer long-term effects from herpes genitalis, but they can be carriers of the organism for an extended period of time. Females with herpes genitalis have an increased risk of cervical cancer and a higher frequency of fetal death or abortion if infected during pregnancy. Approximately 40 per cent of infants delivered through the vagina contract the infection if the mother is infected. The death rate in infected newborns is extremely high. Cesarean section will prevent infection of the infant in a significant number of cases, since no contact is made between the infant and the infected vagina. Unfortunately, there is no effective treatment. Several topical ointments and creams are marketed. These relieve pain but do not inhibit viral growth.

GONORRHEA

The incidence of gonorrhea in the United States has increased from 200 per 100,000 population in 1950 to over 300 per 100,000 in 1980, making it the most common venereal disease and the most prevalent *reportable* communicable disease. Probably only about 30 per cent of the infections are reported, thus tripling the actual number of cases. Males and females in the 15- to 29-year-old age group are most often infected.

The causative agent in gonorrhea is *Neisseria gonorrhoeae,* a gram-negative diplococcus. Contact is usually genital, but oral and rectal transmission is common among homosexuals. In cases involving male-female contact, many authorities blame oral contraceptives for the dramatic increase in incidence. The "pill" prevents conception and probably encourages sexual activity, but it does not provide the protection from infection seen with other forms of contraception.

Pathogenesis   The incubation period for gonorrhea is 2 to 10 days, after which a local tissue infection develops. Males show inflammation of the urethra (urethritis) associated with dysuria, urethral pain, and a yellow, creamy discharge. If treatment is not sought, the infection moves further into the prostate, seminal vesicles, and vas deferens. Chronic inflammation of these structures leads to fibrosis and blockage of sperm transport, a cause of sterility. Females are often asymptomatic, but if symptoms occur, they include urethritis, dysuria, yellowish discharge, and urinary frequency and urgency. Progression of the infection into the fallopian tubes and ovaries is common. The cervix, but not the body of the uterus, is often infected and exquisitely tender to touch.

A common long-term complication to gonorrhea in the female is *gonorrheal salpingitis* (inflammation of the fallopian tube resulting from gonococcal infection). The tube becomes swollen and filled with pus (pyosalpinx). Fibrosis results from the chronic inflammation, and the tube closes and fails to carry the egg to the uterus. Infertility results. Occasionally, the tube is only partly blocked, allowing sperm to move through from the uterus but preventing the fertilized egg from passing through into the uterus for implantation. The result is an *ectopic pregnancy,* with the fertilized egg becoming implanted and growing in the fallopian tube.

Septic gonorrheal infection can occur (1 to 3 per cent of cases), generally causing joint inflammation (gonococcal arthritis) or skin reactions over the joint areas. Women are more prone to septic infection than men, probably because they are more often unaware of the early stages of infection.

Transmission of gonorrhea most often involves sexual contact, but there are two special exceptions. Rubbing the eye with fingers contaminated with urethral discharge can cause *gonococcal conjunctivitis,* a local eye infection. Likewise, infection of newborns with material scraped into the eye from the mother's infected cervix or vagina causes a type of gonorrheal conjunctivitis known as *ophthalmia neonatorum.* At one time, ophthalmia neonatorum was an important cause of blindness in the United States. State laws now require instillation of silver nitrate solution into the eyes of newborns or injection of penicillin after birth to kill any acquired gonococcal organisms.

Gonococci produce a weak endotoxin but cause only a temporary immune response with little or no immunologic memory. For this reason, no immunity develops following infection and a successful vaccine for gonorrhea has therefore never been developed. There are cases on record of individuals having had gonorrhea more than 40 times, with no apparent immunity developing after each infection.

Laboratory Findings   Examination of urethral secretions in males shows the presence of gram-negative diplococci. Organisms are more difficult to recover in females, especially with advanced gonorrhea, and in males with long-standing cases, since the infection goes "underground." If smears are negative but gonorrhea is suspected, culture of urethral or cervical secretions, using Thayer-Martin growth medium, is often successful. Oral or rectal secretions can also be cultured. Since the gonococcal organism has limited antigenicity, antibody response is poor. For this reason no serologic test that is based upon antibody response has been developed for gonorrhea.

Diagnosis   The presence of gram-negative diplococci in urethral or cervical secretions is prime evidence of gonorrhea, since the only other common gram-negative diplococcus infects the central nervous system. (A discussion of *Neisseria meningitidis* infection follows.) Nongonococcal urethritis closely resembles gonorrhea, but organisms other than gonococcus are involved. Herpesvirus usually causes external lesions resembling cold sores. Syphilis causes an external lesion and is detected by serologic tests. Care should be taken to look for additional infections if gonorrhea is found, since they are often transmitted together.

Treatment   Fortunately, many drugs are effective for gonorrhea. Penicillin is the drug of choice and is given by single intramuscular injection of a long-acting form. Probenecid (Benemid) is used prior to injection to delay excretion of the penicillin and increase the blood level. Gonococci are easily killed, in most cases, by brief exposure to high blood levels of most antibiotics. Orally administered ampicillin (Polycillin) is also effective, in conjunction with probenecid pretreatment. For those allergic to penicillin or ampicillin, tetracycline (Achromycin) or co-trimoxazole (Bactrim, Septra) used orally is a good alternative. Resistant cases are treated with intramuscularly administered spectinomycin (Trobicin). Approximately 95 per cent of early cases are cured with such treatment.

If systemic infection is present, treatment is similar to that for early cases but duration of treatment is extended. Failure to cure with penicillin or ampicillin usually occurs because of infection with penicillinase-producing gonococci, which may be treated with the other drugs listed. Single, high-dose penicillin treatment for gonorrhea often also eradicates syphilis before it is clinically apparent.

SYPHILIS   Historically, syphilis is remembered for two things. It earned the name "the great mimic" because it can affect virtually any body system in the late stage, mimicking primary organ disease. Syphilis is also remembered because no country wanted credit for originating this disease, which was always blamed upon whoever was currently invading the country. The French called it the Spanish Disease, the Italians called it the French Disease, and so forth. Spanish explorers are said to have brought smallpox to North America, and this led to decimation of the American Indian population. (The Indians, however, being good traders, gave the men syphilis in return!)

How long syphilis has been around is not known with certainty, but lesions thought caused by syphilis have been found in the bones of mummies. Were it not for the unique method of spread via sexual contact, the disease probably would have disappeared centuries ago because the causative organism does not survive outside the body for any length of time. Currently, syphilis is about one fortieth (1/40) as prevalent as gonorrhea and affects mainly those in the 15- to 20-year-old age group.

Pathogenesis   Contact with a lesion containing *Treponema pallidum* transmits the disease between parties. The incubation period is 2 to 3 weeks. The new lesion (chancre) formed is usually in the genital area at the point of contact. Oral or rectal lesions are also fairly common. Oral lesions resemble herpes lesions (fever blisters). There have been documented cases of transmission of syphilis by oral-to-oral contact. (In one case a man infected seven women by kissing them.) Usually, however, genital contact is involved. Infants can become infected from syphilitic mothers during pregnancy and suffer characteristic birth defects, including deafness, saddle nose deformity (caused by destruction of the nasal bone), and peg-shaped widely spaced front teeth (Hutchinson's teeth). The current practice of testing for syphilis early in pregnancy allows for early treatment of the mother, which normally eliminates these problems.

Unlike gonorrhea, syphilis is associated with a marked immune response, leading to antibody production. This immune reaction forms the basis for serologic tests for syphilis. Unfortunately, extreme sensitization develops to treponemal antigen in late stage syphilis and granulation reactions result, leading to the formation of specific granulomas (called syphilomas or gummas) in a variety of body tissues. It is this reaction that causes the devastation that is characteristic of tertiary syphilis. For some reason, immunologic memory for syphilis is poor, in spite of the powerful immune reaction, and the individual is vulnerable to reinfection after being cured.

Stages of Syphilis   **Primary Stage.** In this stage, a local lesion containing spirochetes forms. Regional lymph nodes are sometimes enlarged, especially in the groin area. Direct contact with the lesion in the primary stage results in disease transmission. Approximately one third of the untreated cases stop at this stage, presumably because of the development of adequate body defenses. The chancre ulcerates and then heals by scar formation.

Secondary Stage. Two thirds of the untreated individuals progress into the secondary stage, often weeks to months after healing of the primary lesion. Healing of the lesion often deludes those afflicted into thinking the disease is cured and they fail to seek treatment. Systemic infection occurs via the blood stream, and the individual develops a widespread rash on the skin and mucous membranes. Warty growths in the genital area or other moist areas of the body may develop. These are called *condylomata lata*. External lesions developing in the secondary stage contain viable organisms and can infect other contacts. In approximately a third of the untreated cases, the disease stops at this stage. The rash clears, and body defenses eradicate the infection.

Tertiary Stage. The remaining third of the untreated cases progress to the tertiary stage. Tertiary syphilis may follow a latent period of several years and is characterized by increasing hypersensitivity to treponemal antigen. Granulation reaction results from this antigen-antibody interaction. Hypersensitivity at this time is curious, since the organism population is lower than during the secondary stage. As a result of granulation reaction, gummas develop in the cardiovascular system, central nervous system, bones, and other body tissues and cause local destruction, leading to a variety of symptoms. Fortunately, the improved diagnosis and treatment measures currently employed have greatly reduced the number of cases reaching the tertiary stage.

Laboratory Findings

Treponemal organisms can be identified from lesion material. Since *T. pallidum* is nearly transparent (*pallidum = pale*), darkfield illumination is required to contrast them against the surrounding medium. Immunofluorescence techniques that outline the organisms more clearly are also available.

Serologic tests for syphilis are of two types:

1. *Nontreponemal antigen test.* The Venereal Disease Research Laboratory (VDRL) test uses beef heart cardiolipin, which has antigenic properties similar to those of treponemal antigen. The VDRL test becomes positive 1 to 3 weeks after the primary lesion appears and measures antibody titer developed against the treponemal antigen. Very early infections or late stage syphilis may produce a negative VDRL result. Decreasing response to the VDRL test during treatment indicates progress in controlling the infection. Since the VDRL is based upon a nontreponemal antigen, it often is positive in other disease states. Lupus erythematosus and rheumatoid arthritis are notorious for causing a false-positive VDRL result, as is mononucleosis.

2. *Treponemal antigen test.* The fluorescent treponemal antibody absorption test (FTA-ABS) uses killed treponemal organisms as a source of antigen. It is a good backup test for positive VDRL results and is more specific, since it utilizes the specific antigen of syphilis. The FTA-ABS test is positive earlier than the VDRL test in syphilis and remains positive in late stage syphilis or after successful treatment. In tertiary syphilis, examination of the spinal fluid for increased protein content, increased cell count, and positive VDRL aids in the diagnosis of *neurosyphilis*. This implies involvement of the central nervous system. Normalization of these findings indicates successful treatment.

Treatment

The treatment of choice in primary syphilis consists of a single intramuscular dose of long-acting penicillin. Erythromycin (Ilotycin) or tetracycline (Achromycin) is also effective in those allergic to penicillin. Syphilis is frequently cured by the treatment given for gonorrhea, often before the primary chancre develops. Late-stage syphilis may require treatment for several weeks to cure.

Complications

Complications to tertiary syphilis are mainly confined to the vascular, skeletal, and nervous systems, although other body areas are occasionally involved. Syphilitic aortitis was a common cause of *dissecting aortic aneurysm* in earlier days. Aneurysm rupture nearly always meant sudden death. *Osteitis* (bone inflammation) can develop as gummas form in bone tissue.

Neurosyphilis includes disorders primarily affecting the brain (meningovascular syphilis) and spinal cord (tabes dorsalis). *Meningovascular syphilis* is caused by meningeal or vascular inflammation in the brain. Headache, partial paralysis and loss of pupillary light reflex result. *Tabes dorsalis* (locomotor ataxia) results from destruc-

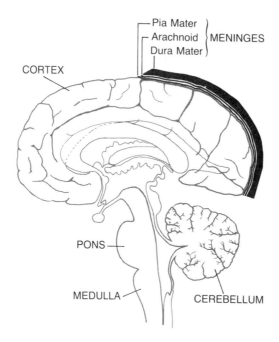

Pia Mater ⎫
Arachnoid ⎬ MENINGES
Dura Mater ⎭

CORTEX

PONS —

MEDULLA —

CEREBELLUM

Figure 9–5. Brain and meninges.

tion of spinal nerve cells and loss of sensation of position of the limbs. Such individuals walk by "planting" the feet and have great difficulty walking in the dark, since they must watch the position of the feet with respect to the ground. Widespread cortical damage in neurosyphilis causes symptoms of mental illness. In past times, "fever therapy" was used as a treatment for mental illness with some success. In the patient population in mental hospitals, about 50 per cent of the so-called "psychotic" individuals actually were suffering from neurosyphilis. Syphilitic patients who were infected with malaria developed high fever that "burned out" the syphilis infection. As a result, about 50 per cent of the population improved with this treatment—the 50 per cent who had neurosyphilis rather than true psychosis!

CENTRAL NERVOUS SYSTEM INFECTION

MENINGITIS

The central nervous system is surrounded by three membranes: the *dura mater* (hard mother), the *arachnoid* (web-shaped), and the *pia mater* (soft mother). These are known collectively as the *meninges* (Fig. 9–5). Their function is to protect the brain and spinal cord from external injury and to form a tight seal so that cerebrospinal fluid (CSF) remains in contact with the nervous tissue. Inflammation of the meninges (*meningitis*) results from infection with bacteria, viruses, or fungi. Meningitis affects all age groups, but infants and small children are the most vulnerable.

Pathogenesis

The condition usually begins as an upper respiratory tract or middle ear infection that travels via the blood stream to the central nervous system. In newborns, the causative organism is usually *E. coli*. *H. influenzae* causes most cases in young children. In teenagers and adults, the cause is usually *N. meningitidis* (meningococcus); in elderly people, it is generally caused by pneumococci. Streptococci, staphylococci, and viruses are less frequent causes of meningitis. Septic infection with meningococci is called *meningococcemia* and often coexists with meningitis. It is also possible to have one without the other.

The tissue reaction to infection is typical of inflammation. Both fluid and cellular exudates are formed and the classic signs of inflammation are present. Edema resulting from inflammation creates additional pressure within the skull and results in well-known disturbances in brain function. Very small children in whom the anterior fontanelle (soft spot above the forehead) has not closed show a bulging of the fontanelle as a result of the increased CSF pressure.

Types of Meningitis   Infection with meningococci (*N. meningitidis* groups A, B, and C), pneumococci, *H. influenzae*, streptococci, staphylococci, or *E. coli* results in pus formation and is called *purulent meningitis*. Infection with *M. tuberculosis, T. pallidum, C. immitis, H. capsulatum,* or *B. dermatitidis* results in granulation reaction and is termed *granulomatous meningitis*. These latter infections are generally seen as complications to systemic infections with the respective organisms and represent local infections that have gotten out of hand. Viruses (especially coxsackievirus and echovirus) cause *aseptic meningitis*, so named because bacteria are absent.

Meningismus is a condition caused by reaction of the meninges to a systemic infection, such as an upper respiratory tract infection. The symptoms and signs resemble those of meningitis, but the meninges are not actually infected.

Symptoms and Signs   High fever, vomiting, delirium, and *nuchal rigidity* (stiff neck) are cardinal signs of meningitis. Nuchal rigidity is part of a larger picture of hyperreflexia caused by meningeal irritation. A common test for the hyperreflexia of meningitis is *Kernig's sign*. Flexion followed by extension of the leg results in contraction and pain in the hamstring muscles (in the thigh). Some individuals with meningitis develop a petechial rash (petechia = flea bite) on the skin and mucous membranes. If the infecting organism produces an endotoxin, severe drop in blood pressure may result (endotoxic shock).

Laboratory Findings   Leukocytosis is seen in most cases of bacterial meningitis but is less marked in tubercular, fungal, or viral meningitis. The most important findings relate to the cerebrospinal fluid. This is sampled from the lower back area (lumbar puncture) and shows increased pressure, increased protein content, leukocytosis (especially granulocytes), and decreased glucose content in bacterial meningitis. The fluid is straw-colored as a result of pus formation and contains organisms that can be identified and cultured on appropriate growth media. In aseptic meningitis, the glucose level is normal; this is important in differential diagnosis.

Diagnosis   The major problem in diagnosis is determination of the specific type of meningitis so that appropriate antibiotic therapy can be instituted. Smears and cultures of the causative organism are of

Table 9–2. DRUG THERAPY OF MENINGITIS

Causative Organism	Drug of Choice
Meningococci	Penicillin, ampicillin, chloramphenicol
Haemophilus	Ampicillin plus chloramphenicol
Escherichia	Gentamicin, kanamycin
Staphylococci	Nafcillin, methicillin
Streptococci	Same as for meningococcal meningitis
Pneumococci	Same as for meningococcal meningitis
Mycobacteria	Isoniazid, rifampin, ethambutol, and streptomycin
Fungi	Amphotericin B
Viruses	No specific drug therapy

greatest benefit. Viral (aseptic) meningitis, while not demonstrable by standard smear and culture methods, is usually milder and does not lower the CSF glucose level. In tubercular, syphilitic, or fungal meningitis, the primary focus of infection should be sought and eliminated, since meningitis is almost always secondary in these cases. Meningismus can resemble meningitis closely but reflects infection elsewhere in the body. Many systemic infections cause a petechial rash, but usually do not also cause the other findings seen in meningitis.

Treatment   Treatment of the various types of meningitis is outlined in Table 9–2. Generally, very large doses of drugs are required, since only a fraction of the administered drug crosses the blood-brain barrier and enters the central nervous system. Drugs are ordinarily given intravenously to ensure the highest possible blood level of drug and hence the highest level in the meningeal area.

A newer method of drug administration consists of placing a cannula through the skull into the brain ventricle (intraventricular injection). Very small doses are needed when using this route of administration, since all of the administered drug enters the brain area and mixes with the CSF.

In addition to treatment of existing cases, a vaccine is available for prevention of meningitis resulting from *N. meningitidis* A and C. This is currently used in crowded areas, such as army camps, where the risk of spread of meningitis is very great. Rifampin (Rifadin) or minocycline (Minocin) can also be given to those at high risk for contracting meningococcal meningitis.

Fluid administration is an important adjunctive treatment in active meningitis, especially if high fever and shock are present.

Complications   Cranial nerve damage, due to fibrosis of brain tissue as a result of inflammation, is a common sequel to meningitis. Deafness or blindness can result. More widespread brain damage causes paralysis or mental impairment. Organization and fibrosis within the brain ventricles may block outflow of CSF and cause a buildup of pressure within the skull. The result is *hydrocephalus* ("water-head"). Treatment is very difficult and involves the insertion of a shunt cannula to bypass fluid around the blocked area and relieve the excessive CSF pressure.

SUMMARY

Infectious diseases represent one of the major reasons for physician visits. Although the location of infection varies with different types of infection, the properties of infecting organisms may be constant. Thus, a staphylococcal skin infection has certain similarities to a staphylococcal pneumonia or a staphylococcal oral infection.

Of great importance in most infections is identification of the causative organism through smear or culture. When the organism is identified, the nature and course of the infection can be determined and appropriate drug therapy instituted.

Acute infections are generally more straightforward and easily treated than chronic infections. Chronic infections result from failure to identify the causative organism, failure to provide appropriate drug therapy, presence of resistant strains, or presence of factors that encourage persistent infection. Only through attention to all of these parameters can chronic infections be cured and their complications prevented.

Questions

1. What is the meaning of the term *opportunistic infection*? How does it relate to mixed pneumonia?
2. Does infection ever occur in the absence of inflammation? Explain.
3. How does knowledge of the properties of an organism help to predict the type and severity of complications from infection with it? Give a specific example.
4. Can miliary spread occur with fungal respiratory infections as it does with tuberculosis? Explain how this might occur.
5. Explain the meaning of the terms *asymptomatic bacteriuria* and *significant bacteriuria*. Would the sex of the patient be important in the implications of each of these findings? How?

Additional Reading

Bergman, H. D.: Drugs for treatment of gram-negative infections. U.S. Pharmacist, 2:60, 1977. (*Good discussion of organisms and drugs.*)

Kory, M., and Waife, S. O. (eds.): *Kidney and Urinary Tract Infections.* Indianapolis, Eli Lilly and Co., 1971. (*Diagnosis and treatment in UTI.*)

Lambert, P. D., and Martin, A.: What you should know about TB. Pharmacy Times, April 1976, p. 50. (*Good overview of tuberculosis for health professionals.*)

Rahal, J. J., and Simberkoff, M. S.: Antibiotics and how to use them. Postgrad. Med., vol. 62, no. 3 (Sept. 1977) to vol. 64, no. 2 (Aug. 1978).

Storch, G., et al.: Acute histoplasmosis—Description of an outbreak in Northern Louisiana. Chest, 1:38, 1980. (*Report on an acquaintance and others who contracted histoplasmosis.*)

CHAPTER **10** CARDIOVASCULAR DISORDERS

Cardiovascular disorders constitute the leading cause of death in the United States and in most other "civilized" countries, surpassing malignant disease, the second major cause of death, by a wide margin. In most underdeveloped areas of the world, infectious disorders and malnutrition are leading causes of death. It might be said that cardiovascular disease is our leading killer by default, since we have largely conquered malnutrition and infectious diseases in the United States. However, there is an additional factor that makes cardiovascular disease especially prevalent in developed countries such as the United States. The process of industrial development that improves our technology regarding food production and control of infection also provides us with a diet that encourages coronary artery disease and relieves us of the need for physical exertion. We are able to afford a high-fat diet that encourages the development of coronary atherosclerosis (formation of an *atheroma* or plaque on the inner surface of an artery). Machines do the physical work for us, including that associated with transportation. The stresses of a highly structured, civilized existence also take their toll.

Great strides have been made in the surgical treatment of congenital heart defects, and thousands of people have been saved through technology who otherwise would die prematurely. Surgery, likewise, helps additional thousands with severe coronary artery disease to live normal lives through coronary bypass operations. However, in the area of prevention of coronary artery disease, our gains have been only modest. The number of deaths from coronary artery disease has declined in the past 10 years, but it is still the single leading cause of death in the United States. The recent interest in exercise and diet modification is largely responsible for this improvement. More needs to be done, though, to slow the process of atherosclerosis.

This chapter deals with several common types of cardiovascular disorders: rheumatic heart disease, coronary artery disease and its widespread clinical manifestations, congestive heart failure, hypertension, peripheral vascular disorders, and cardiac arrhythmias. It will soon become apparent that cardiovascular diseases are often interrelated. Rheumatic heart disease leads to congestive heart failure. Hypertension can also lead to congestive heart failure. Coronary artery disease can lead to cardiac arrhythmias. The process of atherosclerosis that causes artery disease also causes one form of peripheral vascular disease. Therefore, these topics should not be studied as isolated conditions, but with the concept of cause and effect in mind. Sometimes, it is difficult to determine which disorder came first, and a "chicken or egg" situation exists. Usually, though, with careful investigation, we can reveal the initial event that set the disease chain in motion. As mentioned in the introduction of this book, the pathologist can examine the heart of a victim of congestive heart failure and determine that hypertension (or rheumatic heart disease) was the event leading to the later development of congestive heart failure and death. Treatment of the initial condition can often forestall the development of complications and prolong life.

RHEUMATIC HEART DISEASE

The heart is composed of three layers of tissue:

1. The *pericardium* is the thin, almost transparent covering of the heart. Its function is to protect the heart and prevent friction as the heart moves within the chest. Pericardial fluid, secreted by the epicardial layer of the pericardium, lubricates the heart as it contracts within the pericardium.

2. The *myocardium,* or muscular portion of the heart, makes up the bulk of the heart weight and has contractile ability.

3. The inner lining of the heart, or *endocardium,* covers the inside surface of the four heart chambers (right and left atria and ventricles) and includes the four heart valves: the *tricuspid valve,* between the right atrium and right ventricle; the *mitral valve,* between the left atrium and left ventricle; and the *aortic* and *pulmonary semilunar valves,* at the entry to the aorta and pulmonary artery, respectively. The function of the heart valves is to allow blood flow to occur in one direction only: from the right atrium to the right ventricle to the lungs to the left atrium to the left ventricle to the peripheral vascular system.

All three layers of the heart are vulnerable to the destructive effects of rheumatic heart disease. Thus *pericarditis, myocarditis,* and/or *endocarditis* can develop. However, the endocardium is most often affected by the disease process. Among the endocardial components, the mitral valve is the most common site for heart damage (Fig. 10–1).

Rheumatic heart disease is a complication of *rheumatic fever,* which is caused by inflammation often resulting from infection with beta-hemolytic streptococcus group A. Rheumatic fever is most prevalent in the 5- to 15-year-old age group and is uncommon before 4 years and after 50 years of age. Possibly this reflects increased

Figure 10–1. Heart valve damage associated with rheumatic fever. (From the CIBA Pharmaceutical Company, a Division of CIBA-GEIGY Corporation. © Copyright 1969, the CIBA Book Collection, vol. 5, p. 179. From a drawing by Frank B. Netter, M.D. All rights reserved.)

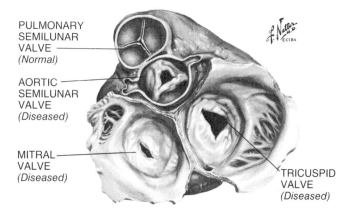

PULMONARY SEMILUNAR VALVE *(Normal)*

AORTIC SEMILUNAR VALVE *(Diseased)*

MITRAL VALVE *(Diseased)*

TRICUSPID VALVE *(Diseased)*

resistance to infection in these extremes of age. The high prevalence in the 5- to 15-year-old age group may be related to the easy transmission of the infection in the crowded school environment. The 5- to 15-year-old age group is also the most vulnerable to rheumatic heart disease, since rheumatic fever is a prerequisite for it. In the 5- to 24-year-old age group, rheumatic heart disease is the most common potentially fatal heart condition.

Pathogenesis

As mentioned, the endocardium and especially the mitral valve are the primary targets for the inflammatory process. The current explanation of the development of endocarditis is that antibodies to the streptococcal antigen form complexes with the antigen as a part of the body's defense to the infection. These complexes then circulate in the bloodstream and attack the endocardial lining of the heart. Chronic inflammation often results, and because it has not been promptly resolved, fibrosis of the endocardial surfaces eventually occurs. This is especially devastating to the heart valves, since even slight changes in the thickness or elasticity of the valve cusps can have drastic effects on valve action. Scarring of the valve cusps results, leading to *regurgitation,* in which the valve fails to close completely and allows blood to leak in the wrong direction, and *stenosis,* in which the valve opening is narrowed by scar tissue formation. In addition, thrombi often form on the valve cusps in response to inflammation. These are called *vegetations,* because of their cauliflowerlike appearance.

Symptoms and Signs

Most cases of rheumatic fever begin with a primary ear, tonsil, or, most commonly, throat infection ("strep" throat). In addition to the symptoms of the primary infection, which include pain, fever, and malaise, there is an extension of the inflammatory component of the infection after 1 to 4 weeks to include the joints, central nervous system, and heart. Thus, the patient may experience a migratory arthritis *(polyarthritis),* which moves among the large joints of the body. Slight inflammation of brain tissue causes *chorea,* consisting of jerking of the limbs, accompanied by facial grimaces and restlessness. Both of these conditions, although quite bothersome, usually resolve completely. The *cardiac manifestations* of inflammation, however, often do not resolve and may even become progressively worse with time.

One obvious sign of heart involvement is a *heart murmur,* or abnormal sound during the cardiac cycle. Murmurs are caused by the movement of blood as it passes through a damaged valve. Some murmurs disappear as the valve inflammation subsides, but many are permanent because the valve damage is often permanent.

Laboratory Findings

Several common laboratory tests are helpful in the diagnosis of rheumatic fever. Since bacterial infection is the initial event in the condition, the white blood cell count is elevated (normal = 5000 to 10,000/mm^3). In the early stages of infection, culture of the throat or other site of infection is useful and will often identify the beta-hemolytic streptococcal organism.

Body response to the infection includes the formation of antibodies to the streptococcal antigen. Thus, the antistreptolysin O

(ASO) titer increases in proportion to the degree of body response (normal = 50 to 150 Todd units per milliter of blood). Since inflammation is a part of the manifestation of rheumatic fever, the erythrocyte sedimentation rate (ESR) also increases (N = 0 to 12 mm/hr for men, and 0 to 20 mm/hr for women).

Cardiac hypertrophy, caused by the effects of impaired valve action and other factors, may develop. This causes a larger cardiac silhouette to appear on chest x-ray films.

Diagnosis   A history of recent streptococcal infection, arthritis, chorea, and evidence of heart involvement are the major diagnostic features of rheumatic fever. Rheumatoid arthritis can mimic exactly the joint manifestations of rheumatic fever. In fact, the name *rheumatoid* means *rheumatic-like* and was coined because of the similarity of the two conditions. However, rheumatoid arthritis is not associated with streptococcal infection and ASO titer and throat culture are thus normal. Other forms of endocarditis are associated with infectious or inflammatory disorders. However, laboratory tests results are different in each case.

Treatment   Prompt treatment of streptococcal infection with penicillin or equivalent drugs will usually prevent rheumatic fever. This is a good reason to treat all suspected streptococcal infections with antibiotics, even though occasionally no treatment is required. The physician who treats suspected "strep" throat in a child with an antibiotic before obtaining culture results is often criticized as practicing "shotgun" medicine. Probably, however, many cases of rheumatic fever are aborted by this early intervention.

If rheumatic fever develops, cure is often difficult. The major thrust of treatment is prophylactic antibiotic therapy to prevent reinfection and exacerbation of endocarditis. Children are often treated until age 25 or so, and adults are treated for a minimum of 5 years, after which time the threat of reinfection is minimal. Penicillin is the drug of choice and is given in a long-acting intra-muscular form each month or as a daily oral dose. For those allergic to penicillin, erythromycin (Ilotycin) or sulfonamides are also effective. By preventing reinfection, the progression of endocarditis may be stopped. However, since endocarditis is an inflammatory process triggered by infection, controlling infection does not always completely halt the progression of the disease. Interestingly enough, anti-inflammatory drugs such as aspirin or corticosteroids are not useful in reducing endocardial inflammation, although they reduce joint inflammation associated with rheumatic fever. Perhaps this is because the effective concentration of drug at the site of endocardial inflammation is relatively small.

As recovery occurs, laboratory values such as ESR, temperature, and ASO titer return to normal. These tests, therefore, can be used to gauge the effectiveness of treatment.

Complications   Although many cases of a rheumatic fever resolve without further difficulty, there is often a long-term risk of reinfection with exacerbation of endocardial damage. This is especially likely following exposure to a person infected with streptococci or after surgery or dental work. Therefore, prophylactic drug therapy in progress at that time is usually increased. This gives additional protection against reinfection.

If significant valve damage occurs as a consequence of endocarditis, the heart loses efficiency and must work harder to satisfy body demands for circulation. In mitral stenosis, blood flow from the left atrium to left ventricle is impeded and right atrial dilation results. If mitral regurgitation is the major problem, leakage occurs from the left ventricle to left atrium during systole and the heart loses pumping efficiency. This can lead to cardiac hypertrophy and eventually to congestive heart failure.

In these severe cases, surgical valve replacement is the treatment of choice. A variety of artificial valves have been employed for replacement, including ball-and-cage–type valves, cusp-type valves made of Dacron, and valves obtained from pig heart that have been treated with radiation to render them nonantigenic to humans. The success rate with this type of surgery is quite good.

CORONARY ARTERY DISEASE

As mentioned, cardiovascular diseases cause the greatest number of deaths among Americans. Of these deaths, coronary artery disease and its complications constitute the greatest single number. In addition, the same process of arterial disease can affect nonheart areas such as the brain with equally harmful consequences. The well-known statement that "you are as old as your arteries" certainly has some validity in that a perfectly healthy 40-year-old man can easily die from an arterial blockage in the heart only a few millimeters long.

Coronary artery disease has been the subject of intensive research and study since the late 1940s. No disease, with the exception of cancer, has had anywhere near the federal and private support, and yet the final answers are still not in. Research has taken several directions, including long-term population studies, experimental artery disease in animals, and attempts to correct, by means of drugs or surgery, advanced artery disease.

A famous long-term study, begun about 1950 in Framingham, Massachusetts, ran for over 20 years and was one of the most thorough and well-controlled of the so-called *prospective* studies. This type of study looks at a problem by controlling all but the desired variables and projects into the future; a *retrospective* study goes from present to past and tries to establish causes for the current problem. In the Framingham study, such variables as diet, smoking habits, and alcohol intake were closely controlled and subjects were categorized as to sex, size, weight, body build, amount of exercise, occupation, and other parameters to see what factors were important in the development of coronary artery disease.

Animal studies have also been performed in which arterial disease could be accelerated by special diets, stress, or other factors, thus providing a research model for human disease. Much work has been done in the area of prevention and treatment through the use of drugs that slow the rate of accumulation of arterial deposits or through special surgical techniques that remove deposits or reroute blood around blocked areas in the coronary arteries.

It would seem, with all that has been done, that it should be easy to pinpoint the cause(s) of coronary artery disease. However, although certain risk factors have been identified, it often is not possible to predict with certainty who will develop coronary artery disease to a symptomatic degree within a lifetime. As with other multifactorial diseases, the control of only one risk factor may not significantly change the course of the disease. Most people are now aware that risk factors such as stress, smoking, obesity, lack of exercise, and high blood pressure may increase the chance of serious artery disease. Nevertheless, many calm, nonsmoking, lean, energetic, normotensive adults develop heart attacks, whereas some "high risk" people escape serious heart disease. It seems that additional, poorly understood factors are at work.

Pathogenesis   A key component of the arterial deposit that leads to coronary artery disease is *cholesterol.* A normal body compound used in the formation of nerve tissue and various hormones, cholesterol deposits on the intimal surface of the arterial wall at a greater rate in some people than in others. This is partly due to the effects of the previously described risk factors in some people, but there is also an inherent tendency for deposition that itself may be an additional risk factor. It is likely that this is largely controlled by heredity and therefore cannot be changed. (Thus the advice to "select your ancestors carefully" may be well taken.)

The normal level of cholesterol in the blood stream is 150 to 250 mg/dl. A high level (hypercholesterolemia) is considered a risk factor for coronary artery disease. Indeed, the Framingham study showed clearly that if a person has a high cholesterol level and other risk factors are matched with those of another person who has a normal or low cholesterol level, the hypercholesterolemic individual has the greater chance of developing significant coronary artery disease.

Early investigators such as cardiologist Paul Dudley White implicated cholesterol as the major culprit in coronary artery disease and other forms of atherosclerosis (Fig. 10–2). They recommended

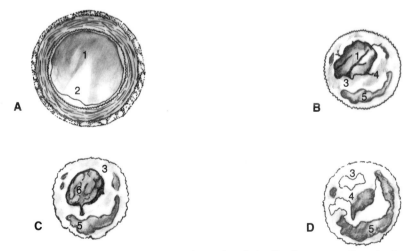

Figure 10–2. Progressive coronary atherosclerosis leading to coronary thrombosis and recovery. *(A)* Minimal plaque. *(B)* Signficant plaque (no symptoms). *(C)* Coronary thrombosis (causes symptoms and myocardial infarction). *(D)* Recovery with scar tissue formation in heart. *1,* Arterial lumen; *2,* early plaque; *3,* advanced plaque; *4,* fatty deposits; *5,* hemorrhage; *6,* thrombus.

Table 10–1. FREDRICKSON-LEES CLASSIFICATION OF HYPERLIPIDEMIAS

Type I	A rare, genetic disorder, usually detected in childhood. There is difficulty in handling chylomicrons because of a lipase deficiency. (Lipase metabolizes fats.)
Type II	There is a defect in the metabolism of beta lipoproteins. Type II exists in A and B subtypes.
Type III	Abnormal beta and pre-beta lipoproteins are present.
Type IV	There is difficulty in metabolizing pre-beta lipoproteins.
Type V	There is difficulty in assimilating triglycerides.

restriction of cholesterol intake in the diet to reduce the level in the blood stream. Thus, the hypercholesterolemic patient was told to avoid eggs, dairy products, shellfish, and other rich sources of dietary cholesterol. It was soon discovered, however, that this did not appreciably help some people to lower their serum cholesterol levels. *Limitation of saturated fat* in the diet and the substitution of *unsaturated products* (e.g., vegetable oil, margarine) for animal fats was more effective for most people than simple restriction of dietary cholesterol. Still, as shown in the Framingham study, there were those who did not respond much to any type of dietary manipulation and they remained at greater risk than those with normal cholesterol levels or those who could be brought to normal through dietary adjustment.

More recently, it has been shown that there are different types of hyperlipidemias—conditions associated with higher levels of certain fatty compounds in the blood stream. Credit for establishing types and subtypes of hyperlipidemias goes to Fredrickson and Lees (Table 10–1). Although cholesterol is certainly an important fatty compound in blood, other fats such as lipoproteins and triglycerides are also important. Moreover, the proportion of each of these varies, depending upon the particular type of hyperlipidemia. Thus, some hyperlipidemias are characterized by high cholesterol levels, some by high triglyceride levels, and others by a combination of high values. Treatments vary, and those effective for one type may not be effective for another type (Table 10–2). The discovery of the different hyperlipidemias has helped to explain earlier discrepancies in treatment response and outcome of patients who were formerly thought to have exactly the same problem.

Table 10–2. DRUG THERAPY OF HYPERLIPIDEMIAS

Drug	Type of Hyperlipidemia
Clofibrate (Atromid S)	III, IV, or V (Slight benefit in II)
Dextrothyroxine (Choloxin)	II (Slight benefit in III)
Cholestyramine (Questran)	II
Colestipol (Colestid)	II
Nicotinic acid	II, III, IV, or V
Probucol (Lorelco)	II

Symptoms and Signs

When enough coronary artery disease occurs so that symptoms develop, the clinical presentation is in the form of one of three conditions: stable angina pectoris (angina = pain, pectoris = shoulder); unstable angina pectoris; or myocardial infarction.

Stable Angina Pectoris. This disorder is characterized by a crushing chest pain that occurs during exertion or excitement and is relieved by rest or with the use of nitroglycerin. The pain radiates from the center of the chest to the left shoulder, left arm, and hand. Occasionally, the jaw or even the right shoulder and arm are involved. The individual typically describes the feeling of the heart being squeezed in a vise. Apprehension and sweating are also often reported during angina attacks. During the attack, the level of cardiac activity is too great for the supply of oxygen reaching the myocardium through the coronary circulation. Ischemia develops, and pain results as it does in any other muscle exercised in the absence of adequate oxygen supply. Rest and/or the use of nitroglycerin (especially in the form of a tablet dissolved under the tongue) improves the ratio of cardiac work to oxygen supply.

In addition to underlying coronary artery disease, some angina sufferers also have signs of hyperthyroidism (enlarged or nodular thyroid gland, protruding eyeballs), hypertension (elevated blood pressure, hypertensive retinal blood vessel pattern), or diabetes mellitus (diabetic retinal blood vessel pattern, elevated blood glucose level). Hyperthyroidism and hypertension increase the workload of the heart and lower the threshold for angina attacks during exercise or excitement, since the basal level of cardiac activity is too high in these cases. Diabetes mellitus accelerates the atherosclerotic process that usually predisposes to angina pectoris.

Unstable Angina Pectoris. Also known as *intermediate coronary syndrome* and *pre-infarction angina,* this condition produces symptoms similar to those of stable angina, but attacks often occur in the absence of exertion or excitement. Nitroglycerin is often ineffective in relieving the anginal pain. Unstable angina often escalates into myocardial infarction and should be carefully observed for this development. The patient should be placed in a coronary care unit and monitored for heart muscle damage (infarction) and/or cardiac arrhythmias for several days. Often, a myocardial infarction occurs in this setting and can be easily treated, thus avoiding needless death from complications.

Myocardial Infarction. Symptoms are similar to those of angina pectoris, but there is detectable permanent heart damage. Damage develops as a result of obstruction of a coronary vessel previously narrowed by atherosclerosis with a thrombus on, or a hemorrhage beneath, the intima of the vessel. The resulting pain builds up in waves and is not relieved by rest or nitroglycerin but is relieved by narcotic drugs, such as morphine. In addition to the pain, which is often mistaken for the pain of indigestion, the individual usually suffers from nausea, vomiting, sweating, and dizziness. Fever, caused by pyrogen released from damaged heart cells, develops 1 to 7 days after the infarct occurs. If severe heart muscle damage occurs, pumping action is impaired and symptoms of congestive heart failure develop. (See the discussion under Complications.)

Prinzmetal's (variant) angina is a form in which ischemia is caused by coronary vasospasm rather than underlying atherosclero-

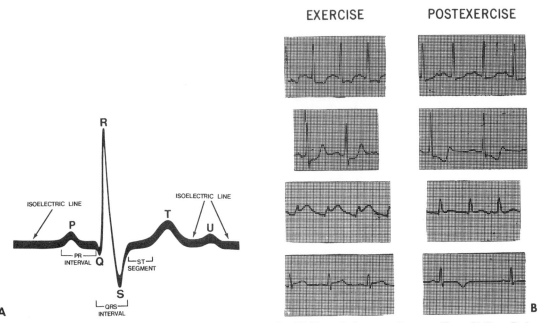

Figure 10–3. Electrocardiographic findings in angina pectoris. *(A)* Normal electrocardiogram. (From Phillips, R. L., and Feeney, M. K.: *The Cardiac Rhythms: A Systematic Approach to Interpretation,* 2nd ed. Philadelphia, W. B. Saunders Company, 1980.) *(B)* Electrocardiogram during an angina pectoris attack. (From Braunwald, E. (ed.): *Heart Disease: A Textbook of Cardiovascular Medicine,* 2nd ed. Philadelphia, W.B. Saunders Company, 1983.)

sis. It is usually worsened by propranolol (Inderal), which ordinarily helps stable angina, but is generally treatable with nifedipine (Procardia) or verapamil (Isoptin, Calan). (See the discussion under Treatment in this section.)

Laboratory Findings

The electrocardiogram (EKG) is the most useful tool in the diagnosis of coronary artery disease. During angina attacks, the characteristic electrocardiographic pattern is a downsloping or depression of the S-T segment, often with flattening or inversion of the T wave (Fig. 10–3). Approximately 25 per cent of the individuals with stable angina show a normal electrocardiogram at rest (resting EKG). Stressing the individual with a treadmill or step test brings out an angina pattern in all but about 10 per cent of the angina patients. The remaining 10 per cent show minimal coronary atherosclerosis, usually involving only one coronary artery. In myocardial infarction, the characteristic EKG finding is called the *Pardee wave,* and consists of S-T segment elevation, prominent Q wave, and T wave inversion (Fig. 10–4). It is helpful to obtain several EKG tracings over a period of days to chart the progress of electrical events following infarction. As the heart muscle heals and scar tissue

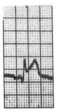

Figure 10–4. Electrocardiographic findings in myocardial infarction (Pardee wave). (From Braunwald, E. (ed.): *Heart Disease: A Textbook of Cardiovascular Medicine,* 2nd ed. Philadelphia, W. B. Saunders Company, 1983.)

forms, the EKG changes toward normal but often a prominent Q wave remains as a sign of an old, healed infarct.

Radioisotope Studies. These studies, which utilize ^{201}thallium, show ischemia occurring during exercise even in the absence of electrocardiographic evidence of angina.

Coronary angiography is a useful and relative safe technique for the diagnosis of coronary artery blockage. In this procedure, a dye is injected into the coronary circulation by means of a catheter and films are taken of the passage of dye through the arterial system. Because the mortality rate for the procedure is about 0.2 per cent, it should be used only on those with a clearly defined need. The largest group of people benefiting from coronary angiography are those with disabling stable angina who do not respond to drug therapy. These people may often be successfully treated with coronary bypass surgery. Coronary angiography will help to decide whether the blockage is in discrete areas (accessible to bypass) or widespread (not accessible to bypass).

Cholesterol and triglyceride levels are often elevated in coronary artery disease, but some individuals have normal levels (normal serum triglyceride level = 75 to 150 mg/dl). In addition, *electrophoresis* of the serum can specifically identify the type of hyperlipidemia. This procedure is based upon the principle that the various lipid fractions (chylomicrons, alpha, beta, and pre-beta lipoproteins) move at different rates in an electrical field and can thus be easily separated. Most serum cholesterol exists in the form of beta lipoproteins, whereas triglycerides are primarily found in the form of pre-beta lipoproteins.

If a myocardial infarction has occurred, the white blood cell count is elevated, presumably because of the inflammation associated with cell necrosis. Cell necrosis occurring after myocardial infarction can be documented with *technetium 99* (^{99m}Tc), an isotope that binds to necrotic tissue.

Damage to cardiac cells results in the leakage into the blood stream of enzymes normally contained within the cells. Glutamic oxaloacetic transaminase (GOT),* lactic dehydrogenase (LDH), and creatine phosphokinase (CPK) are normally present in the serum in small amounts (SGOT = 0 to 15 international milliunits [ImU]/milliliter; SLDH = 0 to 300 ImU/ml; SCPK = 5 to 50 ImU/ml). The serum levels of these increase in proportion to the amount of myocardial damage and can be used to aid in the diagnosis of myocardial infarction. The CPK measurement is especially useful, since the enzyme is found in only a few body tissues and is elevated almost immediately in the serum after heart muscle damage. The GOT and LDH levels also increase in the serum but require 6 to 48 hours before the increase is detectable.

Diagnosis   Many conditions can mimic the symptoms of coronary artery disease. Psychosomatic chest pain (not due to organic heart disease) is extremely common and is brought on by stress. Ulcer, hiatus hernia, and cholecystitis can duplicate the chest pain or pressure associated with coronary artery disease (see Chapter 12). Spontaneous pneumothorax (Chapter 14) often accurately mimics myocar-

---

*Also called aspartate aminotransferase (AST).

dial infarction. Various arthritic conditions of the spine or rib cage create pain misinterpreted as coming from the heart. Diagnosis in these cases is based upon electrocardiographic findings, especially with tracings taken after exercise, serum enzyme levels, and, occasionally, coronary angiography.

Treatment

Stable Angina Pectoris. Stable angina pectoris responds to rest, nitroglycerin, cessation of smoking, and the avoidance of excitement, overeating, and exposure to cold. (Cold constricts peripheral blood vessels, increasing cardiac work.) In addition to nitroglycerin, longer-acting drugs resembling nitroglycerin are available for prevention of angina attacks. These include pentaerythritol tetranitrate (Peritrate), erythrityl tetranitrate (Cardilate), and isosorbide dinitrate (Isordil, Sorbitrate). These drugs act by dilating peripheral blood vessels and reducing resistance to blood flow as well as by dilating coronary arteries and other mechanisms. Propranolol (Inderal) and nadolol (Corgard) reduce cardiac work and excitability, thus increasing the threshold for angina symptoms. A new class of drugs, including nifedipine (Procardia) and verapamil (Isoptin, Calan), reduces cardiac activity through a selective action on intracellular calcium. Control of contributing factors such as hypertension, diabetes mellitus, or hyperthyroidism also increases the success of angina treatment.

Unstable Angina Pectoris. Unstable angina fails to respond to the standard drugs useful for stable angina. Although the attacks are less predictable, it is felt that minimization of contributing factors is a helpful long-term means of reducing the frequency and severity of attacks as it is for stable angina. During an attack of unstable angina, the individual should be hospitalized and monitored for changes in serum enzyme levels and EKG findings that would signify infarction.

Myocardial Infarction. Close monitoring in a coronary care unit is essential. The individual should receive narcotic analgesics such as morphine or meperidine (Demerol) for pain. Oxygen is given during the acute phase of the attack, when cardiac pumping action may be severely impaired. Sodium bicarbonate solution is given intravenously immediately after the infarction to combat the systemic acidosis that develops from impaired cardiac function (retained carbon dioxide in the tissues). Rest is vitally important and should be enforced with the use of sedatives such as diazepam (Valium) or phenobarbital. With time, the area of infarct becomes well defined and the surrounding tissue recovers, leaving only a scar where the infarct occurred.

Follow-Up Treatment

Myocardial Infarction. Many survivors are placed on anticoagulant therapy to reduce the chance of reinfarction. Usually heparin is used initially because it has a rapid onset of action. Warfarin (Coumadin) is started with heparin but takes several days to reach maximum effect, after which heparin is discontinued. The dose is adjusted to give a prothrombin time two to two-and-a half times the normal value of 12 seconds. Studies have shown that the use of aspirin, sulfinpyrazone (Anturane), or propranolol (Inderal) after a myocardial infarction significantly reduces the chance of reinfarction.

Hyperlipidemia. Those individuals with hyperlipidemia (including those who have not had a myocardial infarction) are treated with a diet that emphasizes substitution of unsaturated for saturated fat (margarine instead of butter, fish instead of beef, skim milk instead of whole milk), reduced cholesterol intake (fewer eggs and other rich sources of cholesterol), and reduced sugar intake. (High sugar intake may be a factor in the development of atherosclerosis.) This type of diet will help the individual reach desired weight and eliminate this risk factor for coronary artery disease.

If diet fails to bring serum cholesterol and/or triglyceride levels to within normal range in 3 to 6 months, drug therapy may be added to the treatment program. Drug therapy of hyperlipidemias began about 25 years ago with the use of nicotinic acid and thyroid extract to lower cholesterol levels and has become more refined with the introduction of newer antihyperlipidemic agents such as sitosterols (Cytellin), cholestyramine (Questran), and dextrothyroxine (Choloxin). Clofibrate (Atromid S), used for a number of years, has been severely restricted in use by the Food and Drug Administration because of untoward effects, including increased risk of gallbladder, intestinal, and pancreatic disease and possible malignancy.

There is specialization among the antihyperlipidemic agents as to the type of hyperlipidemia that they will effectively treat. In some cases, diet is more effective than drug therapy. Since no treatment is effective in removing deposits already formed in the coronary arteries, drug therapy is directed toward measures to lower the level of cholesterol, triglycerides, and other lipids in the serum and thus slow the further accumulation of these materials as atheromatous plaques.

There is some evidence that if the levels of serum lipids are kept low for an extended period of time, some of the plaque material may be reabsorbed by the blood stream and the plaque size may actually decrease. This is not a dramatic effect but could be helpful after a period of years.

The drugs currently used to lower serum lipids are outlined in Table 10–2. The newest of this group is probucol (Lorelco), a drug that probably acts by a combination of actions on synthesis and removal of lipids. Other agents that have shown some benefit in treating hyperlipidemias include neomycin and a combination of para-aminosalicylic acid and vitamin C (PAS-C). If diet plus drug therapy does not lower lipid levels at least 10 per cent more than that achieved by diet alone in 1 to 2 months, the drugs should be discontinued.

Surgical Treatment

Surgical intervention in coronary atherosclerosis has progressed from the arterial transplant procedures used by Vineberg in the early 1950s, through endarterectomy, to the current widely used arterial bypass operations.

In the original Vineberg procedure, the internal mammary artery from the chest was transplanted and grafted into a tunnel made in the myocardium. The grafted artery grew new arterial buds and provided an increased blood supply to the ischemic myocardium.

The modern endarterectomy procedure utilizes a stream of high-pressure carbon dioxide gas, which peels away the arterial plaque without damaging the underlying vessel as a scalpel might.

In the coronary artery bypass procedure, a vein borrowed from elsewhere in the body (usually the saphenous vein) is attached to the aorta and sutured into the diseased coronary artery below the area of blockage. All three major coronary vessels can be bypassed during the same operation, if necessary. A patient with localized arterial blockage is a better candidate for surgery than one with widespread coronary atherosclerosis.

Complications

The most common cause of death after a myocardial infarction is ventricular fibrillation or cardiac arrest (40 per cent of deaths). Survival is greatly improved if such patients are monitored in a coronary care unit and if those near them when the attack occurs have knowledge of cardiopulmonary resuscitation (CPR). Other complications include cardiogenic shock (from heart failure), congestive heart failure, and heart block. Myocardial damage is the underlying cause of all these complications. As myocardial cells die during severe ischemia an electrical (injury) current is generated by the leakage of potassium from the cells. This promotes arrhythmias. Damage in the vicinity of the conducting system leads to heart block (to be discussed). Extensive myocardial damage causes loss of pumping action, leading to cardiogenic shock or congestive heart failure. After 2 or 3 days following an infarction, the incidence of complications begins to decrease dramatically.

Cardiogenic shock is treated with peripheral vasodilators, such as sodium nitroprusside (Nipride), which reduce the resistance to cardiac pumping action and improve the circulation of blood. (Treatments of the other complications are discussed later in this chapter.) Cardiac arrest must be treated immediately by pounding the chest, injecting epinephrine into the heart muscle, or applying electrical shock to the heart to establish some circulation so that drug therapy can be instituted.

CONGESTIVE HEART FAILURE

In order to appreciate present-day knowledge of congestive heart failure (CHF), we must go back in time about 200 years. In the 1780s, in rural Shropshire, England, lived a woman who had a reputation as an herbal healer. She collected plants that grew in the wild and concocted teas made from the plant leaves for the treatment of various illnesses. She had particularly good results in treating a condition then known as *dropsy,* in which edema of the ankles and fluid retention were the obvious physical changes. The tea she used for dropsy contained 20 different plant extracts, including the extract of a plant called *Digitalis purpurea,* or foxglove. When the tea was given to a dropsy sufferer, an increased urine volume resulted and the edema was relieved. Since the action of the tea was associated with a fluid loss, she presumed that the tea had a diuretic effect and that dropsy was a result of kidney failure.

William Withering, a physician who lived in the area, became interested in her treatment of dropsy and made a thorough study of the condition and the tea used to treat it. He found that the tea was not effective for all cases of edema. He also found through experimentation that he could omit all ingredients except the digitalis without any loss of effectiveness. Withering published a monograph in 1785 describing in detail his work with digitalis. While he noticed that digitalis affected the action of the heart, he apparently did not

Table 10–3. CAUSES OF CONGESTIVE HEART FAILURE
Aging of Heart Muscle
Coronary Artery Disease
Hypertension
Valve Disease
Cardiac Arrhythmias
Idiopathic

directly relate its action to relieve dropsy with improvement in cardiac function. Later investigators showed that the action of digitalis is directly on the heart and that edema is relieved indirectly through improved cardiac function.

During the past 200 years, tremendous knowledge has been acquired concerning CHF. We now know for certain that the heart is the seat of the problem. We also know much more about the causes of CHF and the factors contributing to the condition (Table 10–3). A few people develop CHF as a result of *aging* and loss of contractile force of the heart as a part of a general deterioration process. Others develop significant *coronary artery disease,* which reduces blood supply to the myocardium and causes reduced force of contraction. Many have a history of *hypertension,* in which the heart has been overworking for years to provide the abnormally high blood pressure, then enlarges (hypertrophy), and finally fails as a result of this overwork. *Valve disease* in the heart, as is seen with rheumatic fever, increases the workload of the heart and leads to cardiac hypertrophy and, ultimately, failure. *Cardiac arrhythmias* reduce the efficiency of the heart and may precipitate CHF. In addition, contributory conditions such as *hyperthyroidism* may increase the body's demand for circulation and contribute significantly to CHF. This is referred to as *high output failure.* Some cases of CHF are not well understood as to cause and are thus labeled *idiopathic.*

Pathogenesis   The initial event in the pathogenesis of CHF is the loss of contractile force by the cardiac muscle fibers. This is caused by a decreased ability of the muscle cells to utilize energy derived from the breakdown of adenosine triphosphate (ATP). Much of the energy is dissipated as heat or otherwise wasted, resulting in decreased energy available for contraction. This one change sets into motion a complex chain of events leading to the clinical manifestations of CHF (Fig. 10–5).

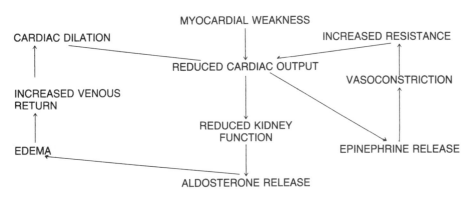

Figure 10–5. Events in congestive heart failure.

As the myocardium becomes weaker and pumps with less force, the cardiac output is reduced and blood that is not completely ejected from the heart chambers is retained, leading to cardiac dilation. The reduced circulation of blood to the tissues caused by left ventricular weakness causes ·hypoxia (reduced oxygen supply) and *cyanosis* (bluish color of the skin) and results in fatigue. In addition, body organs are deprived of adequate circulation and fluid congestion develops in them. The kidneys are particularly affected by this reduced circulation and produce less urine as a result. Whereas the normal urine volume is 1 to 2 liters per day for the average adult, the CHF patient may have a volume of only a few hundred milliliters per day. There are two major reasons for this:

1. Reduced kidney perfusion leads directly to reduced kidney function, since the kidney "processes" less blood.

2. Reduced volume and pressure of renal circulation leads to release of *renin* (an enzyme with a molecular weight of about 50,000) from the kidney. This causes the formation of *angiotensin I* from *angiotensinogen* and leads to release of *aldosterone* from the adrenal cortex. Aldosterone causes retention of sodium and water and reduces kidney output.

Retention of water and sodium results in the formation of *edema* (called *anasarca* in CHF) The renin-angiotensin-aldosterone system has important functions in helping the body to retain fluid in times of severe blood loss or shock, but in this case the results are harmful. Increased fluid volume further loads the heart and increases the failure.

Because blood is not pumped as forcefully by the failing heart, it is retained in the pulmonary system, leading to increased pressure in the pulmonary capillaries. This tends to force part of the fluid portion of the blood through the capillary walls and the fluid accumulates in the interstitial spaces in the lungs, leading to *pulmonary edema* (Fig. 10–6). This capillary leakage is worsened by the hypoxic state of the vascular system, which causes increased capillary permeability. The pressure is transmitted back through the right side of the heart, leading to increased pressure in the venous system which supplies blood to the heart. As venous pressure rises, blood is not returned to the heart from body tissues as rapidly and further edema develops.

In the early stages of failure, the body is able to compensate fairly well for the loss of cardiac output. The hypoxia that develops causes release of epinephrine from the adrenal glands, which increases cardiac rate and force of contraction but which also increases blood vessel resistance through vasoconstriction. Dilation of the right atrium causes reflex stimulation of the heart, which improves cardiac function. These measures fail to compensate for the heart failure as the heart muscle weakness increases, however, and the patient develops worsening symptoms.

Symptoms and Signs   The symptoms and signs of CHF include cough, shortness of breath, difficulty in breathing (dyspnea), difficulty in breathing while lying flat (orthopnea), fatigue, and weakness. Cardiovascular changes include tachycardia and pulsing of the jugular veins because of increased venous pressure (jugular pulse). As the heart catches

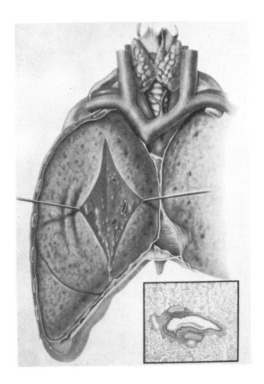

Figure 10–6. Pulmonary edema resulting from congestive heart failure. (Reproduced by permission of Merck Sharp & Dohme, Division of Merck & Co., Inc.)

up with the circulation during sleep, kidney function improves and the patient is awakened by the need to void at night (nocturia). All of the symptoms and signs develop because the contractile force of the heart is too small, and all revert to normal when it is increased.

Laboratory Findings   Most routine laboratory tests are normal in CHF. However, since kidney function is reduced, urine volume is decreased. Specific gravity of the urine is increased because the body must excrete waste material in a smaller volume of urine. In addition, more sodium is retained through increased action of aldosterone. This must be excreted in the urine and adds to the specific gravity. The normal value for specific gravity is 1.015 to 1.025. Chest x-ray films show a larger heart silhouette because of cardiac dilation (Fig. 10–7).

Diagnosis   Symptoms and signs, laboratory tests, and history usually present a clear picture of CHF to the physician. However, respiratory disorders such as bronchial asthma or emphysema may closely mimic the respiratory symptoms of the condition. In fact, the term "cardiac asthma" is sometimes used to describe the respiratory symptoms of CHF. Other conditions associated with edema, such as liver or kidney disease, may confuse the picture as well.

Treatment   The general treatment measures helpful in CHF include rest, light diet with reduced sodium intake, and control or correction of factors contributing to the condition (e.g., hypertension, valve disease).

Drugs are almost always necessary to improve cardiac function and reduce edema. The digitalis compounds increase the contractile

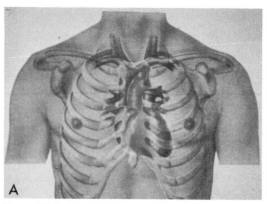 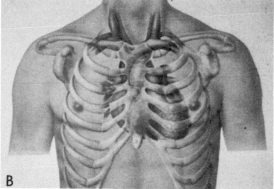

Figure 10–7. Heart size in normal and failing hearts. *(A)* Normal heart. *(B)* Congestive heart failure. (Reproduced by permission of Merck Sharp & Dohme, Division of Merck & Co., Inc.)

force of the heart and indirectly relieve edema through improved blood flow to the kidney. Diuretics are often used in conjunction with digitalis to increase the loss of water and sodium and relieve edema faster. Oxygen is used for severe episodes of dyspnea, but it becomes less needed as cardiac function improves.

Currently, investigative work emphasizes the use of vasodilators, which reduce peripheral resistance and thus reduce the workload of the heart. This would amount to solving the problem from the reverse direction. That is, instead of increasing the contractile force of the heart, vasodilation reduces the resistance against which the heart must pump.

Complications   Some patients become *refractory* to these treatments. It is then necessary to review the drug therapy completely, with special attention to doses, methods of administration, drug dosing schedules, and other factors. It is vitally important that all contributing factors have been controlled as well as possible.

Occasionally, *acute pulmonary edema* develops when cardiac function suddenly decreases, as during a severe arrhythmia. The lungs fill with fluid, and dyspnea and shortness of breath develop. Treatment consists of increasing the doses of digitalis and diuretics already being given, usually by giving the drugs intravenously, along with the administration of oxygen and morphine. Morphine is helpful because it dilates blood vessels in the peripheral areas and helps to relieve the pulmonary edema. Occasionally, tourniquets are applied to the limbs to reduce fluid return to the heart temporarily. These are "rotated" by loosening one tourniquet at a time for a few minutes to prevent ischemia and possible tissue damage. The effect of this treatment is to reduce the load on the heart by temporarily reducing the venous return to the heart and, therefore, its workload.

Prognosis   Most people with CHF do well if the previously described treatment plan is followed carefully and any aggravating factors are controlled. Careful monitoring is necessary, though, to maintain adequate digitalis effect without developing digitalis toxicity. Toxic symptoms include a yellowish or greenish cast to vision, nausea and vomiting, confusion, and a variety of cardiac arrhythmias. Early detection of digitalis toxicity will prevent the development of life-threatening arrhythmias such as ventricular fibrillation.

HYPERTENSION

Normal Blood Pressure Control

Blood pressure control in the normal individual is the result of a complex interaction of physiologic mechanisms. The heart pumps at a variable rate and output against an adjustable resistance created by the peripheral vascular system. Increased heart rate, volume of blood pumped per stroke (stroke volume), or a combination of both causes the blood pressure to increase if the peripheral vascular system does not adjust by providing less resistance to the flow of pumped blood. Likewise, increased peripheral resistance caused by vasoconstriction will increase the blood pressure if adjustments are not made to lower the heart rate and/or stroke volume.

In most individuals, the body is able to maintain blood pressure at a normal level. Thus, the *normotensive* person has a blood pressure of approximately 120 millimeters of mercury (mmHg) over 80 mmHg. The high value (120) is the *systolic* pressure and is generated during the maximum contracting effort of the heart (systole). The low value (80) is the *diastolic* pressure, which is the lowest point the pressure reaches during the rest period (diastole) between systoles. Diastolic pressure is maintained primarily by the elasticity of the peripheral vascular system, which allows the vessels to expand slightly during systole and gradually return to normal during diastole.

Maintenance of normal blood pressure is accomplished through the combined action of *reflex mechanisms,* which return the pressure to normal if it leaves the normal range. Thus, the *carotid sinus reflex* adjusts the heart rate and stroke volume up or down if the blood pressure changes from normal. Pressure-sensitive receptors (baro-receptors) located in the carotid sinuses and in the aortic arch constantly monitor blood pressure and operate through the autonomic nervous system to adjust it to normal.

Receptors in the right atrium respond to stretching caused by accumulation of blood in the heart by increasing the heart rate or stroke volume. This allows the heart to adjust for changes in physiologic function or physical activity.

The kidney senses blood pressure and volume flow by means of specialized receptors and releases *renin* (Fig. 10–8) if blood pressure or blood flow to the kidney decreases, as discussed regarding CHF. Renin causes the conversion of *angiotensinogen* to *angiotensin* I, which is then coverted to *angiotensin* II through the action of an enzyme found in the lungs. Angiotensin II causes arterial constriction, which raises blood pressure. Thus, through the action of these and other control mechanisms, normal blood pressure is maintained under a wide variety of physiologic conditions.

Hypertensive State

In approximately 5 per cent of the population, blood pressure is consistently above normal. These *hypertensive* people, in effect, have blood pressure that has been "set" at a higher level, much as a thermostat can be adjusted to a higher temperature. For some reason, in these individuals, the body reflex mechanisms are "content" to allow blood pressure to remain above normal without readjusting it to normal. Blood pressure values greater than 140/90 mm Hg in a person under 50 years of age are considered hypertensive by most authorities. In older individuals, a somewhat higher pressure is normal because a gradual loss of elasticity associated with aging and hardening of the arteries results in slightly increased resistance and higher pressure. However, the old saying that blood pressure should be "100 plus your age" gives risky approval to those in the 60- to 80-year-old age group, since a systolic pressure of 160 to 180 mm Hg in these individuals is abnormally high.

Pathogenesis

Essential or Primary Hypertension. About 85 per cent of the hypertensives are of a type called *essential* or *primary,* in which no cause for the hypertension can be identified. It assumed that there is some reason why the body sets the blood pressure abnormally high, but at present no physical or chemical basis can be demonstrated. Therefore, no cure yet exists for the vast majority of cases and control of the elevated blood pressure becomes the most important therapeutic goal.

Secondary Hypertension. The remaining 15 per cent of the hypertensive population have *secondary* hypertension, in which there is a demonstrable cause for the condition and the increased blood pressure occurs secondarily. These individuals may be curable if the underlying cause is removed.

Renal hypertension, a type of secondary hypertension, is caused by disease of or damage to the kidney. It results from infection, inflammatory disease, or reduced circulation to the kidney. These factors trigger the renin-angiotensin mechanism (Fig. 10–8), and blood pressure is raised in the body's effort to "protect" the kidney by ensuring adequate blood supply to it. If the underlying kidney condition is corrected through surgery or drug treatment, the blood pressure returns to normal.

Pregnancy or *oral contraceptives* can increase the blood pressure to a mild degree in some women, apparently because of the effects of estrogen in increasing retention of sodium and water. When pregnancy terminates or the oral contraceptive is discontinued, estrogen levels return to normal and blood pressure becomes normal.

Head injuries, brain infections, or *brain tumors* that increase the cerebrospinal fluid pressure cause an elevation of blood pressure that is proportional to the amount of increase in the cerebrospinal fluid pressure. This is a protective mechanism in which the body increases the systemic blood pressure to ensure adequate circulation

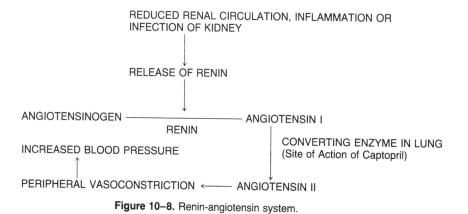

Figure 10–8. Renin-angiotensin system.

to the brain, thus opposing the tendency of the increased cerebrospinal fluid pressure to constrict cerebral blood vessels and impair circulation to the brain. Treatment of the underlying condition will reduce cerebrospinal fluid pressure and cause a reversion of systemic blood pressure to normal.

Rarely, a tumor is found in the adrenal medulla that synthesizes epinephrine and norepinephrine (*pheochromocytoma*). The constant release of the compounds into the blood stream causes the blood pressure to be elevated, since these compounds cause vasoconstriction and increased vascular resistance. Epinephrine also increases heart rate and stroke volume, which prevents the heart from decreasing these parameters to compensate for the increased vascular resistance. Usually, a pheochromocytoma can be removed surgically or its synthetic activity can be blocked with the use of a drug called metyrosine (Demser).

Malignant Hypertension. A severe form of either primary or secondary hypertension, malignant hypertension is characterized by a rapidly increasing blood pressure and early development of complications. It is not associated with cancer, as the name suggests, but is so named for the increased risk to the patient it creates. Without vigorous treatment, it is usually fatal within 2 years. By definition, the term also designates a diastolic pressure of over 130 mm Hg and an elevation or blurring of the optic disc in the retina (papilledema), caused by the vascular effects of extremely high blood pressure.

Symptoms and Signs

Many people with early, primary hypertension are asymptomatic, a fact that often precludes early diagnosis and treatment. The disease continues unabated and complications eventually develop. If symptoms are present, they usually consist of irritability, tiredness, and vague feelings of being unwell (malaise).

Headache, regarded by many as a reliable symptom of hypertension, usually appears later in the course of the disease. Thus, absence of headache does not preclude hypertension. When headache does occur, it is usually felt in the back of the head and is most severe early in the morning after sleeping, presumably due to blood vessel engorgement caused by lying flat during sleep.

If the hypertension is caused by pheochromocytoma, the individual often experiences anxiety, palpitations, sweating, and nervousness, since these are normal effects of epinephrine release. In extremely severe hypertension in which brain damage has occurred, blurred vision, mental confusion, and even paralysis are seen.

In addition to consistently elevated blood pressure, hypertensives may also have changes in the retinal blood vessels caused by the effects of prolonged hypertension. These are called Keith-Wagener (K-W) retinopathies and are designated $K-W_1$ through $K-W_4$ (Fig. 10–9). $K-W_1$ retinopathy demonstrates mild constriction of the retinal blood vessels; $K-W_2$ and $K-W_3$ show added arteriovenous compression (A-V nicking), retinal hemorrhages, exudates, and edema; and $K-W_4$, associated with malignant hypertension, demonstrates papilledema.

Laboratory Findings

Early Hypertension. In mild, early hypertension, laboratory findings are usually normal. However, with increasing severity and

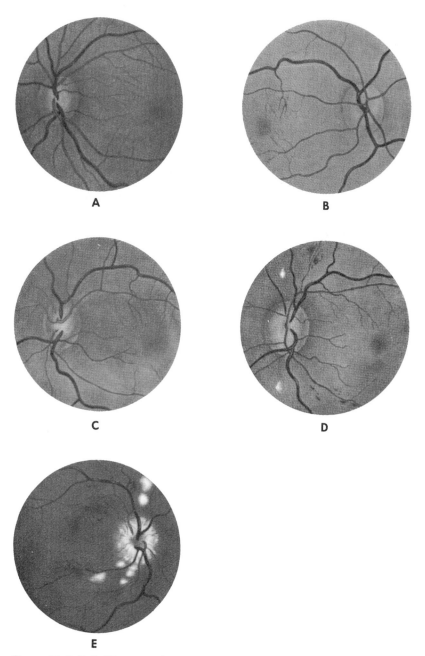

Figure 10–9. Keith-Wagener retinopathy in hypertension. *(A)* Normal. *(B)* K-W₁—mild constriction of blood vessels. *(C)* K-W₂—more severe constriction with arterioventricular nicking. *(D)* K-W₃—severe constriction with arterioventricular nicking, retinal hemorrhages, and exudates. *(E)* K-W₄—severe constriction with arterioventricular nicking, exudates, and edema. (Selected from Scheie, H., and Albert, D.: *Textbook of Ophthalmology,* 9th ed. Philadelphia, W. B. Saunders Company, 1977.)

duration of the condition, kidney damage often occurs, and this is reflected in changes in several common laboratory tests. The specific gravity of the urine may decrease as the kidney fails to remove waste materials as effectively as before. Specific gravity may approach 1.010 if severe renal failure develops. Likewise, materials not as rapidly removed from the blood stream through kidney action tend to accumulate there. The *blood urea nitrogen* (BUN) increases as waste products from protein metabolism accumulate in the blood stream. The normal value for BUN is 8 to 20 mg/dl. Likewise, creatinine, a product of muscle metabolism, accumulates in the face of reduced renal function and the *serum creatinine level* increases (normal = 0.7 to 1.5 mg/dl).

Secondary Hypertension. Laboratory findings may point to the underlying disease process that causes the increased blood pressure. If kidney infection is present, the urine usually contains bacteria, pus, and leukocytes. Abnormalities existing in kidney structure or vascular supply can be identified through a test called an intravenous pyelogram (IVP). This test uses an opaque dye injected into the venous system, with x-ray films taken of the urinary tract as the dye is being excreted by the kidneys. The dye provides a good outline of the urinary tract on the roentgenogram. In cases of pheochromocytoma, the metabolic byproduct of epinephrine and norepinephrine can be measured in the urine. The normal quantity of this compound, vanillylmandelic acid (VMA)—obtained from collecting the urine formed during a 24-hour period, does not exceed 9 mg. Higher values are indicative of increased secretion of epinephrine and norepinephrine and give indirect evidence of pheochromocytoma.

Long-Term Hypertension. In advanced, long-standing hypertension, the heart often enlarges as a consequence of the sustained additional effort involved in constantly maintaining abnormally high blood pressure. The principle is the same as in a weightlifter who develops large muscles from long periods of training. Since the heart does not have the capability of forming additional cells (hyperplasia), it compensates for this overwork by increasing the size of each cell (hypertrophy) and the total muscle mass of the heart increases. A chest roentgenogram of a person with cardiac hypertrophy shows an obvious increase in the size of the heart silhouette. Likewise, the electrocardiogram reflects a change in the mass of muscle through which the axis of electrical depolarization moves. (Electrocardiograms are discussed later in this chapter.) This change can be calculated as to direction (left or right) and angle of deflection from the normal and is called *axis deviation*. In hypertension the deviation is usually to the left, since the left ventricle is responsible for providing the systemic circulation and hypertrophies more than does the right ventricle.

Diagnosis   Hypertension is diagnosed when the blood pressure is consistently elevated above the normal range for the age of the patient. The additional tests previously described help to identify the cause and type of hypertension. In the majority of cases, most test results will be normal because most hypertensives are of the primary type. However, secondary hypertension and advanced primary hypertension may be identified, as mentioned. For most hypertensives, the diagnosis is one of exclusion after failing to find causes or consequences of the condition.

Treatment   General measures that are helpful to all hypertensives include normalization of weight, reduction of excessive stress and nervous tension, and withdrawal of any drugs that might have a hypertensive effect. Drugs such as nasal decongestants and antiasthma products may increase blood pressure markedly, especially in the hypertensive. Any surgically correctable conditions involving the kidney, vascular system, or adrenal glands should be resolved. This often results in complete cure of the hypertension.

For the vast majority of primary hypertensives, drug therapy is the major treatment. Since there is no treatable cause in these cases, complete cure is obtained only rarely. A few very early, mild hypertensives seem to readjust blood pressures after a short period of drug therapy and become normotensive without the further need for drugs. Most, however, require long-term (often lifetime) drug therapy to control their condition. It is important for hypertensive individuals to understand that long-term drug therapy is usually necessary and that they should not discontinue or reduce medication after a short while or because they feel better. The absence of symptoms and the feeling of well-being do not mean that the blood pressure is normal.

Drug therapy of hypertension is quite complex, since there are over a dozen ways in which drugs can lower blood pressure. Most hypertensives receive a "thiazide" diuretic, such as hydrochlorothiazide (Hydrodiuril), as the first step in treatment. Thiazide diuretics reduce excessive extracellular fluid and sodium accumulation and also, more importantly, cause direct dilation of peripheral blood vessels and reduce vascular resistance. Other agents are added in a stepwise manner as needed. Reserpine (Serpasil), methyldopa (Aldomet), prazosin (Minipress), and guanethidine (Ismelin) reduce the nerve stimulation that causes blood vessel constriction in the peripheral circulation. Although there are several different mechanisms of action involved among the different drugs, the end result is an antihypertensive effect with each. Drugs such as propranolol (Inderal), nadolol (Corgard), and metoprolol (Lopressor) reduce cardiac rate and output and thus lower blood pressure from the opposite direction (the heart rather than the peripheral vascular system). A novel approach to severe hypertension is seen with the drug captopril (Capoten), which prevents the conversion of angiotensin I to angiotensin II by inhibiting the converting enzyme (Fig. 10–8).

Attaining the ideal drug therapy program for the hypertensive person requires some experimentation. Many people require two, three, or more drugs for adequate control, and careful attention to dosage and side effects of the drugs is necessary. In severe hypertension, some side effects must often be tolerated in order to maintain good control of blood pressure.

Complications   The major risks of undetected or inadequately treated hypertension are *renal damage, stroke,* and *cardiac hypertrophy.*

Renal damage occurs when the delicate renal blood vessels are progressively destroyed by the mechanical effects of sustained high blood pressure (Fig. 10–10).

Stroke occurs when a blood vessel in the brain bursts (*cerebral hemorrhage*) or when a cerebral vessel becomes obstructed by a thrombus (*cerebral thrombosis*). The brain is most often the site for blood vessel rupture in hypertension, since cerebral blood vessels are poorly supported by surrounding tissues compared with vessels surrounded by other types of body tissues (muscle, bone). (Perhaps the saying that "we are all a little soft in the head" has some basis

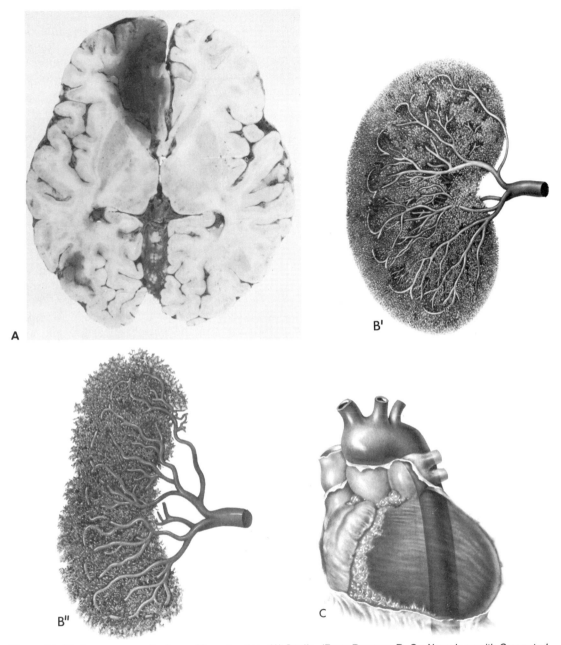

Figure 10–10. Common complications of hypertension. *(A)* Stroke. (From Ramsey, R. G.: *Neurology with Computed Tomography.* Philadelphia, W. B. Saunders Company, 1981.) *(B)* Renal damage. *(B')* Vascular system of normal kidney. *(B")* Vascular system of hypertensive kidney. *(C)* Cardiac hypertrophy. (Reproduced by permission of Merck Sharp & Dohme, Division of Merck & Co., Inc.)

in fact!) When blood pressure increases, the soft brain tissue allows the cerebral blood vessels to bulge and weak areas, or *aneurysms,* can develop. Rupture of an aneurysm causes hemorrhage into the brain tissue, with resulting brain damage (Fig. 10–10).

Cardiac hypertrophy develops as a consequence of prolonged overwork of the heart. If the condition is not treated by lowering the blood pressure, the heart may decompensate into congestive heart failure (Fig. 10–10).

Some hypertensives develop a severe, sudden increase in blood pressure (*hypertensive crisis*), which greatly increases the immediate risk of stroke, renal failure, or congestive heart failure. Vigorous emergency treatment using peripheral vasodilators such as diazoxide (Hyperstat) or sodium nitroprusside (Nipride) is necessary to lower the blood pressure and prevent severe complications.

PERIPHERAL VASCULAR DISORDERS

Disorders of the peripheral vascular system can be divided into two major categories: those affecting the *arterial* circulation *to* the extremities and those affecting the *venous* return *from* the extremities. Arterial disorders usually cause numbness and coolness of the extremity as a result of reduced circulation, whereas venous disorders commonly cause edema of the extremity as a result of poor removal of blood from it. Pain is a frequent finding in most peripheral vascular disorders, since it can be caused by ischemia or edema of the affected area.

Several disease processes are represented by the peripheral vascular disorders. *Occlusive vascular disease* results from an atherosclerotic process. *Raynaud's disease* is a vasospastic disorder. *Thromboangiitis obliterans* and *thrombophlebitis* are associated with inflammation of and clot formation in the peripheral artery and vein, respectively. The etiologic factors responsible for these disorders are also quite varied and range from smoking to hypercholesterolemia to inactivity to effects of hormones (Table 10–4).

Occlusive Vascular Disease

Atherosclerotic involvement of the lower aorta and of the arteries of the legs, feet and, rarely, the arms and hands is seen. The condition is especially common in diabetics and in those with hypercholesterolemia. Often, significant arterial disease of the coronary or carotid (neck) arteries is present as well. The plaques are most common at bends or junctions of vessels where turbulence of the blood is greatest.

Symptoms and Signs

In the typical case, the individual is middle-aged or older and complains about pain and fatigue in the calf muscles (intermittent claudication) while walking. The foot and lower leg area are cool and have reduced or absent arterial pulses. Hair growth is sparse and the extremity easily becomes infected as a result of trivial injury. Ulceration and poor healing of wounds are common because of the reduced circulation.

Table 10–4. PERIPHERAL VASCULAR DISORDERS

Disease	Etiologic Factors
Occlusive vascular disease	Diabetes mellitus, hypercholesterolemia, middle to old age
Thromboangiitis obliterans (Buerger's disease)	Smoking, male sex, Jewish ethnic origin
Raynaud's disease	Exposure to cold, emotional upset, female sex, young age
Thrombophlebitis	Intravenous injection, infection in or around vein, pregnancy, use of oral contraceptives, obesity, inactivity

The atherosclerotic lesion resembles the plaques found in coronary atherosclerosis and consists chiefly of cholesterol and other lipids. As the lesion increases in size, mechanical obstruction of the arterial circulation occurs and symptoms result. Often the plaque increases in size slowly and symptoms gradually worsen over a period of months or years.

Diagnosis

Diagnosis is based upon the history of intermittent claudication or equivalent symptoms, physical examination, and x-ray of the involved artery (arteriography), often with the use of a dye to outline the vessel more clearly. Raynaud's disease and thromboangiitis obliterans also cause peripheral ischemia, but these generally occur in younger people and have distinguishing diagnostic features. In Raynaud's disease, the peripheral pulse is normal between attacks. In thromboangiitis obliterans, the hands and arms are usually also involved and exacerbations and remissions are the rule.

Treatment

Treatment of occlusive vascular disease involves several alternatives: removal of the arterial deposits if possible (endarterectomy) (especially feasible if the carotid arteries are diseased); severing of the sympathetic nerve fibers leading to the affected artery (sympathectomy); or replacement of the diseased segment with a graft made of Dacron. Vasodilator drugs are generally not helpful, since the diseased artery is usually unresponsive to them. Other helpful measures include cessation of smoking, exercising to the point of pain several times a day to improve collateral (side channel) circulation and lowering serum cholesterol level with diet and/or drug therapy.

Complications

Uncontrolled occlusive vascular disease can lead to gangrene and require amputation of the extremity in severe cases.

Thromboangiitis Obliterans (Buerger's Disease)

In 1908 surgeon/pathologist Leo Buerger described a type of peripheral arterial disease characterized by inflammation, thrombosis, and occlusion of the arteries of the feet and hands. Nearly all victims were heavy smokers and most were males and of Jewish ethnic origin. Many physicians originally considered thromboangiitis obliterans (thrombosis, blood vessel inflammation, obliteration) to be a variety of occlusive vascular disease, but it was later shown to be a separate pathologic entity.

Buerger's disease affects males in the 25- to 40-year-old age group and is closely associated with smoking. It is thought that nicotine or some other component in inhaled smoke causes sensitization of the peripheral arteries, resulting in inflammation. Thrombosis, resulting from inflammation and arterial blockage, associated with granulation and abscess formation are eventual consequences. The effects of male hormone and certain genetic traits may cause the predilection for male, Jewish victims. However, females and non-Jews are also affected, although less frequently.

Signs and Symptoms

Signs and symptoms are similar to those of occlusive vascular disease. Intermittent claudication, numbness, and coolness of the affected part are common. However, the symptoms wax and wane as inflammation increases and subsides, whereas occlusive vascular disease is steady and progressive. Raynaud's disease primarily affects females and is not caused by smoking.

Treatment The most effective treatment measure is the *cessation of smoking*. If smoking is continued, the disease inevitably worsens, eventually leading to gangrene, tissue necrosis, and amputation. *Sympathectomy* may be of marginal benefit, as are *vasodilators,* such as nylidrin (Arlidin) or isoxsuprine (Vasodilan). However, since the condition is associated with arterial inflammation and thrombosis rather than arterial spasm, response to these treatments is often poor.

Raynaud's Disease Raynaud's disease primarily affects young women and is not directly related to smoking. There is no ethnic predilection for it. During attacks, spasm occurs in the peripheral arteries, causing numbness and pain in the hands and, occasionally, the feet or tip of the nose. The exact cause is unknown, but exaggerated sympathetic nervous system activity in the extremities is postulated. Attacks usually occur upon exposure to cold, especially in handling ice or cold drinks, or during emotional upset, at which time sympathetic activity is greater. The artery is normal, with no evidence of plaque, thrombus, or inflammatory process, and peripheral pulse and circulation are normal between attacks. Vasospasm is usually symmetric (both extremities are affected equally).

Raynaud's phenomenon occurs as a part of a larger picture of disease, especially in conjunction with systemic autoimmune disorders, such as lupus erythematosus or scleroderma. In these cases, the underlying condition must be controlled.

Treatment Treatment of Raynaud's disease involves avoidance of cold exposure or emotional upset. Smoking, while not a cause, contributes to arterial constriction and should be avoided. Vasodilators, such as isoxsuprine (Vasodilan), nylidrin (Arlidin), nicotinic acid, or long-acting nitrates such as pentaerythritol tetranitrate (Peritrate) are often helpful, since they directly combat the vasospasm that causes symptoms. Nitroglycerin ointment is especially helpful because it can be rubbed directly on the affected area and is well absorbed through the skin. For cases unresponsive to these measures, sympathectomy is often quite useful.

Complications Complications are usually minimal, since arterial circulation is good between attacks and gangrene or necrosis of affected tissues is unlikely.

Thrombophlebitis Vein inflammation (phlebitis) associated with clot formation is a common condition and results from a variety of etiologic factors. Usually, phlebitis develops first and thrombosis occurs as a consequence of the inflammation (Fig. 10–11). Common causes of thrombophlebitis include intravenous injection of irritating drugs or solutions, infection within or near a vein, and high estrogen levels associated with pregnancy or the use of oral contraceptives. Contributing factors include obesity and inactivity, especially the practice

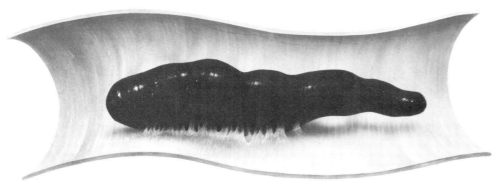

Figure 10–11. Appearance of thrombus in thrombophlebitis. (Reproduced by permission of Merck Sharp & Dohme, Division of Merck & Co., Inc.)

of crossing the legs for long periods of time. When venous circulation is reduced (stasis), platelet aggregation (clumping) occurs and a clot forms, especially in the area of venous injury.

Hospitalized patients are especially prone to thrombophlebitis, since they are relatively immobile and often are being treated with intravenous therapy. This is an important reason for them to become ambulatory as soon as possible.

Thrombophlebitis can affect smaller, surface veins (*superficial thrombophlebitis*) or larger, deeper veins (*deep vein thrombophlebitis*). Symptoms and potential complications are more severe with deep vein thrombophlebitis.

Superficial Thrombophlebitis

Thrombophlebitis of the surface veins produces redness and tenderness of the affected part, especially along the course of the involved vein. Pain is dull and little, if any, swelling occurs. Ischemia and numbness do not develop, as they do with reduced arterial blood supply (described under Occlusive Vascular Disease). About 20 per cent of the individuals with superficial thrombophlebitis have hidden deep vein thrombophlebitis and risk consequences of it.

Treatment. Treatment includes elevation of the affected part (usually leg or arm), application of heat, bed rest, and the use of anti-inflammatory drugs, such as phenylbutazone (Butazolidin). Anticoagulants are used only in those cases in which deep vein involvement also exists. Extensive or recurrent disease may require vein removal (stripping).

Deep Vein Thrombophlebitis

Involvement of deeper veins generally causes symptoms similar to those of superficial thrombophlebitis, but symptoms are more intense and edema of the extremity is present. In about 80 per cent of the cases, the deep veins of the calf are involved (Fig. 10–12). The calf is tender, rigid with edema, and it responds to flexion of the foot with muscle spasm and/or pain (Homans' sign) (Fig. 10–13). In the absence of reliable signs and symptoms, deep vein thrombophlebitis can be diagnosed with the use of an ultrasound blood flow detector (which detects changes in venous blood flow), or phlebography, an x-ray of the vein showing the area of obstruction.

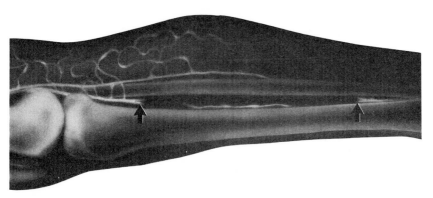

Figure 10–12. Venogram showing deep vein thrombophlebitis involving calf of leg. Clot occupies space between arrows. (Reproduced by permission of Merck Sharp & Dohme, Division of Merck & Co., Inc.)

Deep vein thrombophlebitis is occasionally confused with conditions that produce local edema (infections, injuries) or lymphatic obstruction (tumor, x-ray damage). Systemic conditions causing edema, such as congestive heart failure, kidney disease, or liver disease, produce equal swelling of both legs.

Treatment and Complications. Treatment is similar to that for superficial thrombophlebitis, except that anticoagulants (such as heparin) are used to prevent further clot buildup. Sometimes warfarin (Coumadin) is used following heparin therapy to provide long-term protection against further clotting. In severe cases, when great danger exists from a complication of thrombophlebitis, streptokinase (Streptase) is given intravenously. Streptokinase increases the activity of fibrinolysin, which dissolves the clot. It should be noted that the anticoagulants (heparin, warfarin) do not *dissolve* existing clots but only prevent their further buildup.

The greatest danger with deep vein thrombophlebitis is that as the clot enlarges, a portion can break off and become an embolus. This can then circulate back to the right side of the heart and be pumped into the pulmonary circulation. As the blood vessels become smaller and smaller in the pulmonary arterial system, the clot finally jams (pulmonary embolism). This leads to severe symptoms, including dyspnea and chest pain, with the possibility of death resulting. Emboli from the left side of the heart and its vascular branches can

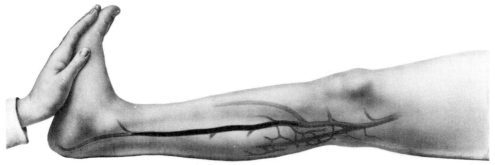

Figure 10–13. Homans' sign in deep vein thrombophlebitis. Pain and/or muscle spasm occurs when the foot is flexed. (Reproduced by permission of Merck Sharp & Dohme, Division of Merck & Co., Inc.)

lodge in the coronary arterial circulation (coronary embolism) and the cerebral arterial circulation (cerebral embolism). In all three cases, local tissue damage (infarction) can result from blocked arterial circulation.

Besides the medical measures outlined for preventing embolism and its consequences, several clever surgical techniques are also employed in severe cases. Partial ligation of the affected vein above the site of clot formation will prevent large clot fragments from returning to the heart. Plastic clips placed around the vein above the clot will allow for circulation of blood but will compress the vein enough to keep clots from passing. A unique *umbrella filter,* developed at the Ochsner Clinic in New Orleans, can be inserted into an accessible vein and passed into the area above the clot, using x-ray guidance. The attached tube is gently pulled forward, opening the umbrella and lodging it in the vein. Holes in the metal umbrella allow blood to pass but not clots. The tube is then unscrewed and removed, leaving the filter in place. With time, the clot fragments contained by these techniques dissolve and the risk of embolus disappears.

CARDIAC ARRHYTHMIAS

Cardiac tissue possesses special properties that uniquely equip it for the task of providing blood circulation without our conscious control. *Excitability,* or the ability to respond to stimulation, is a feature of cardiac tissue as well as other types of muscle.

Heart muscle responds to electrical impulses carried through conducting tissue by contracting. The impulses originate in the *sinoatrial* (SA) *node,* also called the *pacemaker* of the heart. In the resting state, the SA node sends out impulses at the rate of 70 to 80 beats per minute. These spread to the *atrial tissue,* then to the *atrioventricular* (AV) *node,* the *bundle of His, bundle branches, Purkinje fibers,* and *ventricular tissue* (Fig. 10–14). Slowing occurs

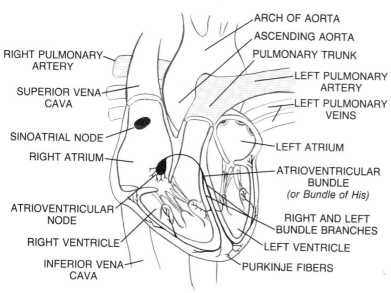

ARCH OF AORTA
ASCENDING AORTA
PULMONARY TRUNK
RIGHT PULMONARY ARTERY
SUPERIOR VENA CAVA
LEFT PULMONARY ARTERY
LEFT PULMONARY VEINS
SINOATRIAL NODE
RIGHT ATRIUM
LEFT ATRIUM
ATRIOVENTRICULAR BUNDLE (or Bundle of His)
ATRIOVENTRICULAR NODE
RIGHT AND LEFT BUNDLE BRANCHES
RIGHT VENTRICLE
LEFT VENTRICLE
INFERIOR VENA CAVA
PURKINJE FIBERS

Figure 10–14. Heart and great vessels.

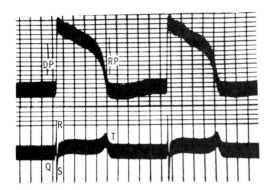

Figure 10–15. Action potential resulting from depolarization of the cardiac cell. DP = Depolarization; RP = repolarization. (From Ganong, W. F.: *Review of Medical Physiology,* 9th ed. Los Altos, Calif., Lange Medical Publications, 1979.)

at the AV node, much like a "bottleneck" on a busy freeway, and then the rate of impulse *conduction* (spread through excitable tissue) increases again as the impulses race through the Purkinje fibers. The entire network of tissue, from SA node to Purkinje fibers, is called the *conduction system* and consists of specialized muscle tissue that behaves like nerve tissue.

Another special feature of cardiac tissue is its ability to spontaneously depolarize and create an electrical impulse. This is called *automaticity* and it gives the heart the ability to drive itself without external control. Even a single cell from any area of the heart kept alive in a physiologic solution will exhibit automaticity.

The key to normal control of the heart by SA node activity is that the SA node normally depolarizes at the greatest rate of any cardiac tissue. The AV node and atrial tissue have an inherent rate of depolarization of 60 to 65 beats per minute and ventricular tissue has an inherent rate of 30 to 40 impulses per minute. The heart follows the SA node, since it has the greatest rate of depolarization. Under special circumstances, when SA node impulses are blocked, another part of the heart can become the pacemaker (e.g., the ventricular tissue in heart block). Ventricular rate then follows the slower stimulus.

Occasionally, another area of the heart begins to depolarize rapidly and supersedes the "leadership" of the SA node. The heart, or a portion of it, then follows the new, faster area. This new area is called an *ectopic pacemaker* (ectopic = out of the normal location). Ectopic pacemakers are important in the generation of arrhythmias.

The *electrocardiogram* (EKG) is an ongoing graphic record of electrical events in the heart. Depolarization of a cardiac cell creates an *action potential* (Fig. 10–15). The EKG is the summation of action potentials from all areas of the heart as the impulse spreads through the conducting system. As the wave of depolarization spreads from SA node to ventricles, it creates a current that, in the main, advances toward the lower, left portion of the body and away from the upper, right portion. If electrodes are applied to the right arm and left leg, the difference in potential generated by the moving electrical wavefront can be measured. This electrode arrangement is referred to as a *lead II* EKG.

In practice, 12 standard leads, represented by different combinations of electrodes, are employed. The electrocardiogram is composed of *P, QRS,* and *T* portions, along with the interval representing the distance between the beginning of P and the beginning of the QRS complex (PR interval) (Fig. 10–3*A*). The *S-T segment* is the distance between the end of the S wave and the beginning of the T wave. Since the EKG is a moving record of electrical activity, "distance" is recorded as "time" and values are expressed in seconds rather than in terms of length of paper traveled.

The P wave consists of electrical activity associated with atrial depolarization, the QRS complex represents ventricular depolarization, and the T wave represents ventricular repolarization. Atrial repolarization occurs during ventricular depolarization and is obscured by the QRS complex. Note that depolarization (an electrical event) is not identical to contraction (a mechanical event). Occasionally, a ventricular depolarization complex occurs that is too weak to initiate ventricular contraction.

Even though the heart is capable of maintaining contractions without outside influences, it is partly controlled by sympathetic nerve fibers, which increase the rate and force of contraction of the heart, and by parasympathetic fibers, such as the vagus nerve, which have the opposite effect. Compounds such as epinephrine that are circulating in the blood stream also influence the rate and force of contraction of the heart. The final result is a composite of several different influences on cardiac function.

Theories of Arrhythmia Formation

Two major theories are used to explain the generation of most cardiac arrhythmias. The *ectopic focus theory* (Fig. 10–16*B*) states that increased automaticity in certain areas of the heart causes one or more small areas to act as pacemakers. If one ectopic focus is active, it may add its influence to that of the SA node and create additional atrial or ventricular contractions. These extra contractions are called *extrasystoles.* If SA node and ectopic influences alternate, the condition is referred to as *bigeminal* (twin) *rhythm* or *coupling.* If multiple ectopic areas form in the ventricles, the heart attempts to respond to all of them plus the SA node and a chaotic pattern results in which the heart quivers like a "bag of worms." This is *fibrillation.* Factors such as myocardial damage, blockage of normal SA node impulses, or the effects of certain drugs increase the tendency for the formation of ectopic foci.

The other major theory of arrhythmia formation states that under certain conditions, an impulse can travel in a circular manner and re-enter the area it left a short time before. This is the *circus* or *re-entry theory* (Fig. 10–16*A*). Under conditions similar to those that facilitate the formation of ectopic foci, an electrical impulse "chases its tail" in a circle, restimulating the same area each time it passes through. The mental picture is one of a traveling salesman or circuit preacher. Circus movement can occur at a rate greater than the rate of SA node firing and can then supersede the control normally held by the SA node. This is the explanation given for the development of *paroxysmal atrial tachycardia,* a common arrhythmia that consists

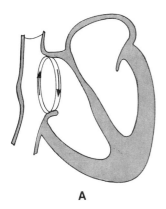 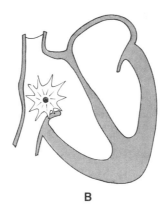

A   B

Figure 10–16. Theories of arrhythmia formation. *(A)* Circus (re-entry) theory. *(B)* Ectopic focus theory.

of attacks (paroxysms) of rapid atrial (and ventricular) rate. Usually, the impulse travels through the AV node and circles back through the atrial tissue to re-enter the node. The cycle is repeated over and over. Conditions that block impulse transmission in one direction favor development of circus activity. Note that the two theories do not compete with each other but may each be used to explain the development of different arrhythmias.

Types of Arrhythmias

Arrhythmias are categorized as to tissue of origin and particular malfunction demonstrated:

1. *Sinus arrhythmias* originate in the SA node and consist of sinus tachycardia (rapid rate) and sinus bradycardia (slow rate).

2. *Atrial arrhythmias* originate in atrial tissue and consist of atrial premature beats, paroxysmal atrial tachycardia, atrial flutter, and atrial fibrillation.

3. *Ventricular arrhythmias* originate in the ventricular tissue, bundle of His, bundle branches, or Purkinje system. As with atrial arrhythmias, ventricular premature beats, paroxysmal ventricular tachycardia, ventricular flutter, and ventricular fibrillation can occur.

Flutter is a very rapid *regular, coordinated* contraction of atria or ventricles (250 to 350 beats per minute); *fibrillation* is a very rapid *irregular, uncoordinated* contraction of atria or ventricles (400 to 600 beats per minute). *Tachycardia* is a rapid, regular contraction of the atria or ventricles like flutter, but the rate is between 100 and 240 beats per minute. At any rate above 200 beats per minute, the atria and ventricles do not have adequate time for refilling between contractions, since a minimal time is needed for the movement of blood into the heart chambers. As a result, cardiac output begins to fall as the rate exceeds 200 beats per minute. At extremely high rates, as in flutter, almost no blood is pumped, since filling time is extremely short. Excessive heart rate also shortens the rest period (which occurs during diastole) and causes fatigue of cardiac muscle, leading to heart failure if not reduced.

Sinus Tachycardia

Conditions that increase the rate of SA node firing cause sinus tachycardia. By definition, the rate is between 100 and 180 beats per minute. The EKG shows a rapid, regular pattern (Fig. 10–17). Fever, shock, exercise, emotional upset, overactive thyroid gland, and the effects of certain drugs are common causes.

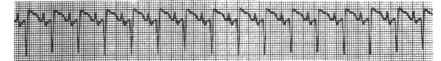

Figure 10–17. Sinus tachycardia. (From Braunwald, E. (ed.): *Heart Disease: A Textbook of Cardiovascular Medicine,* 2nd ed. Philadelphia, W. B. Saunders Company, 1983.)

In fever, the condition is caused by the demands of increased circulation associated with attempts at heat removal. Sinus tachycardia in shock is due to the *carotid sinus reflex,* which triggers sympathetic stimulation of the heart as compensation for low blood pressure. Exercise or emotional upset causes increased release of epinephrine, which increases SA node firing rate. Thyroid overactivity (hyperthyroidism) causes increased production of the thyroid hormones thyroxine and triiodothyronine, which increase SA node activity. Stimulant drugs, including amphetamines, decongestants, and antiasthma preparations (bronchodilators) often increase the rate of SA node discharge.

Treatment. Treatment of sinus tachycardia is directed toward removal of the underlying cause.

Sinus Bradycardia

Sinus bradycardia is caused by increased vagal slowing effect on the heart and is characterized by a rate of less than 50 beats per minute (Fig. 10–18). It can be a normal finding, especially in young people with good cardiac function, and is common in runners who have conditioned the heart to pump more blood per stroke and thus require fewer strokes per minute. In long-distance runners, rates of 40 to 50 beats per minute are common at rest. Sinus bradycardia can also occur if coronary artery disease is present and often is seen after myocardial infarction.

A variation of sinus bradycardia, in which both bradycardia and tachycardia occur, is known as *sick sinus syndrome.* It may be due to abnormal variations in vagal control over the SA node. Bradycardia leads to reduced perfusion of the brain and other vital organs, while tachycardia increases the risk of more serious arrhythmias, such as atrial fibrillation.

Treatment. Treatment is accomplished with atropine, which blocks vagal slowing effects on the SA node, or ephedrine, a drug that increases SA node activity. In severe cases, an artificial pacemaker may be required. Newer *demand pacemakers* operate only when heart rate reaches a pre-set low point, and they become inactive at normal or elevated heart rates. If both sinus bradycardia and tachycardia are present, a pacemaker can be used to treat the bradycardia, while a cardiac depressant drug, such as quinidine (Quinidex), can be used to control the tachycardia.

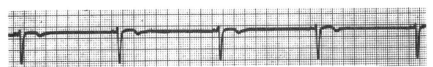

Figure 10–18. Sinus bradycardia. (From Braunwald, E. (ed.): *Heart Disease: A Textbook of Cardiovascular Medicine,* 2nd ed. Philadelphia, W. B. Saunders Company, 1983.)

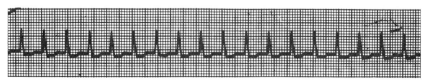

Figure 10–19. Paroxysmal atrial tachycardia. (From Braunwald, E. (ed.): *Heart Disease: A Textbook of Cardiovascular Medicine,* 2nd ed. Philadelphia, W. B. Saunders Company, 1983.)

Atrial Premature Beats

Atrial premature beats occur commonly in normal as well as in diseased hearts and are caused by an ectopic focus operating in atrial tissue. The ventricles respond prematurely to the ectopic impulse conducted through the AV node, and this is followed by an abnormally long pause until the next regular contraction. This is often reported by the patient as a "skipped beat" but is merely a syncopation of the rhythm. Atrial premature beats generally disappear on exercise and are not considered important unless severe heart disease or drug toxicity (e.g., digitalis) is present.

Paroxysmal Atrial Tachycardia

Sudden attacks of tachycardia originating from an atrial circus activity are termed paroxysmal atrial tachycardia (PAT). The rate is 140 to 240 beats per minute, and all impulses pass through the conducting system and initiate ventricular contractions (Fig. 10–19). The rapid ventricular rate is felt by the person, who also frequently complains of tightness in the chest or dyspnea (labored breathing). The problem is only rarely due to organic heart disease and is usually a *functional* disorder. Nervous tension, fatigue, or excessive use of nicotine, alcohol, or caffeine triggers the attacks in susceptible people. Occasionally, medicinal drugs may be the cause, for example, in hypokalemia caused by diuretic administration. The condition can usually be controlled by the elimination of factors that bring on attacks.

Treatment. Treatment of the acute attack involves procedures that increase vagal activity and reduce heart rate or drugs that directly slow the heart. Massaging the carotid sinus areas in the neck, coughing, holding the breath, or vomiting all increase vagal activity. Drug therapy includes the use of quinidine (Quinidex), procainamide (Pronestyl), or propranolol (Inderal) to slow the heart and prevent attacks. Digitalis will partially block the AV node and prevent atrial impulses from reaching the ventricles. This generally does not convert the rapid atrial rate to normal but prevents its action on the ventricles. Tachycardia of only the atria with a controlled normal ventricular rate is asymptomatic and relatively unimportant. Verapamil (Isoptin, Calan) blocks the excitation induced by calcium uptake of cardiac cells and is also an effective treatment. Besides drug therapy, electrical shock to the heart often abolishes the circus activity that perpetuates the arrhythmia.

Atrial Flutter

Atrial flutter is uncommon and is thought to be caused by ectopic foci operating in the atrial tissue. The rate is 250 to 350 beats per minute, and blockage of half of the impulses at the AV node (2:1 block) commonly occurs (Fig. 10–20). The AV node cannot respond at the high rate and every other impulse fails to excite it, resulting in a regular ventricular rate at half the atrial rate.

Figure 10–20. Atrial flutter. Electrocardiogram tracing shows block varying between 2:1 and 4:1. (From Braunwald, E. (ed.): *Heart Disease: A Textbook of Cardiovascular Medicine,* 2nd ed. Philadelphia, W. B. Saunders Company, 1983.)

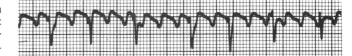

Most patients with atrial flutter have underlying heart disease, especially coronary artery disease or rheumatic heart disease.

Treatment. Several measures are employed for the treatment of atrial flutter. Electrical shock to the heart (using chest paddles) usually abolishes the flutter activity. For control of recurrent attacks of atrial flutter, digitalis is the drug of choice, followed by propranolol (Inderal) or metoprolol (Lopressor).

Atrial Fibrillation

Many factors are associated with atrial fibrillation, the most common chronic arrhythmia. It is seen in heart conditions such as rheumatic heart disease or coronary artery disease or in conjunction with hyperthyroidism, infections, or physical trauma in the absence of heart disease. The cause is ectopic atrial activity, creating an atrial rate of 400 to 600 beats per minute. The AV node cannot respond to impulses entering it at that frequency; partial conduction block thus occurs, resulting in a ventricular rate of 80 to 160 beats per minute (Fig. 10–21). Ventricular rate is irregular, since impulses do not arrive at the AV node at a regular frequency. Some peripheral pulses are strong because the timing is such that complete filling of the ventricles occurs, whereas others are weak or absent, because the ventricles contract before becoming completely filled with blood.

Treatment. Atrial fibrillation occurs on a paroxysmal or chronic basis. Single attacks of atrial fibrillation can be treated by electrical shock to the heart or with digitalis or verapamil (Isoptin, Calan). Chronic, refractory atrial fibrillation is treated similarly with shock, digitalis, verapamil, propranolol (Inderal), or metoprolol (Lopressor). The drugs all act to slow and regulate the ventricular rate. This "protects" the ventricle from chaotic atrial influences and improves the pumping action.

Ventricular Premature Beats

Like atrial premature beats, ventricular premature beats are not dangerous in themselves but may be related to a pathologic state of the heart. They are caused by ectopic activity in the ventricle and result in an early contraction, followed by a *compensatory pause* until time for the next regular beat (Fig. 10–22). The individual often reports this as a "skipped beat," as with atrial premature beats, but again it represents only a syncopation of heart rhythm. In normal individuals, premature ventricular beats are common, are

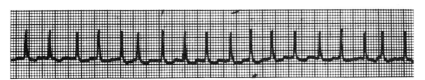

Figure 10–21. Atrial fibrillation. (From Braunwald, E. (ed.): *Heart Disease: A Textbook of Cardiovascular Medicine,* 2nd ed. Philadelphia, W. B. Saunders Company, 1983.)

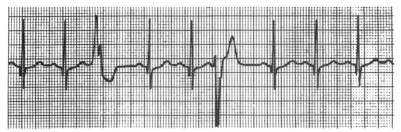

Figure 10–22. Ventricular premature beats. (From Braunwald, E. (ed.): *Heart Disease: A Textbook of Cardiovascular Medicine,* 2nd ed. Philadelphia, W. B. Saunders Company, 1983.)

harmless, and usually disappear with exercise. In people with heart disease, hypokalemia, or digitalis toxicity, they may signify the beginning of a serious arrhythmia.

Treatment. Treatment depends upon the cause. In normal individuals, no treatment is usually given unless the irregularity causes great concern. Digitalis toxicity is treated by reduction in dosage until the rate becomes normal. If hypokalemia is present, potassium compounds (e.g., Kaon) can be given. In the presence of heart disease or occasionally in normal individuals who worry excessively about the irregularity, quinidine (Quinidex), procainamide (Pronestyl), propranolol (Inderal), disopyramide (Norpace), and verapamil (Isoptin, Calan) are drugs of choice.

Paroxysmal Ventricular Tachycardia

Although rare in normal individuals, paroxysmal ventricular tachycardia (PVT) occurs often after myocardial infarction or as a result of digitalis toxicity. The rate is 160 to 240 beats per minute, regular, and maintained by ectopic activity in the ventricle (Fig. 10–23). The presence of PVT is ominous, since it is almost always associated with a serious heart condition, in contrast to PAT, and since it can easily escalate into ventricular fibrillation. Occasionally, it may reoccur on a chronic basis and require intensive treatment.

Treatment. PVT usually responds to electrical shock to the heart, which abolishes the ectopic pacemaker activity. Drugs of choice include lidocaine (Xylocaine), procainamide (Pronestyl), quinidine (Quinidex), and disopyramide (Norpace). Phenytoin (Dilantin) is useful if digitalis toxicity is the cause of the arrhythmia. Some patients with chronic recurrent ventricular tachycardia can be cured by surgical removal of the small area of myocardial tissue that is the ectopic focus, provided that it can be precisely located.

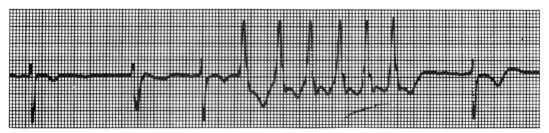

Figure 10–23. Paroxysmal ventricular tachycardia. (From Braunwald, E. (ed.): *Heart Disease: A Textbook of Cardiovascular Medicine,* 2nd ed. Philadelphia, W. B. Saunders Company, 1983.)

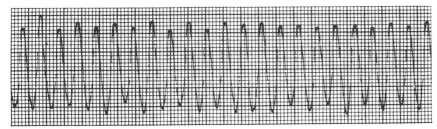

Figure 10–24. Ventricular flutter. (From Braunwald, E. (ed.): *Heart Disease: A Textbook of Cardiovascular Medicine,* 2nd ed. Philadelphia, W. B. Saunders Company, 1983.)

Ventricular Flutter and Fibrillation

These two conditions are considered together, since cardiac pumping action virtually ceases in both cases. Ventricular activity is regular in flutter, but the rate is too rapid and the contractions too small for any effective circulation of blood (Fig. 10–24). In fibrillation, the activity is irregular and, again, no pumping results (Fig. 10–25). Both conditions occur as an escalation of a lower-grade arrhythmia, such as PVT, especially following myocardial infarction or digitalis toxicity. Since there is no circulation of blood, serious brain damage will occur in 5 to 10 minutes.

Treatment. Intravenous drugs are ineffective unless some semblance of a pumping action is restored. Treatment consists of electrical shock to the heart or striking the chest to break up the ectopic ventricular activity, followed by the intravenous administration of lidocaine (Xylocaine) after pumping action is established. Cardiopulmonary resuscitation (CPR) is extremely useful for maintaining the victim until medical treatment can be obtained and has resulted in the saving of many lives.

Heart Block

Heart block generally affects the AV node, bundle of His, or bundle branches. Impulses are slowed or prevented from passing through the blocked area. Heart block occasionally occurs because of an anatomic aberration (e.g., presence of the bundle of Kent, which bypasses impulses around the AV node at the wrong time). However, it is usually due to myocardial damage or the effects of certain drugs, such as propranolol (Inderal) or quinidine (Quinidex), which slow impulse conduction. A common clinical situation is the development of heart block following a myocardial infarction, in which case the infarct area encroaches upon the specialized conducting tissue. Occasionally, this is temporary, if the infarct does not destroy the tissue but merely causes local inflammation in its vicinity. In these cases, temporary pacing of the heart with a removable pacemaker inserted into the ventricle plus the use of anti-

Figure 10–25. Ventricular fibrillation. (From Braunwald, E. (ed.): *Heart Disease: A Textbook of Cardiovascular Medicine,* 2nd ed. Philadelphia, W. B. Saunders Company, 1983.)

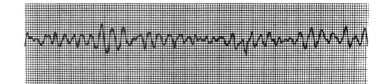

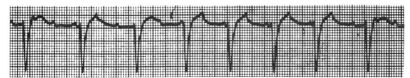

Figure 10–26. First-degree atrioventricular block. (From Braunwald, E. (ed.): *Heart Disease: A Textbook of Cardiovascular Medicine,* 2nd ed. Philadelphia, W. B. Saunders Company, 1983.)

inflammatory drugs may tide the patient over until good conduction is re-established.

There are three basic types of heart block.

First-Degree AV Block. This type consists only of slowing of conduction through the AV node with no skipped ventricular beats. This is shown electrocardiographically by a prolonged PR interval (Fig. 10–27).

Treatment. First-degree block may require no treatment but can be treated with drugs such as ephedrine or isoproterenol (Isuprel) that increase AV conduction.

Second-Degree AV Block. Some impulses do not reach the ventricles in time to initiate ventricular depolarization and ventricular beats are skipped. If ventricular beats are skipped without a prolonged PR interval, the condition is termed *Mobitz Type II* block (Fig. 10–27). If there is a progressive prolongation of the PR interval leading to a skipped ventricular beat, this is called *Mobitz Type I* block (Wenckebach phenomenon) (Fig. 10–28).

Treatment. Second-degree block of both types may respond to the drugs used to treat first-degree block or it may require the installation of a permanent pacemaker in the ventricle. A pacemaker can drive the ventricle at a pre-set rate and supersede the conducting system.

Third-Degree (Complete) AV Block. No impulses reach the ventricle. The ventricle reverts to its inherent rate of 30 to 40 beats per minute (idioventricular rhythm). The EKG shows a normal atrial rate and a slow ventricular rate with complete dissociation of the two events (Fig. 10–29). Often, during the attack, the individual loses consciousness or becomes faint because the heart stops for a few seconds as block occurs before reverting to the idioventricular rhythm. This is called a *Stokes-Adams attack.* Frequently, the slow ventricular rate is not adequate for normal activities and the individual is alive but bedridden.

Treatment. Drugs are usually ineffective in improving conduction, and a pacemaker is required. This can be of the demand type, which engages only when the heart rate drops below the pre-set level.

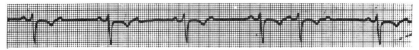

Figure 10–27. Mobitz type II block (second-degree atrioventricular block). (From Braunwald, E. (ed.): *Heart Disease: A Textbook of Cardiovascular Medicine,* 2nd ed. Philadelphia, W. B. Saunders Company, 1983.)

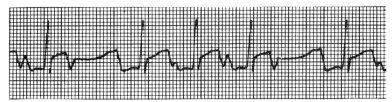

Figure 10–28. Mobitz type I block (second-degree atrioventricular block). (From Braunwald, E. (ed.): *Heart Disease: A Textbook of Cardiovascular Medicine,* 2nd ed. Philadelphia, W. B. Saunders Company, 1983.)

SUMMARY

In most developed countries of the world, cardiovascular disorders represent the most frequent cause of death. The same technology that improves the quality of life for us also demands less of us physically and promotes cardiovascular disease through a less healthful diet and the stresses associated with a "civilized" existence. Cardiovascular disorders are often interrelated and multiple disorders or cardiovascular complications are common in the same person. They should be studied, therefore, with the idea of cause and effect in mind.

Several disease processes are represented in the spectrum of cardiovascular disorders, including inflammation, infarction, atherosclerosis, thrombosis, embolism, myocardial degeneration, abnormal sympathetic blood vessel control, and electrical disturbances of cardiac tissue. Thus, the disorders are interesting from a pathophysiologic as well as symptomatic standpoint.

Treatments often involve removal of the cause of the disorder, but since it is not always possible to accomplish that, they may consist of measures to control the disorder or its major signs and symptoms. Prevention, although not as well-defined as treatment in most cases, is certainly as important. Advances in prevention of cardiovascular disease probably represent the major goal of future research.

Questions
1. Explain why atherosclerotic deposits are usually larger at bends or junctions of arteries. Why do you think that certain arteries, such as the coronary arteries, are affected more than most other arteries in the body?
2. Explain why digitalis would not be effective in "dropsy" caused by liver or kidney disease rather than congestive heart failure.
3. What is the difference between congestive heart failure and "high output" failure? Is digitalis equally effective for both?
4. Do you think that essential hypertension really has no cause? What are some possible causes for it that could not be detected with our existing technology?

Figure 10–29. Third-degree atrioventricular block.

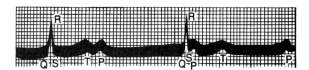

5. If you had to have an arrhythmia, which one of each pair would you pick? Give the reasons for your choice in each case.
   a. Sinus tachycardia or sinus bradycardia.
   b. Paroxysmal atrial tachycardia (PAT) or paroxysmal ventricular tachycardia (PVT).
   c. Ventricular fibrillation or atrial fibrillation.

Additional Reading　　Bergman, H. D.: Congestive heart failure and its treatment. Southern Pharmacy Journal, 69:22, 1977. (*Good overview of congestive heart failure.*)

Bergman, H. D.: Hypertension and its treatment. Southern Pharmacy Journal, 73:22, 1981.

Colby, A. O.: What does smoking really do to the heart? Modern Medicine, 45:53, 1977.

Ferguson, G. G.: New developments in the treatment of coronary heart disease. Southern Pharmacy Journal, 73:37, 1981. (*Newer approaches to the treatment of coronary artery disease.*)

Gessner, F. B.: Hemodynamic theories of atherogenesis. Circ. Res., 33:259, 1973. (*Interesting theories concerning plaque formation.*)

Henahan, J.: Regression of atherosclerosis: Preliminary but encouraging news. J.A.M.A., 246:2309, 1981.

CHAPTER 11

RENAL DISORDERS

Three major tasks are performed by the normal kidney:

1. *Maintenance of water balance.* In this way, the body can adjust to variations in intake of water along with changing environmental conditions. Water balance is largely controlled by the action of antidiuretic hormone (ADH, vasopressin) on the collecting duct, triggered by osmoreceptors located in the hypothalamus (see Chapter 7).

2. *Maintenance of acid-base balance.* The kidney can alter urine pH and affect the systemic pH by varying the amount of hydrogen ion secreted and sodium ion reabsorbed, largely through the action of carbonic anhydrase. In addition, the kidney provides for excretion of water formed from the breakdown of carbonic acid and thus aids in the operation of the carbonic acid–bicarbonate buffer system (see Chapter 8).

3. *Removal of waste materials.* In this capacity, the kidney functions like a highly sophisticated filter, holding back larger molecules and particles and allowing smaller molecules to pass into the urine. The body produces a constant stream of chemical compounds as a result of metabolic activity, including acids and bases, water, urea, creatinine, and drug metabolites. The kidney filters these into the urine and prevents their accumulation in the blood stream (Fig. 11–1).

The functional unit of the kidney is the *nephron* (Fig. 11–2), which consists of the *glomerulus,* the *proximal convoluted tubule,* the *loop of Henle,* the *distal convoluted tubule,* and the *collecting duct.* There are approximately one million nephrons in each normal kidney.

Glomerulus. The glomerulus is a twisted mass of capillaries that is an extension of the renal arteriole. It provides a large capillary surface area for filtration. A key component of the glomerulus is the *basement membrane,* which serves as the "filter paper" of the kidney. Alteration of the basement membrane by inflammation or other disease processes drastically changes the nature of the filtrate and the type and quantity of material retained in the blood stream.

Proximal Convoluted Tubule. This structure begins with Bowman's capsule, which collects the filtrate that has passed through the basement membrane. Throughout the length of the tubule, water and electrolytes—such as sodium, potassium, hydrogen, and chloride ions—are moved into or out of the tubule across the tubular membrane. Osmosis is the prime mover here, but active transport is also employed for movement of electrolytes, such as sodium ion. Surrounding the tubule is a capillary network that picks up any molecules that move across the tubular membrane and leave the tubule.

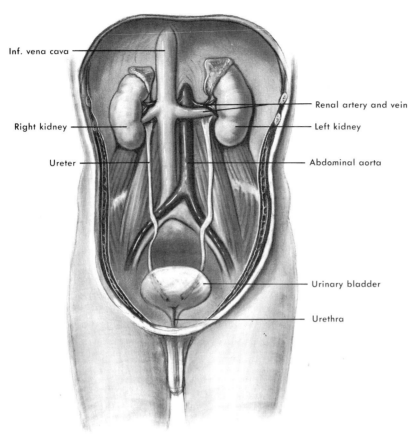

Inf. vena cava

Right kidney

Ureter

Renal artery and vein

Left kidney

Abdominal aorta

Urinary bladder

Urethra

Figure 11–1. The urinary system. (From Dienhart, C. M.: *Basic Human Anatomy and Physiology,* 3rd ed. Philadelphia, W. B. Saunders Company, 1979.)

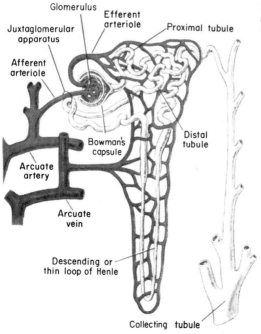

Glomerulus

Efferent arteriole

Juxtaglomerular apparatus

Proximal tubule

Afferent arteriole

Distal tubule

Bowman's capsule

Arcuate artery

Arcuate vein

Descending or thin loop of Henle

Collecting tubule

Figure 11–2. The nephron. (From Guyton, A. C.: *Textbook of Medical Physiology,* 6th ed. Philadelphia, W. B. Saunders Company, 1981.)

Loop of Henle. This is an extension of the proximal convoluted tubule that dips from the cortex (outer portion) deep into the medulla (inner portion) of the kidney. Its action is similar to that of the proximal convoluted tubule, except that the membrane is impermeable to water in the ascending limb but freely permeable to water in the descending limb. The osmotic effect caused by sodium leaving the ascending limb and remaining temporarily in the space between the two limbs (interstitial space) results in water being pulled through the membrane of the descending limb. The net result of this action is to decrease the water content within the loop of Henle and therefore to increase the concentration of dissolved materials in the fluid within the loop of Henle. More water is reabsorbed by the body, and the urine eventually formed is more concentrated. This phenomenon is called the *countercurrent multiplier effect* and allows the relatively small kidney of a human being to do a job that would require a much larger organ in the absence of this capacity.

Distal Convoluted Tubule. This structure is a further extension of the loop of Henle. Here aldosterone acts to regulate sodium reabsorption and potassium secretion. Carbonic anhydrase, formed in the distal tubular cells, regulates the formation of hydrogen ion, which exchanges for sodium ion in the distal convoluted tubule. Thus, the distal tubule is important from the standpoint of electrolyte and acid-base balance.

Collecting Duct. The final link in the nephron chain, the collecting duct (tubule) is the site of action of ADH. Antidiuretic hormone increases the pore size in the duct membrane and allows water to leak out, thus promoting water reabsorption via the surrounding capillary network.

The kidney utilizes a complex mixture of *filtration* (passage through the basement membrane), *reabsorption* (movement *out of* the tubular system into the capillary network), and *secretion* (movement *into* the tubular lumen from the capillary network via the tubular cells). Generally, molecules are filtered and then partially reabsorbed, often in conjunction with secretion at another point in the tubular system. The final disposition, therefore, depends upon the relative degree to which these processes operate. The time required for a compound to drop to one half of its original blood level is called the *half-life* and depends upon many factors, including the three listed.

Some molecules are not filtered to any extent, since they are too large to pass through the basement membrane. Albumins and globulins, large proteins found in the blood stream, generally do not pass at all or pass only in trace amounts. The same is true for red blood cells. The finding of significant amounts of proteins and red blood cells in the urine, therefore, signifies damage to the basement membrane and is an important diagnostic indicator of kidney disease. Likewise, the failure to remove compounds normally filtered by the glomeruli and/or secreted by the tubular system also signifies kidney disease.

Two common tests for reduced kidney filtering ability are *blood urea nitrogen* (BUN) (normal = 8 to 20 mg/dl), and *serum creatinine level* (normal = 0.7 to 1.5 mg/dl); BUN measures the concentration of nitrogen as urea in blood, formed largely through protein metabolism. Creatinine is primarily a by-product of muscle metabolism. Values for both tests are elevated if reduced filtration is present. *Creatinine clearance* is the amount of blood theoretically "cleared" of creatinine in one minute by filtration (normal = 90 to 130 ml/min). In reality, the kidney does not completely clear one segment of blood but removes some creatinine from all blood it receives via the circulation. Thus, the concept of clearance is a theoretical one, but it is useful because it allows for mathematical expression of kidney function. Creatinine clearance decreases if renal filtration is impaired, since less blood is cleared (theoretically) of creatinine by the kidney.

Urinary tract disease causes about 35,000 deaths per year in the United States, a small number when compared with the number of deaths due to heart disease or cancer. However, urinary tract disease is a significant cause of morbidity (nonfatal disease). Approximately 20 per cent of American women suffer from urinary tract infection at least once during their lives, and 1 per cent of the American population develop renal stones during their lives. Chronic renal disorders cause great suffering, disability, and expense to those afflicted. This chapter considers some of the more common renal disorders. Urinary tract infection (UTI) was covered in Chapter 9 but is mentioned again in relation to certain renal disorders.

GLOMERULO-NEPHRITIS

Inflammation of the glomeruli—glomerulonephritis—is a common clinical finding. Most significantly affected is the basement membrane, resulting in alterations in filtration of blood to form tubular fluid. In common forms of glomerulonephritis, an immune process seems responsible for the inflammation of and damage to the basement membrane.

Pathogenesis

The immune process that characterizes most forms of glomerulonephritis is of two types. In the most common type (*immune complex disease*), antigen-antibody complexes (immune complexes) are trapped by the glomeruli as they circulate in the blood stream. These are not directed at the kidney but are formed in response to bacterial or viral infection (or possibly autoimmune reaction). These damage the kidney as they are retained by the glomeruli, in a manner similar to that of immune complexes depositing on the heart valves in rheumatic fever. The term "innocent bystander" is often used to describe the kidney's role in the process. In the most common situation, the individual first has a streptococcal infection of the throat, followed by the formation of antibodies to the streptococcal antigen (poststreptococcal glomerulonephritis). Immune complexes form and damage the glomeruli, as described. Occasionally, infection with staphylococci or other bacteria represents the initial event in the development of glomerulonephritis. Often, bacterial infection cannot be documented through culture or symptom history and viral infection or autoimmune reaction is assumed.

In the second type of glomerulonephritis in which an immune reaction is seen, antibodies are formed against an infectious agent (usually a virus) that has the same antigenic properties as the basement membrane tissue. Thus, the antibodies attack not only the causative virus but also the basement membrane (*antiglomerular basement membrane disease*). The most common form of this is called *Goodpasture's syndrome* and is characterized by a viral respiratory infection resembling viral pneumonia, followed by the development of glomerulonephritis.

Sometimes glomerulonephritis is associated with a much more widespread disease and represents only a part of the total picture. In systemic lupus erythematosus, a generalized inflammatory disorder (see Chapter 17), glomerulonephritis often develops in conjunction with systemic inflammatory changes in the skin and connective tissue. A variety of antibodies against DNA, erythrocytes, and leukocytes are formed in this condition and it is thought that immune complexes formed from these deposit in the glomeruli. Again, the kidney is an innocent bystander to immune complexes formed elsewhere in the body (immune complex disease).

Acute Poststreptococcal Glomerulonephritis

The most common infection antecedent to glomerulonephritis in adults and children over 6 years of age is streptococcal pharyngitis ("strep" throat), caused by infection with group A beta-hemolytic streptococci. In children under 6, impetigo (a local skin infection), often caused by the same organism, is the most common cause. Antibody formation occurs 1 to 4 weeks after exposure, and the immune complexes formed are deposited in the glomeruli. The antigen in this case is streptolysin O and the antibody formed is antistreptolysin O (ASO). The level of antibody found in the blood stream is called the *ASO titer* and is an important diagnostic indicator of streptococcal immune disease. (See Chapter 10 regarding rheumatic fever.)

Symptoms and Signs

Usually, symptoms of the antecedent infection have subsided by the time glomerulonephritis develops. Common findings in glomerulonephritis include headache, fatigue, weakness, and fever (presumably related to tissue damage and pyrogen release). Flank pain and puffiness around the face (facial edema) are indications that kidney inflammation is present. In mild cases, often no symptoms are present. Oliguria (scanty urine) and hematuria (blood in the urine) are common signs of kidney inflammation. Hypertension develops in severe glomerulonephritis as a result of release of renin by the damaged kidney (see Chapter 10).

Laboratory Findings

Hematuria, usually reported as bloody, brown, or coffee-colored urine, is a common finding and results from failure of the damaged basement membrane to retain erythrocytes in the blood stream. Various test strips are available for determining the presence and quantity of blood in the urine (e.g., Hemastix).

Proteinuria results from glomerular leakage primarily of albumin (a slightly smaller molecule than globulin). Proteinuria is commonly designated as 1+ (0.5 to 1 gm/liter), 2+ (1 to 5 gm/liter), 3+ (5 to 10 gm/liter) and 4+ (10 or more gm/liter).

Urine *specific gravity* is usually increased, since the volume is reduced. *Erythrocyte sedimentation rate* (ESR) is elevated in proportion to the amount of inflammation present. *ASO titer* is increased relative to the quantity of streptococcal antigen present.

Various types of *casts* are found in the urine. These are formed around small renal structures, much as a cast is shaped to fit a broken arm, and are composed of an assortment of materials, including protein, wax, or deteriorated cells.

If severe renal damage is present, BUN and serum creatinine levels are elevated and the creatinine clearance is decreased.

Diagnosis

Diagnosis of glomerulonephritis is based upon the preceding findings, plus a history of suspected or confirmed streptococcal infection several weeks previously. The condition should be differentiated from *pyelonephritis* (caused by direct infection of the kidney) and conditions in which it is only part of a systemic disease (e.g., systemic lupus erythematosus). Specific diagnostic tests for lupus erythematosus are available (see Chapter 17), and pyelonephritis can usually be detected by the finding of large numbers of bacteria in the urine along with pus.

In difficult cases, diagnosis can be facilitated through the use of a *renal biopsy,* in which a "core sample" is removed from the kidney through the skin with a long needle. Renal biopsy is especially helpful in separating the many subtypes of glomerulonephritis.

Treatment

Penicillin is the drug of choice for existing streptococcal infection and should be given in full doses for 10 to 14 days. Usually, however, the primary infection has resolved by the time glomerulonephritis develops and the problem has become an immune one. Antibiotics may be ineffective at this point but should be tried anyway. The problem is similar to that of rheumatic fever.

Anti-inflammatory drugs, such as corticosteroids, are ineffective in relieving the glomerular inflammation and merely add to the sodium and fluid retention already present. If renal damage has caused secondary hypertension, sodium and fluid retention will further aggravate it.

Antihypertensive drugs and diuretics are helpful in these cases. Analgesic drugs, such as propoxyphene (Darvon) or codeine may be needed for kidney pain. Supportive measures include bed rest, restricted fluid intake if oliguria is present, and sodium restriction if severe edema develops. Dietary protein intake should be restricted if BUN is elevated and encouraged if BUN is normal to prevent depletion of blood proteins.

Complications

Hypertension and its attendant risks constitutes the biggest danger in glomerulonephritis. Antihypertensive drugs and diuretics help to normalize blood pressure. Hypertensive crisis can be treated with intravenous vasodilators, such as sodium nitroprusside (Nipride) or diazoxide (Hyperstat), to greatly reduce the risk of stroke, renal failure, or congestive heart failure. Edema caused by reduced renal function causes overloading of the heart, leading to congestive heart failure. This improves with the use of diuretics, such as hydrochlorothiazide (Hydrodiuril), that mobilize edema fluid. Infection, especially with streptococci, can reactivate quiescent glomerulonephritis. Long-term prophylactic drug therapy is not recommended, but prompt treatment of infections with antibiotics may prevent reactivation.

Prognosis   Approximately 90 per cent of individuals with acute poststreptococcal glomerulonephritis recover completely. The remainder develop *latent* or *chronic* disease, which causes progressive renal damage and complications. Many of these eventually develop chronic renal failure.

Chronic Glomerulonephritis   Long-term glomerulonephritis may be asymptomatic for an extended period of time. The person continues to excrete protein and erythrocytes in the urine, usually accompanied by casts, with a progressive worsening of the condition.

Treatment   Infections should be promptly eradicated with antibiotics and vaccinations should be avoided, since they result in the formation of additional immune complexes. Acute flare-ups are treated as acute attacks and dietary intake of water, sodium, and protein must be adjusted according to existing conditions.

Complications   Many people with chronic glomerulonephritis live 20 to 30 years but usually develop nephrotic syndrome, which progresses to chronic renal failure and is often associated with renal hypertension (Fig. 11–3). Renal dialysis and/or kidney transplant then become the only treatment alternatives.

PYELONEPHRITIS   Pyelonephritis is an inflammatory disease of the kidney pelvis (pyelo = pelvis) and parenchymal area that is usually caused by bacterial infection. Infectious pyelonephritis is referred to as an *upper tract* infection, as opposed to *lower tract* infection involving

Figure 11–3. Chronic glomerulonephritis. The glomeruli are infiltrated with hyaline material, eventually leading to renal failure. (From Robbins, S. L., and Cotran, R. S.: *Pathologic Basis of Disease,* 2nd ed. Philadelphia, W. B. Saunders Company, 1979.)

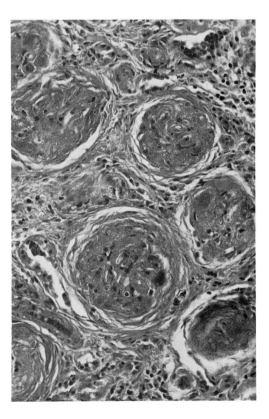

the bladder or urethra. (See the discussion of UTI in Chapter 9.) Infection usually results from ascending spread, whereby organisms introduced into the bladder migrate up the ureter to the kidney. Occasionally, hematogenous spread is the cause (see Chapter 9).

In contrast to glomerulonephritis, the causative organism in pyelonephritis is usually a gram-negative rod (coliform) rather than a gram-positive coccus. In pyelonephritis, inflammation is caused by the presence of large numbers of bacteria, not by the effect of immune complexes on the kidney. In other words, the kidney is not an innocent bystander but is the focus of infection. Severity of infection depends upon the type and number of organisms present. In addition, the glomeruli (which are located primarily in the renal cortex rather than in the pelvis) are relatively unaffected and the tubules are the major victims of the infection.

Pathogenesis   The most common infecting organism in pyelonephritis is *Escherichia coli,* which exists in many strains. Other common coliform pathogens are Proteus, Enterobacter, Klebsiella, and Pseudomonas. Infection occurs because of ascending spread from the bladder or, occasionally, hematogenous spread.

Acute   Symptoms and signs in acute pyelonephritis may be minimal,
Pyelonephritis   but they usually consist of fever, chills, backache, and/or abdominal pain (kidney pain is interpreted both ways). Nausea and vomiting are common, presumably from toxic effects of the infection. Pus entering the bladder from the kidney via the ureter irritates the bladder wall, causing urinary frequency and urgency. In severe infections, urine output may be reduced. The urine is generally dark-colored because of reduced volume and the presence of pus.

Laboratory Findings   Significant bacteriuria (see Chapter 9), pyuria, proteinuria, and, occasionally, hematuria are findings upon urinalysis. Hematuria and proteinuria may be caused in part by glomerular membrane leakage but are probably mostly due to damage to renal tissue by the infection. Culture of the urine usually reveals a coliform (especially *E. coli*) as the causative agent. Occasionally, more than one pathogen is identified. Leukocytosis is present, since active bacterial infection exists (Fig. 11–4).

Most individuals with acute pyelonephritis have normal urinary tracts, but anatomic or functional defects in the urethra, bladder, ureter or kidney can promote urine retention and infection. An intravenous pyelogram (IVP) will identify stones, constrictions, or other abnormalities causing urinary obstruction. Generally, an IVP is done if there is recurrent or chronic kidney infection.

Diagnosis   The presence of gram-negative bacteria, pus, and erythrocytes in the urine, along with symptoms referable to the kidney strongly supports a diagnosis of acute pyelonephritis. Glomerulonephritis causes increased ASO titer (usually) and bacteria are in minimal numbers or absent from the urine. A history of "strep" throat is often obtained in glomerulonephritis, whereas prior instrumentation or infection of the lower tract is common in acute pyelonephritis.

The pain from ureteral stone is intense and not usually confused

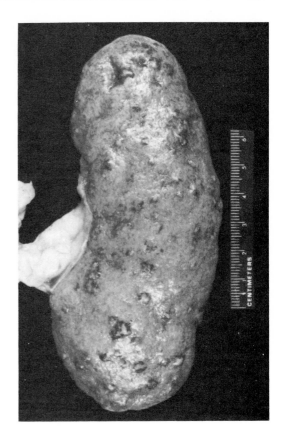

Figure 11–4. Acute pyelonephritis. Kidney shows multiple areas of infection. (From Robbins, S. L., and Cotran, R. S.: *Pathologic Basis of Disease,* 2nd ed. Philadelphia, W. B. Saunders Company, 1979.)

with that from acute pyelonephritis, although stones within the kidney could produce a similar kind of pain. Infection in the latter case would be secondary, as a result of renal obstruction.

Treatment The treatment of acute pyelonephritis (outlined in Chapter 9) consists of drug therapy in conjunction with measures designed to prevent infection. The drugs of choice are co-trimoxazole (Bactrim, Septra), sulfisoxazole (Gantrisin), and nitrofurantoin (Macrodantin). Cinoxacin (Cinobac), tetracycline (Achromycin), and ampicillin (Polycillin) are also generally effective.

Duration of treatment is 10 to 14 days. If recurrence develops, culture of the urine is required to establish organism identity and to select the appropriate anti-infective agent. Further recurrence requires the use of longer treatment periods and careful examination for any anatomic or functional defects in the urinary tract.

Additional fluid intake aids in flushing bacteria from the kidney but will dilute anti-infective drugs if fluid intake is excessive.

Chronic Chronic pyelonephritis occurs as a complication of acute pye-
Pyelonephritis lonephritis that is resistant to drug therapy or that is facilitated by the presence of factors that prevent complete resolution (e.g., reinfection and anatomic or functional defects). Long-term infection often results in scarring and atrophy of the affected kidney tissue, associated with reduced renal function (Fig. 11–5). However, many individuals live a long time with chronic pyelonephritis with minimal symptomatology and little or no residual kidney damage. If symp-

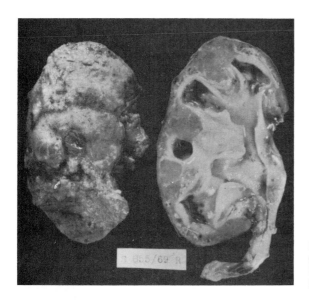

Figure 11–5. Chronic pyelonephritis. Extensive kidney damage is present. (From Robbins, S. L., and Cotran, R. S.: *Pathologic Basis of Disease,* 2nd ed. Philadelphia, W. B. Saunders Company, 1979.)

toms do exist, they resemble those of acute pyelonephritis but are generally less pronounced.

Laboratory Findings   The major laboratory finding is significant bacteriuria that perists or recurs after treatment. The BUN and serum creatinine levels become elevated as renal damage increases. Creatinine clearance is reduced in proportion to decreased excretory ability of the kidneys. As further renal damage develops, the urine becomes more dilute, because concentrating mechanisms are impaired.

Treatment   Full-dose treatment with an appropriate anti-infective agent (determined by culture and sensitivity tests) for 4 weeks will often eradicate chronic pyelonephritis. If this fails, long-term suppressive treatment is indicated (see Chapter 9). Drugs of choice are nitrofurantoin (Macrodantin) and methenamine derivatives (Mandelamine, Hiprex). Cinoxacin (Cinobac), a newer drug, is also effective in most cases. Careful attention to contributing anatomic or functional disorders and their surgical correction, along with drug therapy, may result in complete cure. Good personal hygiene and avoidance of instrumentation or catheterization of the urinary tract is important in complete recovery from infection.

Complications   Progressive renal damage leading to renal failure occurs frequently in chronic pyelonephritis that continues uncontrolled for long periods of time. Hypertension, resulting from release of renin by the damaged kidney, is another common long-term complication. Although these conditions can be partly controlled through drug therapy, elimination of chronic pyelonephritis and prevention of these complications are much preferred when possible.

NEPHROTIC SYNDROME (NEPHROSIS)   The consequence of a variety of glomerular lesions is the nephrotic syndrome. As the name implies, more than one causative factor is present and the condition is not a true disease but a symptom complex. The key features of nephrotic syndrome are proteinuria, edema, hypoalbuminemia, and hyperlipidemia.

In the majority of cases of nephrotic syndrome, the condition results from long-standing glomerulonephritis. In 20 to 30 per cent of adults and 80 per cent of children with nephrotic syndrome, the underlying cause is *lipoid nephrosis,* a type of glomerulonephritis in which minimal damage occurs to the glomeruli.

Other forms of glomerulonephritis (generally more severe) are also important causes of nephrotic syndrome. Less common causes include diabetes mellitus, systemic lupus erythematosus, or exposure to certain drugs (gold salts, trimethadione). It should be noted that immune complexes are not found in the basement membrane in nephrotic syndrome, whereas they are in glomerulonephritis.

Pathogenesis   Damage to the basement membrane or associated structures as a result of one of the underlying conditions previously discussed causes leakage of protein into the urine in large amounts. Albumin is lost in larger amounts than globulin because it is a smaller molecule and leaks out more easily. The preferential leakage of plasma albumin over plasma globulin causes a change in the proportion of albumin to globulin in the plasma (A to G ratio). This is normally 1.5:1 to 2.5:1 but drops to less than 1:1 in severe nephrotic syndrome. Loss of plasma albumin causes reduced osmotic pressure of the serum and allows water to leave the capillaries more easily. Normally, the blood pressure tends to squeeze water through the capillary walls (hydrostatic pressure), but this is opposed by the osmotic effect of proteins and other materials within the capillaries (serum oncotic pressure). Depletion of plasma albumin (hypoalbuminemia) results in an unbalancing of these two opposing forces, and water is forced through the capillary walls by the then stronger hydrostatic pressure (Fig. 11–6). Accumulation of water in the interstitial spaces results, causing generalized edema (anasarca). The liver responds to hypoalbuminemia by attempting to synthesize larger amounts of albumin but apparently also synthesizes lipoproteins in large amounts (primarily pre-beta and beta lipoproteins). This leads to *hyperlipidemia.*

Lipiduria results as some of the excess lipid is excreted in the urine. Often, lipid deposits on tubular epithelial cells, which are then shed and excreted in the urine. These cells are called *oval fat*

Figure 11–6. Edema development in nephrotic syndrome.

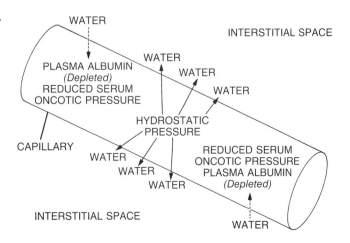

bodies and are characteristic of nephrotic syndrome. The high serum lipid levels (especially cholesterol) increase the risk of coronary atherosclerosis in long-standing nephrotic syndrome.

Symptoms and Signs   Edema, associated with fluid accumulation in the chest (hydrothorax) and in the abdominal cavity (ascites), is the most common symptom of nephrotic syndrome. Often, tissue stretching due to edema causes the formation of *striae* (stretch marks), similar to those seen during pregnancy. Since erythrocytes may be lost in addition to protein by the damaged glomerular membranes, anemia often develops and causes a pale appearance to the skin (pallor). Hypertension, along with hypertensive retinopathy, is seen in some cases.

Laboratory Findings   Massive proteinuria (2+ to 4+) is common, consisting mostly of albuminuria. Hypoalbuminemia (normal = 3.5 to 5.5 gm/dl) results from the tremendous loss of albumin in the urine. Hyperlipidemia is present and the cholesterol level is usually above 300 mg/ dl. The urine contains free fat, oval fat bodies, and fatty casts, along with a significant number of erythrocytes. If glomerular damage is extensive enough so that large quantities of globulins are lost, *hypoglobulinemia* develops. This may increase the risk of infection, since globulins are needed for normal resistance to infection. Renal biopsy will help to differentiate nephrotic syndrome from other renal conditions and will aid in monitoring progress toward recovery or advancing pathologic changes.

Diagnosis   The findings of edema, massive proteinuria, hypoalbuminemia, and hyperlipidemia are characteristic of nephrotic syndrome, but these can occur to some extent in other conditions. Acute poststreptococcal glomerulonephritis can usually be differentiated from nephrotic syndrome by the history of recent infection, elevated ASO titer, and the absence of hyperlipidemia. Pyelonephritis generally causes bacteriuria and pyuria as well as proteinuria and hematuria. Renal biopsy is especially helpful in differentiating among the several renal conditions that may produce overlapping symptoms.

Treatment   No effective treatment exists for nephrotic syndrome. Many individuals, especially children with lipoid nephrosis, recover spontaneously. Corticosteroids (e.g., prednisone) given for several months may be helpful in lipoid nephrosis, but they are less effective in other forms of the condition. Corticosteroids are often given on an *alternate-day* basis (twice the daily dose every other day) to reduce the severity of side effects. The beneficial effect seems as good as with daily therapy. Diuretics, such as hydrochlorothiazide (Hydrodiuril), may be useful to reduce edema.

A high-protein diet is recommended to replace protein lost in the urine unless the BUN is elevated. In that case, a normal or low-protein diet is necessary.

Recent evidence indicates that immunosuppressive drugs, such as azathioprine (Imuran), plus corticosteroids may be effective in severe forms of nephrotic syndrome.

Prognosis   Approximately half of the children with lipoid nephrosis recover without serious consequences. Adults (who less commonly have lipoid nephrosis) have more frequent and severe consequences. If recovery does not occur, a downhill course, with increasing BUN, hypertension, and eventual renal failure, is likely.

RENAL FAILURE   Inability of the kidney to perform its usual tasks of maintaining water, electrolyte, and acid-base balance and of removing waste materials is termed renal failure. It can occur on a short-term basis (acute) or a long-term basis (chronic). Sometimes the term *chronic renal insufficiency* is applied, since the kidney in chronic failure is impaired in function but may not yet have failed completely. *End-stage kidney* refers to a kidney in the throes of complete failure.

The consequences of renal failure are varied and often severe because of the central position of the kidney regarding acid-base balance, water and electrolyte concentrations, and waste removal. In addition, the kidney is indirectly involved in calcium metabolism and erythrocyte production and these parameters are adversely affected by renal failure.

Accumulation of nitrogenous wastes in the blood stream is called *azotemia*, reflected in an increased BUN and serum creatinine level and in a decreased creatinine clearance. The whole picture of azotemia with cardiovascular, neurologic, gastrointestinal, and metabolic disturbances, along with their characteristic types of symptoms, is called *uremia*, and usually represents end-stage renal failure.

Acute Renal Failure   Acute renal failure is a sudden, short-term, often reversible form of renal failure most commonly caused by *acute renal tubular necrosis*, a condition in which the renal tubular cells die and are sloughed off and replaced in 1 to 4 weeks with new cells. *Reduced renal circulation*, as often occurs in shock, is a common cause of acute renal tubular necrosis. *Drugs*, such as gentamicin (Garamycin) and amphotericin B (Fungizone), or *poisons*, such as mercury or arsenic compounds, carbon tetrachloride, or ethylene glycol (found in antifreeze), can also damage the renal tubule and cause acute renal failure. A few *infections*, notably yellow fever, also cause acute renal tubular necrosis, resulting in acute renal failure.

Pathogenesis   As the tubular cells die, debris (dead cells, protein, casts) accumulate in the tubular lumen and cause obstruction. This leads to reduced urine output (oliguria) and to accumulation of materials in the blood stream (especially potassium and nitrogenous compounds). The first phase of acute renal failure is thus termed the *oliguric phase*. Later, as the tubular epithelium regenerates and debris is cleared from the tubules, urine volume dramatically increases. The new tubular cells formed to replace the damaged ones cannot reabsorb water effectively at first and diuresis results. This is called the *diuretic phase*.

Symptoms and Signs   In addition to reduced urine volume, the chief symptoms are loss of appetite, nausea, and lethargy. Later, if improvement in renal function does not occur, symptoms of chronic renal failure may develop. These include, in addition, vomiting and headache.

Laboratory Findings   Urinalysis reveals the presence of brown granular casts, erythrocytes, protein, and tubular epithelial cells. Specific gravity is usually 1.015 or less, with a volume of 200 ml/day or less. As more time elapses, BUN and creatinine levels increase, as do serum potassium, phosphate, and sulfate ion levels. When the diuretic phase begins, urine volume increases to 1 liter/day and above. However, BUN and creatinine levels may remain high until nearly complete restoration of renal function occurs.

Diagnosis   Acute renal failure usually occurs immediately after some event that causes acute renal tubular necrosis. A history of surgery, blood loss, shock, infection, or the exposure to certain drugs or poisons aids greatly in diagnosis. Urinary obstruction and bladder rupture are easily confused with acute renal failure, but the conditions can be corrected surgically. Acute glomerulonephritis can sometimes develop suddenly enough to cause symptoms similar to those of acute renal failure.

Treatment   If shock is the cause, blood pressure should be restored to a normal level and maintained to prevent further tubular cell damage. Any suspected toxic agents should be immediately discontinued. The patient should be monitored carefully for elevation in BUN, serum creatinine level, and potassium level. Water intake should be restricted during the oliguric phase to prevent overhydration, edema, and overloading of the cardiovascular system (about 400 ml/day is the recommended intake). A diet containing no protein is recommended during the oliguric phase to prevent elevation of BUN and other compounds derived from protein sources. Dialysis (via kidney machine or using fluid injected into and removed from the peritoneal cavity) is often necessary during the oliguric phase. Treatment during the diuretic phase consists of protein restriction until BUN levels return to normal and close observation for signs of sodium and chloride ion retention (hyperreflexia, confusion).

Prognosis   Prognosis is good with good supportive care, since regeneration of tubular cells is usually possible. Overhydration and potassium or (later) sodium intoxication are common causes of complications.

Chronic Renal Failure   Chronic renal failure develops slowly with progressive worsening of function over months or years. It usually results from long-standing *inflammation* of the kidney (especially glomerulonephritis), *infection* (especially chronic pyelonephritis), *diabetes mellitus,* or *hypertension.* In the latter two cases, renal vascular damage, occurring as a complication to the underlying disease, is the cause of renal failure. Occasionally, drug ingestion (especially phenacetin) and gout (gouty nephropathy) are causes. As mentioned, chronic renal failure is a complex disorder, since so many physiologic parameters are disturbed, and treatment therefore must be multifaceted.

Pathogenesis   A wide variety of renal lesions are seen in chronic renal failure, depending upon the cause. In general, scarring, reduced size and weight, and loss of tubules occur in the affected kidney. Blood vessels are thickened or obstructed and the glomeruli are infiltrated with hyaline material (clear connective tissue). Often, there is a mixture of pathologic changes in the kidney that makes exact assignment of cause impossible. For example, hypertension can *cause* chronic renal failure or it can *result* from it. Again, the "chicken or egg" dilemma exists.

Symptoms and Signs   Fatigue, malaise, headache, nausea, vomiting, and loss of appetite are common symptoms of chronic renal failure. The urine volume is increased (polyuria), resulting in dehydration and itching. Blood pressure is often elevated, probably because of release of renin by the damaged kidney (see Chapter 10). Pallor, primarily due to anemia, is also present. Physical examination shows hypertensive or diabetic retinopathy, if these conditions are involved in chronic renal failure.

Laboratory Findings   It is helpful to think of chronic renal failure as primarily a tubular disorder, although this is not entirely correct. Most of the abnormal laboratory findings can be explained on the basis of tubular malfunction (Table 11–1). *Hyponatremia, hyperkalemia,* and *hypocalcemia* occur. The tubules normally reabsorb sodium and calcium, but they fail to do this as completely in chronic renal failure. Conversely, the tubules normally secrete potassium but fail to remove it as rapidly in the failure state.

Metabolic acidosis develops for several reasons. The kidney loses sodium and bicarbonate ion, which buffer acid, and fails to secrete organic acids produced as a result of metabolic activity. Formation of ammonium ion, an important route in the removal of hydrogen ion, is decreased. Calcium is lost in larger amounts, and phosphate ion is not secreted as well. These two latter malfunctions also result in increased release of parathormone from the parathyroid gland and depletion of calcium from the bones to raise the blood calcium level. Various skeletal disorders result, including osteoporosis (reduced bone density) and osteomalacia (softening of bone). Bone disease associated with renal failure is termed *renal osteodystrophy.*

The urine volume is high in chronic renal failure because of reduced tubular reabsorption of water and the specific gravity is low (1.010 or less), since waste materials are not as completely removed from the body. (In some end-stage patients, urine volume may be *reduced*, resulting in edema.) The BUN and serum creatinine levels increase in proportion to the reduction in waste removal.

Table 11–1. LABORATORY FINDINGS IN CHRONIC RENAL FAILURE

Hyponatremia
Hyperkalemia
Hypocalcemia
Metabolic acidosis
Renal osteodystrophy
Anemia
Large urine volume (except in end-stage disease)
Reduced specific gravity of urine

Table 11–2. **TREATMENT OF CHRONIC RENAL FAILURE**

Elimination of kidney infection
Control of diabetes mellitus, hypertension, and/or gout
Discontinuation of renotoxic drugs
Careful monitoring of physiologic parameters and normalization
  of them if possible
Restriction of protein intake
Adequate water intake
Replacement of sodium and calcium
Lowering of serum levels of potassium and phosphate
Blood transfusions
Renal dialysis
Renal transplantation

Anemia develops partly as a result of loss of erythrocytes in the urine but, more importantly, because of reduced renal secretion of *erythropoietin* into the blood stream. Erythropoietin acts on the bone marrow to stimulate erythrocyte formation. Consequently, erythrocyte count and hemoglobin and hematocrit values are below normal. The urine contains erythrocytes and several types of casts, especially a large *broad renal failure cast.*

Diagnosis   As mentioned, renal failure often exists in a setting of hypertension, diabetes mellitus, inflammatory kidney disease, or infection. Renal failure itself is the nonspecific result of many long-term disease processes. In general, the presence of acidosis, anemia, azotemia, large-volume dilute urine, and electrolyte abnormalities should be adequate for diagnosis.

Treatment   Every effort must be made to eliminate treatable causes of chronic renal failure (Table 11–2). Diabetes mellitus, hypertension, and gout can be controlled, and infection can often be cured with long-term treatment. *Renotoxic drugs* can be discontinued and their damaging effects halted.

The remainder of the treatment program consists of careful monitoring of electrolytes, BUN, serum creatinine level, serum pH, and other parameters and maintaining these as close to normal as possible. *Protein* intake should be restricted to keep BUN levels near normal. Adequate *water* replacement should be given to counteract the polyuria that usually develops, or water restriction should be instituted if oliguria develops. *Sodium* (as $NaCl$-$NaHCO_3$ mixture) and *calcium* (as calcium lactate) replacement helps to correct the low levels of these electrolytes in the serum. *Restriction of potassium* intake is helpful in preventing hyperkalemia. *Phosphate* levels can be lowered by the administration of aluminum hydroxide (a common antacid), which binds phosphate in the gastrointestinal tract and prevents its absorption. *Vitamin D* supplements help to promote recalcification of bone tissue and combat renal osteodystrophy. *Blood transfusions* are needed in severe anemia, since red blood cell synthesis is impaired. *Iron* compounds or other "blood builders" are generally ineffective. Hypertension is treated in the usual way, with combination drug therapy. Occasionally, in complete renal failure, kidney removal (*nephrectomy*) is necessary to prevent severe renal hypertension and its complications.

Renal dialysis is a life-saving measure in end-stage renal failure and can be continued indefinitely in many cases, even with the use of a home unit. A current alternative to the use of *hemodialysis* (use of a kidney machine) is *ambulatory peritoneal dialysis.* The patient attaches a plastic bag containing dialysis fluid to a permanent cannula in the abdomen and elevates the bag to drain the contents into the abdominal (peritoneal) cavity. The patient then folds up the bag (still attached) and puts it into a pocket. After several hours of normal activity, the patient unfolds the bag and lowers it to drain the dialysis fluid from the abdominal cavity (cannula still attached). The fluid has dialysed against membranes within the abdomen and has removed waste materials from the blood stream. A new bag is attached, and the process is repeated. The advantages of ambulatory peritoneal dialysis over hemodialysis are that it is simpler, much less expensive, and generally nonrestrictive to normal activities.

Renal transplantation has become a successful alternative to long-term dialysis for many patients with end-stage renal failure. Although donor kidneys from identical twins are the best for transplantation, kidneys with a close tissue match (similar antigens of the HLA system) from living donors or cadavers also often work well. Immunosuppressive drug therapy, with compounds such as azathioprine (Imuran), is usually necessary to prevent tissue rejection and transplant failure.

Prognosis　　Long-term prognosis for the renal failure patient is usually good, since dialysis or renal transplant can generally be used. A number of problems attend long-term hemodialysis, including damage to red blood cells from passage through the machine, but the 1-year survival rate on dialysis is 87 per cent and the 6-year survival rate is 60 per cent, a wonderful improvement over the essentially 0 per cent survival rate in end-stage renal failure.

URINARY CALCULI
(STONES)　　Stone formation in the urinary tract is relatively common, especially in the desert environment of Iran, Lebanon, and Saudi Arabia. Presumably the dehydration and resulting concentrated urine brought on by the climate are important, perhaps in conjunction with dietary and hereditary factors. In other parts of the world, urinary stones also occur for a variety of reasons. In some cases, there is excessive formation of a relatively insoluble compound that crystallizes out in the urine (gout, hypercalcemia, cystinuria). Bone disease or hyperparathyroidism often causes hypercalcemia. In other cases, overingestion of foods containing a compound relatively insoluble in urine (e.g., spinach or rhubarb, which contain large quantities of oxalate ion) results in stone formation. In addition, reduced urine volume or changes in pH may promote precipitation of stone-forming compounds. Particles within the urinary tract can serve as a nucleus for stone formation. These can include clots, clumps of bacteria or dead cells, or foreign materials (e.g., a broken-off tip of a catheter).

An unusual situation associated with stone formation occurs in the treatment of malignant diseases, such as leukemia, with anticancer drugs. Massive numbers of cells are killed by the treatment, and the metabolic pathway for uric acid is flooded with precursor

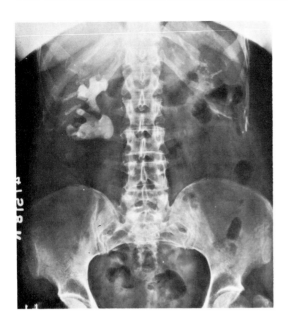

Figure 11–7. Staghorn calculus of kidney. Antlerlike stone appears in upper left (right kidney). (From Griffiths, H. J., and Sarno, R. C.: *Contemporary Radiology: An Introduction to Imaging.* Philadelphia, W. B. Saunders Company, 1979.)

compounds (purines) derived from the killed malignant and normal cells. The purine compounds are converted into uric acid, and urinary stones often form from the relatively insoluble uric acid as it is excreted by the kidney. (See discussion of gout in Chapter 17.)

In addition to these causes, deformities or obstructions in the urinary tract favor stone formation because of stagnation of urine. An example of this is "horseshoe" kidney, a congenital deformity that is often associated with urinary stones.

Urinary stones are formed from three major compounds: uric acid, calcium phosphate, and calcium oxalate. A mixture of calcium phosphate and calcium oxalate stones (mixed stones) is common. Occasionally, cystine stones are found in patients with cystinuria, a metabolic disorder. Calcium-containing stones are visible on x-ray examination, whereas uric acid and cystine stones are usually translucent and poorly visible with this method. Urinary stones are also subdivided as to their location: kidney, ureter, or bladder.

Kidney Stones

Stones formed within the kidney usually produce a dull flank pain, nausea, and vomiting, associated with hematuria. Bacteriuria, leukocytosis, and pyuria, along with chills and fever, occur if secondary infection is present. Often, no symptoms are present, and the stone is found upon routine x-ray examination.

The size of kidney stones varies, from those small enough to pass through the ureter to huge stones that occupy the entire renal pelvis and have roughly the shape of a deer antler (staghorn calculus) (Fig. 11–7). Most suspected stones can be identified with the use of an IVP, which will also rule out tumor, deformity, or obstruction of the kidney.

Treatment

The treatment of kidney stones lies in control of the underlying condition. In some cases, calcium intake or the intake of oxalate-containing foods is restricted. Gout is controllable with several types of drugs (see Chapter 17). Contributing factors, such as UTI, can usually be controlled. Increased water intake is usually helpful in solubilizing stone-forming compounds or in flushing out small stones from the kidney. A urine output of more than 2 liters/day is advisable. Large stones will not pass and may require surgical removal.

Ureteral Stones

Ureteral stones are formed in the kidney but are small enough to pass into the ureter. The inner mucosa of the ureter is irritated by the sharp edges of the stone and the smooth muscle of the ureter contracts, causing a knife-like pain in the back or abdominal area on the side of the stone (ureteral colic). Rigidity of back or abdominal muscles results, associated with nausea and vomiting.

Diagnosis

X-ray film or IVP shows the location of obstruction. The ureter is dilated above the stone (hydroureter) because of pressure from urine formed by the kidney, and frequently the kidney is also distended with retained urine (hydronephrosis). Leukocytosis, pyuria, and bacteriuria are common, since secondary infection occurs easily in the presence of urinary obstruction. Crystals of the stone material are often found in the urine, permitting exact identification. Stones that pass out of the urinary tract through the urethra should be saved for analysis.

Treatment

Most small ureteral stones will pass if fluid intake is increased and drugs are used to relax the ureteral spasm (e.g., atropine). Morphine or meperidine (Demerol) relaxes the ureteral spasm and relieves pain and is much welcomed by the patient. Antibiotics are generally given to control or prevent the infection that so often follows ureteral trauma and obstruction. Stones that do not pass must be removed surgically, either with an instrument that is threaded up the ureter through the urethra and bladder or via direct incision of the ureter. The follow-up treatment is similar to that for renal stones.

Vesicular (Bladder) Stones

Stones arising in the bladder are usually associated with obstruction, infection, or the presence of foreign material in the bladder. A common situation is prostatic hypertrophy in an elderly male. The reduced urine flow and retention of stagnant urine favor precipitation of stone-forming compounds. Inflammation and infection of the bladder also foster stone formation, as does spinal cord damage that reduces bladder motility (neurogenic bladder).

Symptoms and Signs

Common symptoms are urinary frequency and urgency, dysuria, and a feeling of obstruction within the bladder. Often, even large stones produce no symptoms. Secondary infection is common, and leads to the findings of pyuria, bacteriuria, and hematuria.

Diagnosis

X-ray exam or IVP often shows the outline of the stone(s) in the bladder and demonstrates hydroureter and/or hydronephrosis when present. Direct examination of the bladder through the urethra (cystoscopy) allows for visualization of the stone(s) and exclusion of other conditions producing similar symptoms (e.g., bladder tumor).

Treatment   Only the smallest bladder stones pass through the urethra. Most must be removed surgically. Small to medium-sized stones can be removed through the urethra after crushing them with an instrument called a *lithotrite* (litho = stone). Large stones require removal from the bladder through the abdominal wall (suprapubic lithotomy). If prostatic hypertrophy is present, a transurethral resection (TUR) of excess prostate tissue is often done at the same time. Antibiotic coverage to control or prevent infection is recommended. The drugs are similar to those used to treat acute UTI.

Complications   Infection and urinary obstruction (hydroureter, hydronephrosis) are the common complications to urinary calculi. Early stone removal usually prevents these entirely or greatly reduces their severity. Prolonged hydronephrosis eventually leads to renal tissue damage and failure.

SUMMARY

The kidney has a major function in the maintenance of water balance, maintenance of acid-base balance and in the removal of wastes. Through a unique system of filtration, reabsorption, and secretion, the kidney retains materials needed to maintain homeostasis and eliminates chemical compounds that are toxic in large amounts. Filtration, reabsorption, and secretion are in the domain of the glomerulotubular system, all parts of which are vulnerable to disease.

Glomerular inflammation is referred to as glomerulonephritis and results primarily in disturbances in filtration functions. Pyelonephritis is inflammation of the kidney pelvis and parenchymal area, usually as a result of infection. Nephrotic syndrome is a nonspecific disorder characterized by edema, proteinuria, hypoalbuminemia, and hyperlipidemia. Renal failure results primarily from loss of tubular function and consists of reduced urine concentrating ability, acid-base and electrolyte imbalance, impaired waste removal, and other abnormalities.

Urinary calculi are composed of a variety of compounds, including calcium oxalate, calcium phosphate, and uric acid. They form in the kidney, ureter, or bladder and are influenced by an assortment of metabolic, dietary, and pathologic conditions.

Renal disorders result from inflammatory, infectious, metabolic, or other disease processes. In all cases, the underlying condition must be treated, if possible, through drug therapy, surgery, or diet modifications before permanent cure can be expected.

Questions   1. Why do you think the kidney goes to the trouble of filtering great quantities of water and other compounds at the glomeruli, only to reabsorb most of the material in the tubular system? Isn't this a wasteful system? What are the advantages of this type of system?
2. Why don't all individuals with beta-hemolytic streptococcal infection develop glomerulonephritis? What is meant by the term "innocent bystander" as it applies to the kidney?
3. Compare and contrast acute glomerulonephritis and acute pyelonephritis as to causes, clinical and laboratory findings, and long-term complications.

4. Explain the significance of oval fat bodies and broad renal failure casts in renal disorders. How are they formed?
5. How would you differentiate among calcium phosphate stones in the kidney, ureter, and bladder, based upon symptoms, laboratory findings, and contributing factors? How would the treatments of these three conditions be similar? Different?

Additional Reading   Brenner, B. M., and Rector, F. J., Jr. (eds.): *The Kidney.* Philadelphia, W. B. Saunders Company, 1976.

Broadus, A. E., and Thier, S. O.: Metabolic basis of renal-stone disease. N. Engl. J. Med., 300:839, 1979.

Ferguson, G. G.: Common renal disorders and their treatments. Southern Pharmacy Journal, 69:13, 1977. (*Overview of renal disorders.*)

Kory, M., and Waife, S. O. (eds.): *Kidney and Urinary Tract Infections.* Indianapolis, Eli Lilly and Co., 1971. (*Diagnosis and treatment in UTI.*)

Popovich, R. P., et al.: Continuous ambulatory peritoneal dialysis, Ann. Intern. Med., 88:449, 1978. (*Discussion of new, simplified technique of dialysis in renal failure.*)

CHAPTER 12

DIGESTIVE DISORDERS

Digestion begins in the oral cavity and continues throughout most of the gastrointestinal tract (Fig. 12–1). Food taken into the mouth is mixed with saliva, which contains *ptyalin,* an enzyme that hydrolyzes starches, and *mucin,* a glycoprotein whose action is primarily as a lubricant. Mastication (chewing) of large food particles helps to mix these with saliva and form a bolus that is easily swallowed.

Swallowing (deglutition) consists of voluntarily pushing food material into the pharynx (upper throat) using the back of the tongue, followed by reflex contraction of the pharyngeal muscles. The food bolus is forced into the upper esophagus, where it is carried through by the peristaltic action of the esophageal musculature. During swallowing, the vocal cords close and respiration stops to prevent aspiration of food materials. Occasionally, a mistake is made, especially when talking or laughing while eating, and swallowed material enters the larynx, leading to violent coughing and expulsion of the material from the respiratory tract.

At the lower end of the esophagus, the food bolus encounters the *cardiac sphincter,* a circular muscle that opens to admit food or liquid into the stomach. At times other than during swallowing, the cardiac sphincter is closed, keeping stomach contents from entering the esophagus and causing local irritation. Food material in the stomach is acted upon by *gastric juice,* which contains hydrochloric acid (pH 1 to 3), secreted by the gastric parietal cells; mucus and various digestive enzymes, such as pepsin (three types); and lipase. The gastric parietal cells also secrete intrinsic factor, a substance needed for the absorption of cyanocobalamin (vitamin B-12). The churning action of the stomach aids in breaking up remaining food particles and mixing them with gastric juice. Material thus liquefied is squirted, little by little, into the duodenum (first portion of the small intestine). This is accomplished by contraction of the lower part of the stomach (antrum) in conjunction with opening of the *pyloric sphincter.* Contraction of the duodenum follows and the liquefied material is propelled through the small intestine.

The *sphincter of Oddi* is an opening in the duodenum that connects to the *common bile duct* (Fig. 12–2). Through this duct a mixture of bile and pancreatic juice is admitted to the duodenum. Bile is secreted by the liver through hepatic ducts that connect with the common bile duct. It is stored in the gallbladder so that large amounts can be released upon demand to aid in the digestion of fats. Pancreatic juice is secreted by the pancreas into the *pancreatic duct,* which joins with the common bile duct near the sphincter of Oddi. The pH of the duodenum is slightly alkaline, largely because

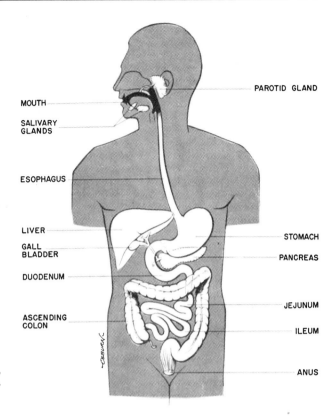

Figure 12–1. The digestive tract. (From Guyton, A. C.: *Textbook of Medical Physiology,* 6th ed. Philadelphia, W. B. Saunders Company, 1981.)

of secretion of bile and pancreatic juice, whereas the adjacent stomach is strongly acidic.

Duodenal contents are propelled through the duodenum into the *jejunum* and *ileum,* and absorption of digested materials occurs at all three portions of the small intestine. The terminal end of the ileum joins to the *cecum* (blind end of the large intestine), marking the beginning of the large intestine (colon). The *appendix,* an organ causing little joy and much consternation, is an outgrowth of the cecum (Fig. 12–3). It is vestigial in man and apes but has digestive functions in some birds. Lymphoid tissue in the appendix and in other areas of the gastrointestinal tract is a source of B lymphocytes (Chapter 2).

Figure 12–2. Relationship of pancreas, ducts, and duodenum.

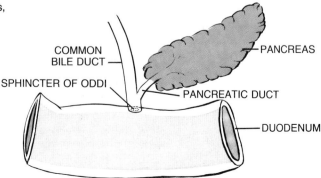

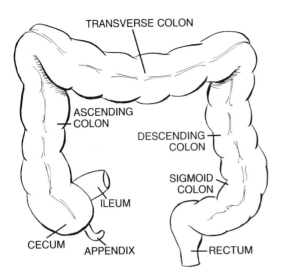

Figure 12–3. Parts of the human colon.

The colon consists of four sections (ascending, transverse, descending, and sigmoid) and terminates in the rectum (Fig. 12–3). The colon has little digestive function; it is concerned mainly with absorption of water and electrolytes and in thus converting its liquid contents into semisolid feces. The colon contains *coliforms* (Chapter 2), bacteria that have important functions in the synthesis of vitamins. Fecal material is propelled through the colon primarily by peristaltic action. It is then stored in the lower colon and eventually released by contraction of the colon and rectum in conjunction with relaxation of the anal sphincter.

A number of regulatory processes control gastrointestinal activity in humans. *Histamine* causes secretion of gastric hydrochloric acid by the parietal cells. *Gastrin* also stimulates gastric acid secretion as well as the secretion of pepsin. Cholecystokinin (CCK) causes contraction of the gallbladder, thus releasing bile into the duodenum, and secretion of pancreatic juice into the duodenum. Release of these hormones is affected by the presence of food in the mouth or stomach, emotional state, or even the sight, smell, or thought of food. Alcohol, nicotine, and caffeine stimulate gastric acid secretion and are important in the development or persistence of ulcer.

The common disease processes affecting the gastrointestinal tract are inflammation, infection, and neoplasia. Neoplastic disease of the colon and rectum, a common malignancy, is discussed in Chapter 21.

ULCER   *Peptic ulcer* refers to ulceration of any part of the digestive tract that comes in contact with gastric juice (containing pepsin), including the stomach, duodenum, and esophagus. The stomach is normally resistant to the effects of gastric juice, partly because of a protective mucous barrier coating the gastric mucosa. However, ulceration can occur. The duodenum and esophagus are not "designed" for operation in the presence of gastric juice. Passage of gastric juice into the upper part of the duodenum or lower part of the esophagus results in inflammation and, eventually, ulceration. Not surprisingly, most ulcers in the duodenum and esophagus occur in the portion immediately adjacent to the stomach, where spilled gastric juice would be the most concentrated and therefore the most irritating. Ulceration is really a process of self-digestion, in which the mucosa is eroded, and the process often extends to the muscle layer below the mucosa.

Acute ulcers are often shallow and represent only minimal erosion of the mucosa. They occur as a result of ingestion of irritating foods, (e.g., peppers) or drugs (aspirin, alcohol, indomethacin [Indocin], phenylbutazone [Butazolidin]). Acute ulcers also form after burns, surgery, or other traumatic conditions and are called *stress ulcers,* since stress is the common denominator in those cases. Healing of acute ulcers occurs quickly when the cause of ulceration is removed and is usually complete.

Chronic ulcers are generally deeper and represent a long-term inflammatory process. Healing is slower and is often accompanied by scar formation. The healed area remains vulnerable to subsequent ulceration.

Malignant ulcers are rare in the duodenum or esophagus but represent 5 to 10 per cent of the gastric ulcers. There is no evidence that a benign ulcer becomes malignant; rather, malignant ulcers start out that way.

If surgery is performed for severe, intractable ulcer, often the lower portion of the stomach is removed and connected to the duodenum or jejunum (gastroenterostomy). This removes the pyloric sphincter and a large portion of the acid-secreting cells of the stomach. Interestingly enough, ulceration often occurs at the junction of the remaining stomach and intestine. This is referred to as a *stomal* or *marginal ulcer* and its frequency is 35 to 75 per cent following gastroenterostomy.

Duodenal Ulcer   Ulceration of the duodenum is approximately five times as common as gastric ulcer and affects males and females in a ratio of 4:1. Ninety-five per cent of duodenal ulcers occur within the first 2 inches of the duodenum below the stomach. Because the incidence of malignant duodenal ulcer is extremely low, concern about cancer is slight if a duodenal location of the ulcer is confirmed.

Pathogenesis   Some authorities identify an "ulcer personality" as being a risk factor in the development of ulcer. Individuals of this type are perfectionistic and striving. We think of the hard-driving executive or sales manager as being typical ulcer patients. Yet, personality type is only one factor and many calm, easy-going people also develop ulcers. There is always the question, though, of whether the "easy-going" person is really that way inside or merely gives the appearance of calmness to the outside observer.

Studies of individuals with gastric fistulas (outside openings permitting observation of the stomach) have demonstrated the effect of emotions on gastric function. The same has been done using gastroscopy (insertion of a tube into the stomach through the esophagus). Anger or stress causes the stomach to secrete more acid, and the gastric tissue becomes hyperemic, even if there is little noticeable outward response.

With the advent of changing sexual roles and the increased number of women in executive roles, the incidence of ulcer is increasing in women. This is interesting, since the traditional role as homemaker is often considered at least as stressful as a "high pressure" executive position.

Factors such as diet, alcohol consumption, and the use of irritating medicinal drugs seem important in the pathogenesis of duodenal ulcer. Often, the ulcer patient gives a history of an unusual, restricted diet or of infrequent eating. Excessive alcohol intake increases acid secretion and directly irritates the gastrointestinal mucosa. In addition, the heavy drinker often follows a poor or erratic diet. Digestive juice secreted in anticipation of a normal time for eating may find no food to digest and may then act on mucosal tissue. Drugs taken for legitimate purposes (e.g., aspirin) may be ulcerogenic or may promote continuation of an established ulcer.

Examination of the ulcer crater in duodenal ulcer shows a clearly defined erosion extending through the mucosa and often into or through the muscular layer of the duodenum (Fig. 12–4). Tissue surrounding the crater shows signs of chronic inflammation, often with fibrosis. When the ulcer heals, a base of granulation tissue forms over the crater, followed by regeneration of the mucosal layer (Fig. 12–5). In cases in which healing is delayed, fibrous tissue often forms in the crater and remains, preventing regeneration of the mucosa. This is equivalent to scar formation in the skin in healing by secondary intention.

Symptoms and Signs

Most duodenal ulcer sufferers complain of a gnawing or burning pain in the center of the abdomen just below the lower tip of the rib cage (xiphoid process). Heartburn is often present, reflecting reflux of gastric juice into the lower end of the esophagus as well as spillage into the duodenum. Nausea and vomiting are common. Symptoms are most severe about 1 hour after eating, when food has been digested and gastric juice is operating on the ulcerated area. Pain and feelings of hunger are also common at night and often awaken the individual from sleep. Temporary relief is obtained with food, milk, or antacids, but the problem reoccurs every hour or so.

Laboratory Findings

Many, but not all, duodenal ulcer patients have excessively high acid levels in the stomach. This is assumed to be part of the problem, but the relationship is by no means clear-cut. Symptoms may occur during sleep, when acid production is usually reduced. Many indi-

Figure 12–4. Ulcer crater.

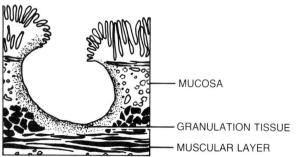

— MUCOSA

— GRANULATION TISSUE
— MUSCULAR LAYER

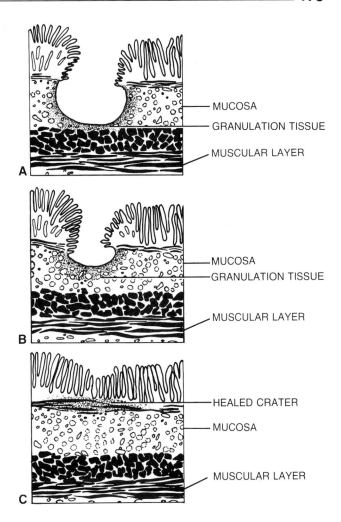

MUCOSA

GRANULATION TISSUE

MUSCULAR LAYER

A

MUCOSA

GRANULATION TISSUE

MUSCULAR LAYER

B

HEALED CRATER

MUCOSA

MUSCULAR LAYER

Figure 12–5. *(A–C)* Healing of ulcer.   C

viduals with excessive acid production do not develop ulcers. If hyperacidity is found in an ulcer patient, however, attempts should be made to normalize it if possible.

Bleeding ulcers result in occult blood in the feces (detected with Occultest or a similar test) and may result in anemia (shown by reduced erythrocyte count, hemoglobin, and hematocrit values). This is a common cause of anemia in adult males, who are not generally prone to anemia.

X-ray examination of the esophagus, stomach, and duodenum after barium swallow (upper GI series) shows ulcer in 50 to 70 per cent of the cases but fails to locate some ulcers. Small ulcers or those hidden from x-ray by ribs or other structures may not be visible. In these cases, a lighted flexible tube (fiberoptic duodenoscope) can be passed into the duodenum through the mouth and esophagus and direct observation can be made. This technique also permits visualization of minor eroded areas of the duodenum, stomach, or esophagus, anatomic abnormalities, or tumors in the area.

Diagnosis   Patients with typical symptoms are easily diagnosed. Atypical cases must be differentiated from gastric ulcer or tumor of the duodenum or stomach. Inflammation without deep ulceration (duodenitis, gastritis) produces similar symptoms. In equivocal cases, where x-ray findings are inconclusive, duodenoscopy is especially helpful.

Treatment   General measures in the treatment of duodenal ulcer include rest; reduction of stress (work, home); and the avoidance of alcohol, caffeine, and nicotine. Any drugs that cause gastrointestinal irritation should be discontinued or substituted with nonirritating drugs if possible. The diet should emphasize a wide variety of foods, and meals should be regular and moderate in size. Overeating or skipping meals encourages increased acid irritation. Although this is not the best time to explore all of the spicy food restaurants in town, the diet does not have to be bland and dull, as was the case in the past.

Several types of drugs are useful in the control of ulcer symptoms and may promote faster healing of the lesion.

Antacids. Antacids, such as magnesium and aluminum hydroxides (Maalox, Gelusil), are useful for buffering excess acid. These should be taken hourly at first and then four to six times per day as healing progresses. Finally, they can be used as needed. In severe cases, suspensions of these drugs are given by gastric drip into the ulcer area.

Anticholinergic Drugs. These agents (e.g., propantheline [Pro-Banthine]) reduce gastric acid secretion and gastrointestinal motility and may relieve ulcer symptoms.

Antianxiety Drugs. These drugs (e.g., diazepam [Valium]) may reduce the effects of stress or anxiety and promote faster healing of the ulcer.

Blocking Agents. A welcome addition to the therapeutic armamentarium against ulcer is *cimetidine* (Tagamet). Cimetidine blocks histamine receptors in the gastric mucosa that trigger acid production (histamine H_2 receptors). These are different from the type (H_1) associated with allergic responses. Cimetidine is given four times daily for 6 weeks, during which time the ulcer usually heals. Rebound reactivation is prevented by giving a single dose at bedtime after healing has occurred.

Complications   In addition to failing to heal, duodenal ulcers may hemorrhage, perforate, penetrate, or cause pyloric obstruction.

Hemorrhage. The ulcer erodes through a blood vessel in the duodenum or because of bleeding granulation tissue in the ulcer crater. Blood loss may be minimal or life-threatening and can be assessed by stool examination; severity of vomiting of blood (hematemesis), if present; or decreases in erythrocyte count, hemoglobin, and hematocrit values.

Perforation. The ulcer erodes completely through the duodenal wall, and intestinal contents spill into the abdominal cavity. Laboratory findings include characteristic filling of the perforation with leakage of barium contrast medium through the hole and an elevation of the diaphragm on the affected side as a result of pressure from gas escaping into the abdominal cavity. Although perforated ulcers used to be the death knell for the victims, the outlook is now much brighter with the advent of improved surgical and antibiotic treatment.

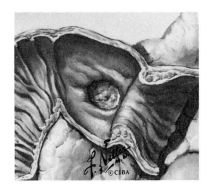

Figure 12–6. Penetration of duodenal ulcer with attachment to pancreas. (Copyright, 1969, CIBA Pharmaceutical Company, Division of the CIBA-GEIGY Corporation. Reprinted with permission from the CIBA Collection of Medical Illustrations, illustrated by Frank H. Netter, M.D. All rights reserved.)

Penetration. The ulcer extends through the duodenal wall and continues into a nearby organ (pancreas, liver) (Fig. 12–6). There is no leak of duodenal contents into the abdominal cavity, as with perforation, but there may be additional organ damage from the effects of the duodenal materials on the adjacent tissue. Surgical treatment is usually required.

Pyloric Obstruction. This results from scar tissue formation (fibrosis) caused by chronic inflammation or from edema and pylorospasm associated with inflammation of the area. If surgery is required, an operation called a pyloroplasty (repair of the pyloric area) is done.

Prognosis

The outlook is generally good with duodenal ulcer. Approximately 25 per cent of ulcer sufferers develop complications, but only 5 to 10 per cent require surgery. Reactivation is common and can often be controlled by attention to the nonsurgical means of treatment and control previously discussed.

Gastric Ulcer

The stomach is also a common site for ulceration, although less so than the duodenum. Hyperacidity appears less important in the pathogenesis of gastric ulcer than with duodenal ulcer and it is likely that reduced tissue resistance (perhaps reduced protection by mucus) is more important. Most gastric ulcers occur in the lower part of the stomach, within a few inches of the pyloric sphincter (Fig. 12–7).

Symptoms and Signs

Symptoms and signs are similar to those of duodenal ulcer but are often less intense. Bleeding, with resulting anemia, is fairly common and can be detected in a similar way to duodenal bleeding.

Laboratory Findings

Gastric acid level is usually normal and responds to drugs such as betazole (Histalog) that increase acid secretion. This finding is important because gastric acid levels are often low and nonresponsive to drugs if there is extensive malignancy of the stomach (when parietal cells have been replaced with nonfunctional tumor cells).

Diagnosis

Upper GI series and gastroscopy are useful in the diagnosis of gastric ulcer. Since 5 to 10 per cent of gastric ulcers are malignant, gastroscopy with biopsy of the affected area is frequently done to rule out malignant gastric ulcer. Other conditions producing similar symptoms include duodenal ulcer, gastritis, or duodenitis.

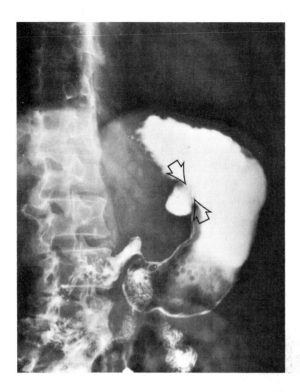

Figure 12–7. Gastric ulcer as seen in upper gastrointestinal tract series. (From Griffiths, H. J., and Sarno, R. C.: *Contemporary Radiology: An Introduction to Imaging.* Philadelphia, W. B. Saunders Company, 1979.)

Treatment   Treatment of gastric ulcer is similar to that of duodenal ulcer. Failure of response should be investigated carefully, perhaps by exploratory surgery, if malignant gastric ulcer cannot be completely ruled out. Follow-up gastroscopy is helpful in the observation of treatment response or failure to respond adequately.

Complications   The complications of hemorrhage, perforation, penetration, and pyloric obstruction are also common in gastric ulcer and often require surgical treatment.

Prognosis   The outlook is usually favorable in benign gastric ulcer, since benign ulcers do not become malignant. Reactivation is common but can generally be handled with medical, rather than surgical, treatment.

ULCERATIVE COLITIS   The colon is also subject to ulceration, although the clinical condition of ulcerative colitis is quite different from gastric or duodenal ulcer. Gastric juice is not a contributing factor in this case, since the colon is a great distance anatomically from the stomach. Therefore, the term "peptic ulcer" does not apply.

In spite of the name, ulcerative colitis occasionally affects the lower ileum, a portion of the small intestine. This is seen as an extension of colon disease. In addition to ulceration of the intestinal mucosa, there is chronic inflammation, especially in the left portion of the colon, sigmoid area and rectum. The onset is commonly in adolescence or young adulthood, with slightly greater incidence in females and whites. A similar condition, *regional enteritis* (Crohn's disease), affects the colon and small intestine but frequently skips over areas of normal intestine. Regional enteritis affects the muscular and submuscular layers of the affected intestine, whereas ulcerative colitis primarily involves the mucosal layer.

Pathogenesis

The cause of ulcerative colitis is unknown, and the disorder is therefore labeled *idiopathic*. There are several interesting theories regarding its etiology, including infection with mycobacteria or viruses, allergy to milk or gluten (a component of wheat and corn), or autoimmune mechanisms. Although all of these theories have some experimental support, no one is completely convincing. Many ulcerative colitis patients have an "ulcer personality" (characterized by perfectionism and excessive dependence on others), but the idea that the disease represents strictly a psychosomatic reaction has not been widely accepted. It is possible that there are several causes and that the condition should be more properly called a syndrome.

Chronic inflammation of the colonic mucosa leads to ulceration, hyperemia, petechial hemorrhage, and the formation of pseudopolyps (Fig. 12–8). Pseudopolyps result from attempted regeneration of mucosal tissue and stand out against adjacent ulcerated areas. The mucosa is friable (crumbles easily upon touch). Pathologic changes are most noticeable in the lower colon and rectal area but can occur in the upper colon or lower ileum, as mentioned.

Symptoms and Signs

The chief complaint with ulcerative colitis is diarrhea, with passage of blood and mucus in the stool. Fecal incontinence often occurs, but occasionally constipation is a major problem because of

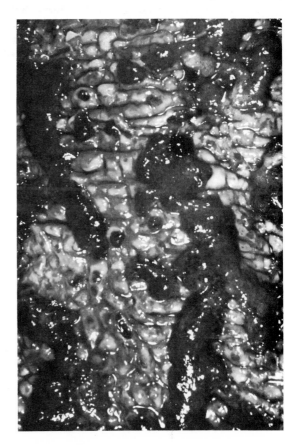

Figure 12–8. Appearance of colonic mucosa in ulcerative colitis. (From Robbins, S. L., and Cotran, R. S.: *Pathologic Basis of Disease,* 2nd ed. Philadelphia, W. B. Saunders Company, 1979.)

sustained cramping of the lower intestine. There is generally loss of appetite (leading to loss of weight), fever, and abdominal tenderness during the active phase. In most cases, milk products aggravate the symptoms. Weakness and malaise, resulting from anemia due to chronic blood loss, are also common symptoms. Symptoms usually develop gradually and worsen with time, although occasionally the onset of disease is more dramatic.

A fulminant form of disease exists in which symptoms worsen very quickly, leading to acute dilation and congestion of the large intestine (acute toxic megacolon). This is a life-threatening condition, since perforation of the intestine and peritonitis often result. In most cases, though, the condition undergoes less severe exacerbations and remissions and follows the pattern of many other inflammatory disorders.

Laboratory Findings   Stool examination shows blood, mucus and, occasionally, pus, but no pathogenic organisms. Sigmoidoscopic examination of the colorectal area (using a lighted tube inserted into the rectum) reveals the pathologic changes previously discussed (Fig. 12–8). Hypochromic anemia, due to chronic blood loss, is usually present (low erythrocyte count and reduced hemoglobin and hematocrit values). Barium enema, followed by x-ray examination, often shows evidence of intestinal cramping and an irregular mucosal surface.

Diagnosis   *Regional enteritis* produces symptoms similar to those of ulcerative colitis but has an erratic distribution, often skipping over areas of the intestine. It commonly affects the small as well as the large intestine, frequently causing perforation or penetration of the intestinal wall. *Parasitic infection* of the colon (amebiasis, certain bacterial infections) causes similar symptoms but shows organisms in the stool and is curable with appropriate drug therapy. *Functional diarrhea* (no pathologic condition present) can cause similar symptoms but would show relatively normal sigmoidoscopic findings. *Tumors* of the lower gastrointestinal tract could produce similar symptoms but would present different sigmoidoscopic and x-ray findings (see Chapter 21).

Treatment   General helpful measures include the avoidance of roughage (nuts, raw fruits and vegetables) and milk products in the diet to reduce irritation of the inflamed mucosa. Anti-inflammatory corticosteroids or corticotropin (ACTH) help to reduce the severity of colitis during exacerbations of symptoms. Corticotropin must be injected but corticosteroids can be given orally. Corticosteroids of choice include prednisone (Meticorten) and hydrocortisone (Cortef). Another useful route of administration of hydrocortisone is via enema, in which the drug is mixed with vegetable oil or used in the form of a commercially available enema (Cortifoam, Cortenema).

Prevention or control of infection is also important. Although ampicillin (Polycillin) and cephalosporins (e.g., cephalexin [Keflex]) are effective, the drug of choice is sulfasalazine (Azulfidine) and the other drugs are used in those allergic to sulfa drugs.

Surgery is required for severe ulcerative colitis to eliminate badly diseased tissue. Either resection of involved areas of the colon is performed, or the entire colon is removed (total colectomy) and the ileum is attached to the abdominal wall (ileostomy). In the latter case, a plastic bag is used to collect discharged fecal material.

Complications   Long-term inflammation of the colon leads to fibrosis, with possible stricture formation, development of a fistula (pipelike communication of colon with other tissue), abscess, or perforation of the colon as a result of acute toxic megacolon. In some patients, ocular or joint lesions also develop, suggesting a more general immune response resembling that seen with rheumatoid arthritis or lupus erythematosus (see Chapter 17).

The risk of malignancy of the colon is always present in ulcerative colitis, presumably because of the chronic inflammation and attempts at repair by the body. Eventually the tissue may undergo malignant degeneration, rather than just repair. Risk of cancer is greater in extensive and long-standing disease (5 to 10 per cent after 15 years; 40 to 50 per cent after 25 years of extensive disease). Repeated sigmoidoscopic examination is necessary to detect early malignant lesions in the colorectal area. Total colectomy is often performed in long-standing cases, not only to relieve symptoms but also to avoid the development of cancer.

Prognosis   Individuals with mild to moderate disease, especially with limited involvement of the colon, often do well with medical management. Exacerbations and remissions are common, as mentioned, and drug therapy must be continually adjusted to keep symptoms under control. Severe disease is often not well controlled and carries the increased risk of cancer, frequently requiring surgery for prevention and cure.

DIVERTICULITIS   The intestinal tract is vulnerable to herniation of the muscular wall and the formation of pouches of mucosa. These are termed *diverticula,* since they represent a diversion in the direction the normal bowel takes, and the condition is called *diverticulosis.* If digestive products enter the diverticula and cause inflammation and/or infection, the disorder is then called *diverticulitis.*

Approximately 8 per cent of the healthy United States population have diverticulosis and the incidence increases to 30 to 35 per cent in the population group over 60. The lesions in these cases are called *silent diverticula,* since symptoms are absent. Colonic diverticula are the most common, especially in the sigmoid colon, but diverticula of the small intestine are also frequently seen. Only in the rectum do they fail to develop.

Pathogenesis   Constipation is a contributing factor in diverticulosis and diverticulitis. The increased force necessary to propel a hard fecal mass along the intestinal tract favors herniation of the muscular tissue of the intestinal wall. In addition, it tends to force fecal material into previously formed diverticula, fostering impaction, inflammation, and infection. The diet in the United States and in most other "civilized" countries is blamed for the unusually high incidence of diverticulosis and diverticulitis in these areas. We eat too little bulk and too much processed food that leaves a small, compact residue.

The intestinal tract must work too hard to digest the compact food mass. Members of certain African tribes, in which the incidence of diverticular disease (and appendicitis and colorectal cancer) is extremely low, live on a diet with considerably more bulk (raw fruit, vegetables, and grains) than ours. They produce a fecal mass roughly three times the bulk of ours that passes through the digestive tract in a quarter of the time ours does. A high-residue diet is, therefore, probably a protective factor against diverticular disease.

Symptoms and Signs

Left lower-quadrant abdominal pain that is steady or intermittent but severe in intensity, along with constipation or diarrhea, is usually seen in diverticulitis. Diverticulosis is usually asymptomatic, but low-grade, chronic symptoms of constipation and lower abdominal discomfort sometimes occur. There may be a history of "irritable colon" or other poorly defined digestive complaint. If infection develops in impacted diverticula, chills and fever often result. Perforation, which develops only occasionally, leads to internal bleeding and shock in severe cases, or, more commonly, to rectal bleeding or occult blood in the feces.

Laboratory Findings

Routine laboratory tests are of little help unless anemia is present because of blood loss. Leukocytosis is seen if infection or severe inflammation develops. Barium x-ray exam shows the characteristic pouches filled with barium contrast medium (Figure 12–9) and often suggests the presence of inflammation or abscess. Sig-

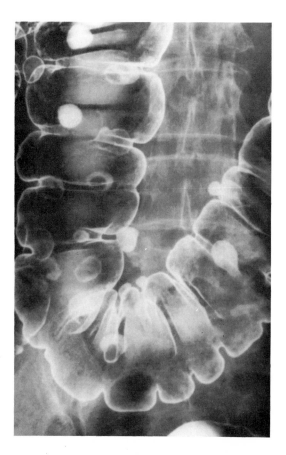

Figure 12–9. Diverticulitis as seen in barium enema x-ray film. (From Laufer, I.: *Double Contrast Gastrointestinal Radiology: With Endoscopic Correlation.* Philadelphia, W. B. Saunders Company, 1979.)

moidoscopy identifies disease in the lower colon but might miss disease higher up in the digestive tract.

Diagnosis   It is important to rule out cancer of the colon because it is a common form of cancer and has a higher incidence in middle-aged or older people, as does diverticulitis. Appendicitis can produce similar symptoms, but the pain is usually on the right side, although it is occasionally central or, rarely, on the left side.

Treatment   A high-residue diet (containing a large amount of dietary fiber) will help to prevent diverticular disease by providing a bulky fecal mass that retains water and is thus soft and easy to propel through the digestive tract. This probably helps to prevent diverticulosis and to prevent the development of diverticulitis in those with existing diverticulosis. In addition to the liberal ingestion of raw fruits, vegetables, and nuts, bran can be added to the diet as a cereal or suspended in fruit juice. Commercial bulking agents, such as Metamucil, are also helpful. (Note that the diet for *ulcerative colitis* emphasizes the avoidance of rough bulky foods.) In existing diverticulitis, foods containing seeds or nuts may be contraindicated, since these particles may enter the diverticula and cause further irritation. Anticholinergic drugs (e.g., propantheline [Pro-Banthine]) help to reduce cramping, and mild laxatives (mineral oil, olive oil) relieve constipation.

To treat or prevent infection associated with diverticulitis, ampicillin is the drug of choice and penicillin/streptomycin or cephalothin (Keflin) is also helpful. Hemorrhage may require blood transfusion and, occasionally, surgical intervention to control the bleeding.

Surgery is not usually required for diverticulitis but may be needed for the complications of perforation, penetration, or hemorrhage. Occasionally, a pouch-ridden segment of intestine is removed to eliminate a constant source of discomfort to the patient. There is no increased risk of bowel cancer in diverticular disease, and "preventive" removal of the colon is not necessary as it often is in ulcerative colitis.

Prognosis   The outlook is usually good with diverticulitis, and individual attacks generally respond well to the treatment outlined. Preventive dietary measures often reduce the frequency and severity of diverticulitis. It is quite likely that these same measures could prevent much of the diverticulosis and therefore greatly decrease the incidence of diverticulitis in the American population.

APPENDICITIS   Although the vermiform (wormlike) appendix is clearly part of the digestive tract (Fig. 12–3), it has no apparent digestive function in man. In birds and some mammals, the appendix seems to be functional. Since the appendix of young people contains a large amount of lymphoid tissue, it has been proposed that it represents an equivalent in humans to the bursa of Fabricius found in birds (see Chapter 4). B lymphocytes are thought to mature in lymphoid tissue in the digestive tract, possibly including the appendix. However, older individuals have little if any lymphoid tissue left in the appendix, yet retain B lymphocyte activity. Removal or absence of the appendix has no effect upon the immune response. Any role played by the appendix in B lymphocyte activity must be supportive, at best.

The appendix is usually located on the right side and represents an outgrowth of the cecum (Fig. 12–3). Great variation exists as to the exact location of the organ. It can be found much higher or lower than the normal location in some individuals and is occasionally found on the left side.

The major disease of the appendix is acute inflammation. Chronic inflammation is rare and usually represents repeated acute attacks. Tumors or cysts are occasionally found in the appendix, where they may cause symptoms of appendicitis. The most common tumor of the appendix is an intermediate tumor (between benign and malignant) that secretes histamine and other compounds. This is called a *carcinoid* (carcinomalike) *tumor.* Multiple tumors of this type cause symptoms of flushing, abdominal cramps, and wheezing, although single tumors of the appendix usually cause obstruction and inflammation of the organ without other symptoms.

Appendicitis can affect all age groups of either sex but is especially common in males in the 10- to 30-year-old age group.

Pathogenesis   Although tumors or foreign bodies in the appendix can initiate inflammation, the most common situation is impaction of fecal material into the appendix from the cecum. Sometimes hard, stone-like fecal particles (fecaliths) (-lith = stone) become trapped in the appendix and cause obstruction and inflammation. Appendicitis is much less common in countries in which the diet contains a large amount of fiber or bulk, as previously mentioned. As with diverticulitis, it seems that the extra force required of the intestine in digesting and propelling the fecal mass may favor impaction and result in inflammation. Once the appendix is obstructed, circulation of blood to it is reduced (ischemia) and the typical signs of inflammation appear. Infection develops because of ischemia and the tissue necrosis that results from it. Infecting organisms are usually coliforms, especially *Escherichia coli,* presumably derived from the normal bacterial flora of the colon.

Symptoms and Signs   Typical appendicitis begins with central abdominal pain in the umbilical or epigastric area that localizes within a few hours to the right lower quadrant. Movement usually increases the steady pain and the abdominal muscles react to the local inflammation by contracting, especially during physical examination (rebound spasm and tenderness). Intestinal tract function is generally reduced, resulting in constipation, although occasionally diarrhea results. Nonspecific additional symptoms include loss of appetite, malaise, and fever.

Unfortunately, typical signs and symptoms of appendicitis are often absent or distorted, especially in elderly people, the obese, or those with abnormal locations of the appendix. Atypical cases, therefore, can be real diagnostic nightmares.

Laboratory Findings   Leukocytosis (up to 20,000/mm³), often with a shift to the left, is the most reliable laboratory finding in appendicitis. Occasionally, appendicitis can be identified by x-ray examination of the right lower quadrant. In these cases, a fecalith or foreign body is visible. Most often, however, x-ray methods are not helpful.

Diagnosis   Acute gastroenteritis (usually caused by food poisoning) frequently produces symptoms resembling those of acute appendicitis. However, symptoms often subside in a few hours. Mesenteric adenitis (inflammation of the lymph nodes in the nearby mesentery) can mimic appendicitis, but it usually occurs following a respiratory infection as a complication. Gastric or duodenal ulcer, kidney stones, or various gynecologic conditions can mimic the abdominal pain of appendicitis. Generally, the pain from appendicitis will localize in the right lower quadrant in a few hours and rebound muscle spasm and tenderness will occur, permitting more accurate diagnosis. A policy of "wait and see" (for 6 to 8 hours) often results in more definitive signs with little additional risk.

Treatment   Penicillin/streptomycin, tetracyclines, or cephalosporins will often cause acute appendicitis to subside. However, repeated attacks are the rule and such medical treatment usually only buys more time for the individual. This is acceptable if good facilities are not available and the person must be taken elsewhere.

Surgery (appendectomy) is the only real cure for appendicitis and should be performed in all suspected cases. Since in 95 per cent of the cases perforation will occur in the absence of treatment, surgery is warranted even in cases in which the diagnosis is not completely certain. The operative risk in the early stages of acute appendicitis is extremely low. Laxatives should be avoided, even though constipation is often present, since they may cause perforation by increasing bowel motility.

Complications   *Perforation* is the most common complication to acute appendicitis. Observation for longer than 8 to 12 hours increases the risk of perforation. If perforation occurs, intestinal contents and products of infection leak into the area around the appendix.

If the leak is slight and is walled off by the resulting inflammatory reaction, an *appendiceal abscess* results. This can be treated with antibiotics in conjunction with drainage prior to eventual appendectomy.

More extensive leakage involves the peritoneal cavity, resulting in *peritonitis*. Peritonitis is more serious than appendiceal abscess and was a common cause of death in earlier times. (Houdini, the great magician, died of peritonitis caused by a perforated appendix.) However, it can be treated with modern antibiotics and supportive measures and is not always the death knell it used to be.

Prognosis   Prognosis in acute appendicitis is usually excellent, since surgery is both safe and curative.

HIATUS (HIATAL)   The term *hiatus* means a gap or opening. For example, anes-
HERNIA   thesia is sometimes described as a hiatus in consciousness. Likewise, a hiatus can occur in body tissues, in which the tissue fails to fill in the normal space. Hiatus (hiatal) hernia refers to a condition in which a portion of the stomach protrudes into the chest cavity

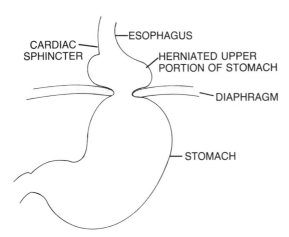

Figure 12–10. Hiatus hernia (sliding type).

through a hiatus in the diaphragm. Approximately 5 per cent of the population have hiatus hernia, but over half have no symptoms. Obese, elderly females have the highest frequency of the condition.

Pathogenesis   Hiatus hernia is of two general types. In the *sliding* type (85 to 90 per cent), the upper portion of the stomach slides up and down through the opening in the diaphragm. A congenitally short esophagus or an esophagus shortened by stricture formation (as with scarring) pulls the stomach up through the diaphragm (Fig. 12–10).

In the *rolling* type (10 to 15 per cent), the upper portion of the stomach is forced alongside the esophagus above the diaphragm (Fig. 12–11). The result of displacement of the upper stomach, in both types, is malfunction of the cardiac sphincter, allowing gastric juice to reflux into the esophagus. As is the case with the duodenum, the esophagus is not designed to handle the acid and enzymes contained in gastric juice and inflammation (esophagitis) results. In more severe cases, esophageal ulceration occurs. Obesity and prone position aggravate hiatus hernia because these conditions increase the abdominal pressure, which forces the stomach through the diaphragmatic hiatus.

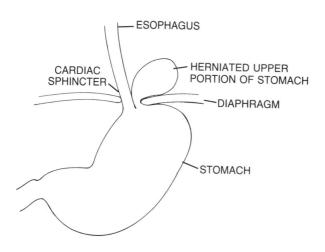

Figure 12–11. Hiatus hernia (rolling type).

Symptoms and Signs Heartburn (pyrosis), a feeling of pressure and pain behind the sternum, and palpitations (throbbing or fluttering of the heart) are common symptoms of hiatus hernia. Heartburn is a symptom of esophagitis, caused by gastric reflux into the lower esophagus. Pain and pressure in the chest result partly from gastric reflux and partly from pressure of the upper stomach against structures within the chest. If herniation is moderate to severe, the upper stomach may press against the heart, causing palpitations and suggesting a cardiac disorder to the patient. Symptoms are generally worse when lying down or after a big meal, when the production of gastric juice is increased (big meal) or the position favors gastric reflux (lying down).

Laboratory Findings Most routine laboratory tests are not helpful in the diagnosis of hiatus hernia. An exception is the finding of anemia and occult blood in the feces if chronic esophageal or gastric bleeding occurs. A chest x-ray exam is the most useful tool for diagnosis. Some hernias can be visualized with a standing chest roentgenogram. Occasionally, a "feet up" chest x-ray (feet above the head) is needed to demonstrate the sliding nature of the hernia. Often a circular contraction is visible at the gastroesophageal junction (esophageal ring), and this is highly suggestive of hiatus hernia. Direct observation of the esophagus with a lighted instrument (esophagoscopy) is also helpful in questionable cases. It should be pointed out that hiatus hernia can exist without producing symptoms and the typical symptoms can exist in the absence of hiatus hernia.

Diagnosis The major conditions to rule out in the diagnosis of hiatus hernia are cardiac diseases (angina pectoris, myocardial infarction, arrhythmias), gastric or duodenal ulcer, and esophageal cancer. An electrocardiogram will rule out heart disease, usually to the great relief of the patient. Ulceration below the esophagus can usually be detected with an upper GI series, gastroscopy, and/or duodenoscopy. Esophagoscopy permits elimination of malignant disease as a possibility.

Treatment Eighty-five to 90 per cent of hiatus hernia sufferers respond to conservative medical treatment. Most of those requiring surgery have the rolling type, which is more prone to complications than the sliding type. General measures include weight reduction to normal, avoidance of overeating and lying down after meals, and elevation of the head of the bed 8 to 10 inches. These factors reduce the production of gastric juice or its reflux into the esophagus. Antacids (Maalox, Gelusil) are useful in neutralizing acid in the upper stomach and lower esophagus and reducing heartburn.

There is debate over the use of anticholinergic drugs, such as propantheline (Pro-Banthine) for esophagitis caused by hiatus hernia. Although the drugs reduce acid production, they relax the cardiac sphincter and may actually facilitate gastric reflux into the esophagus.

Complications Esophageal ulceration is the most frequent complication of hiatus hernia and is especially common in the rolling type. Gastritis is also common in the trapped upper portion of the stomach.

Bleeding, occasionally severe, is always a possibility in these cases, as it is with ulceration of other parts of the gastrointestinal tract.

Prognosis

Most individuals do well with conservative medical management. Surgery is needed only if intolerable symptoms or severe complications develop.

HEMORRHOIDS

Of all human ills, hemorrhoids probably cause the greatest ratio of suffering to sympathy. (That is, they may be extremely painful and uncomfortable to the sufferer, but the poor victim receives little sympathy and even mild ridicule from peers. Much better to have a cold or minor cut, for which the measure of sympathy is rather large.)

Hemorrhoids represent varicosities (bulging and weakness) of the internal hemorrhoidal veins. Approximately 5 per cent of the population is afflicted and pregnant women have an especially high incidence. In others, the incidence increases considerably above age 30.

Pathogenesis

It is likely that some individuals have an inherited tendency toward hemorrhoids, possibly due to weakness in the venous walls, just as is the case with varicose veins of the leg. In addition, etiologic factors that increase pelvic venous pressure promote hemorrhoid formation. These include pregnancy (pressure of the uterus on blood vessels), prolonged sitting (as with desk workers and truck drivers), and chronic constipation with straining. The lesions protrude beneath the thin mucosa of the rectal area. Varicosities contained within the rectum are called *internal* hemorrhoids and produce partial obstruction of the rectum. Those visible below the anal opening are referred to as *external* hemorrhoids. Commonly, both types exist together (combined hemorrhoids).

Symptoms and Signs

Bleeding, mucous discharge, and rectal discomfort and pain, especially during defecation, are common clinical findings. Discharged blood is usually bright red, since it is coming from the extreme lower portion of the digestive tract and is not altered much by exposure to air or intestinal contents. Blood from high up in the digestive tract is often dark red or black when it reaches the rectal area. Bulging of hemorrhoids to the outside during straining is also common.

Laboratory Findings

Routine laboratory tests are not generally helpful in the diagnosis of hemorrhoids, except when bleeding is present. Then, occult blood (or obvious bleeding) can be detected and the erythrocyte, hemoglobin, and hematocrit values are decreased, reflecting anemia due to blood loss. Barium enema outlines irregularities in the rectal wall caused by the bulging hemorrhoidal veins.

Sigmoidoscopy is especially useful for diagnosis, since it permits direct inspection of the lesions and allows for examination to detect ulcerative colitis or colorectal cancer at the same time. This is important, since it is common for an individual to have hemorrhoids as well as more serious intestinal disease simultaneously.

Diagnosis Ulcerative colitis, colorectal cancer, polyps of the colorectal area, and rectal fistula or abscess can produce symptoms resembling those of hemorrhoids. Sigmoidoscopy, in conjunction with barium enema, is useful for differentiating among the several conditions. Bleeding, pain, and mucous discharge should not be attributed to hemorrhoids until other, more serious conditions have been ruled out. Occasionally, hemorrhoids represent a complication of liver disease that is more commonly seen in the esophagus. (See the discussion of esophageal varices in Chapter 13.)

Treatment Most hemorrhoidal conditions do not require surgery. The use of a low-roughage diet reduces irritation to the inflamed tissues (although it may promote constipation). Mineral oil or other mild laxatives help to prevent constipation with associated straining and worsening of symptoms. Anti-inflammatory suppositories (Anusol, Preparation H) reduce pain and discomfort. Warm water (sitz) baths sooth inflamed hemorrhoidal tissue. Surgery is required for severe cases or for certain complications. Hemorrhoidectomy (removal of both internal and external hemorrhoids) is most often quite successful, although painful in the postoperative period.

Alternatives to surgical incision for hemorrhoidectomy include the use of freezing probes (cryosurgery) and the novel use of rubber bands. Rubber bands placed around the hemorrhoids will cause necrosis of the tissue as a result of ischemia and the hemorrhoids will eventually drop off with little or no bleeding.

Complications Thrombosis of blood trapped within hemorrhoids, prolapse, and strangulation occur in more severe cases. Surgery is usually eventually required for cure.

PANCREATITIS The pancreas is both an endocrine and an exocrine organ, since it secretes insulin into the blood stream (endocrine function) and pancreatic juice into the duodenum (exocrine function). Insulin is produced by *beta cells,* located in the islets of Langerhans; pancreatic juice is secreted by *acinar cells,* which make up small glands (acini) comprising the bulk of the pancreas. The most important digestive enzymes secreted in pancreatic juice are *amylase,* which digests starches, and *lipase,* which digests fats. Pancreatic juice is secreted into the pancreatic duct, which connects to the common bile duct near the sphincter of Oddi (Fig. 12–2).

Pancreatitis is seen in about 0.2 per cent of hospitalized patients. It is especially common after middle age, in alcoholics, and in those with liver or gallbladder disease. The disease is characterized by inflammation of the pancreas with escape of cellular contents of the pancreatic tissues (both insulin and pancreatic juice). Since lipase digests fats, the fatty tissue around the pancreas is usually damaged, as are portions of the normal fatty tissue of the pancreas. In severe cases, the pancreas becomes greatly damaged and necrotic.

Pathogenesis Several theories are proposed to explain the development of pancreatitis. *Bile reflux*—whereby bile backs up the pancreatic duct, damages the pancreas and allows for leakage of cellular contents— has been suggested. This may apply in certain cases of biliary obstruction. *Hypersecretion of the pancreas,* with intra-organ damage and resulting obstruction, has also been proposed. *Effects of alcohol* are also considered important, since the condition favors heavy users of alcohol. Perhaps alcohol relaxes the sphincter of Oddi and allows duodenal contents to enter the pancreas through the pancreatic duct, thus causing organ damage.

Duodenal reflux, with or without the effects of alcohol, is currently the most widely accepted etiologic factor in pancreatitis. Approximately half of the patients with acute pancreatitis develop the condition after a heavy meal or overuse of alcohol, supporting the idea that duodenal reflux initiates the disease. Since bile is released following fat intake, attacks following a heavy meal also implicate the biliary system in the development of pancreatitis. However, at least one fourth of those with acute pancreatitis have no known predisposing factor for the condition. These cases are termed idiopathic.

Acute Pancreatitis

Acute pancreatitis causes severe, sudden epigastric pain radiating to the right or left or into the back area. Indigestion, intestinal cramping, nausea, vomiting, and constipation are often seen, largely related to a lack of pancreatic juice reaching the duodenum. Malaise, prostration, and sweating are also common. Jaundice is a fairly common finding, attributed to pressure on the bile duct by the edematous adjacent pancreas causing biliary obstruction (reduced bile removal). If blood vessels in the pancreas or nearby tissue are damaged, hemorrhage and shock can result, leading to loss of consciousness and pallor.

Laboratory Findings

Leukocytosis, due to inflammation, tissue necrosis, and/or infection, is seen. Hyperglycemia, resulting from the loss of insulin normally secreted into the blood stream, is common. The normal fasting blood sugar (FBS), the value obtained after an overnight fast, is 60 to 110 mg/dl. Much higher values are seen in acute pancreatitis, since insulin destined for the blood stream leaks out of the damaged pancreatic cells and is destroyed by enzymes released from other damaged pancreatic cells. In severe cases, glucose appears in the urine (glycosuria), representing a "sugar spill" resulting from failure of the kidneys to reabsorb all the glucose that has been filtered. The blood glucose level is so high that not all filtered glucose can be reabsorbed. Usually, the blood glucose level must be over 170 mg/dl for this to happen. (See discussion of glycosuria in Chapter 16.)

The serum amylase level is also elevated (normal = 60 to 180 Somogyi units/100 ml), since amylase leaks from the damaged pancreatic cells and is absorbed into the blood stream by surrounding blood vessels instead of being secreted into the duodenum in pancreatic juice. The same situation exists with lipase (normal = 0.2 to 1.5 units/ml), and its level is increased in the blood stream.

Serum bilirubin and liver enzymes are often elevated, primarily because of bile duct obstruction caused by pressure from the swollen pancreas, as previously mentioned. (See Chapter 13 for a discussion of normal values.)

X-ray examination is not especially useful in pancreatitis, since the organ is fairly well hidden, but it may show gallstones or other factors contributing to its development.

Diagnosis   Many intra-abdominal conditions can mimic the pain and some of the laboratory findings of acute pancreatitis. Perforated ulcer, bile duct obstruction (especially at the sphincter of Oddi), acute cholecystitis (see Chapter 13), and a host of other conditions produce similar findings. It is important, however, for the physician to make an accurate diagnosis, since some of the conditions require immediate surgery to prevent complications and must be distinguished from pancreatitis, which is not generally treatable surgically.

Treatment   General treatment measures include a low-fat diet and strict avoidance of alcohol to prevent recurrence of the attack. Relief of pain with meperidine (Demerol) is welcomed during the acute attack. Antibiotic therapy is usually recommended to prevent or control infection resulting from tissue necrosis. Anticholinergic drugs, such as atropine, may help to relieve associated intestinal cramping.

Surgery is not indicated for most cases of acute pancreatitis, but it may be required to drain resulting abscesses or to debride (remove) necrotic tissue from the pancreas. Surgical investigation (laparotomy) is often performed, however, since the diagnosis is frequently in doubt.

Complications   Abscess and hemorrhage are the most common complications of acute pancreatitis. Abscesses are treated with antibiotics and by surgical drainage. Hemorrhage and the shock that sometimes results may require blood replacement and the use of plasma expanders (e.g., Dextran) or vasopressor agents such as levo-norepinephrine (Levophed). In rare cases, diabetes mellitus develops after pancreatitis because of destruction of beta cells and loss of insulin secreting capacity.

Prognosis   The rate of recurrence of acute pancreatitis is high, with resulting attacks of pain and disability. Death results from severe hemorrhage from extensive pancreatic necrosis. Respiratory distress syndrome (shock lung) sometimes develops, probably caused by destruction of surfactant material in the lung by absorbed pancreatic juice. Long-term respiratory therapy may be required in these cases.

Chronic Pancreatitis   Chronic pancreatitis is more properly called *chronic relapsing pancreatitis,* since it is a series of acute attacks resulting in progressive fibrosis and organ damage. The condition is most often seen in alcoholics and in those with certain types (I, IV, and V) of hyperlipidemia (see Chapter 10).

Symptoms and Signs   Symptoms are similar to those of acute pancreatitis. Exacerbations and remissions are the rule.

Laboratory Findings   Laboratory findings are similar to those of the acute condition during attacks, including elevated serum amylase, lipase, bilirubin, and glucose levels, along with increased liver enzyme levels in the serum.

Treatment   A low-fat diet and avoidance of alcohol, along with administration of anticholinergic drugs, are recommended. Narcotics are
avoided in pain control, since narcotic addiction develops rapidly in
the face of such chronic, severe pain. Pancreatic enzyme preparations
(Pancrease, Ilozyme) help to supplement the subnormal levels produced by the damaged organ. Surgery is useful only to drain an
abscess or to correct biliary tract disease that may be contributing
to the problem.

Complications   Chronic pain, digestive disturbances, and debility often result
from chronic pancreatitis. These can be partly alleviated but not
generally eliminated. Pancreatic abscess often occurs as it does with
acute pancreatitis. Diabetes mellitus is more common in chronic
than in acute pancreatitis and requires treatment using diet, insulin,
or oral hypoglycemic drugs. In severe diabetes resulting from pancreatitis, oral hypoglycemic drugs are ineffective, since there are
virtually no functioning beta cells remaining for the drugs to stimulate. Insulin is required in these cases.

SUMMARY

Digestion is a complex process, requiring the interaction of
enzymes, gastric acid, bile, chewing, and peristaltic action for
completion. The digestive tract, being a complicated organ system,
is prone to several types of disease process, including inflammation,
infection, and neoplastic growth.

Most common digestive disorders result from inflammation of a
portion of the digestive tract, often associated with infection as a
complicating factor. Pancreatitis, appendicitis, diverticulitis, and
ulcerative colitis are good examples. In gastric ulcer, duodenal ulcer,
or hiatus hernia, inflammation of the affected area caused by gastric
juice is the major problem. Hemorrhoids begin as varicosities of the
hemorrhoidal veins but usually become inflamed or even infected
with time.

A variety of measures are used in the treatment of digestive
disorders, including diet, drugs, surgery, and control of causative
factors such as stress. Preventive therapy is especially important in
diverticulosis to prevent worsening of the condition and the development of diverticulitis. Probably, attention to the preventive aspects
of therapy would reduce the incidence of other digestive disorders
as well.

Questions   1. How are appendicitis and diverticulitis similar? Different? Describe the
etiology, pathogenesis, clinical findings, and complications of each
disorder.
2. Compare and contrast ulcerative colitis with regional enteritis (Crohn's
disease).
3. Why is surgery performed frequently on patients with ulcerative colitis
but only occasionally on those with diverticulitis?
4. Give the function of each of the following in the process of digestion:
mucin, ptyalin, amylase, lipase, bile, histamine, gastrin, CCK.
5. Define the following terms and explain the pathophysiologic processes
involved in each case: perforation, penetration, pyloric obstruction (as
applies to gastric or duodenal ulcer).

Additional Reading   Almy, T. P., and Howell, D. A.: Diverticular disease of the colon. N. Engl. J. Med., 302:324, 1980.

Bergman, H. D.: Peptic ulcer and its management. Southern Pharmacy Journal, 69:32, 1976.

Blackwood, W. S. et al.: Prevention by bedtime cimetidine of duodenal ulcer relapse. Lancet, 1:626, 1978.

Goligher, J. C.: Cryosurgery for hemorrhoids. Dis. Colon Rectum, 19:213, 1976.

Kirsner, J. B.: Observations on the medical treatment of inflammatory bowel disease. J.A.M.A., 243:557, 1980.

Law, D. et al.: The continuing challenge of acute and perforated appendicitis. Am. J. Surg., 131:533, 1976.

CHAPTER 13

HEPATIC AND BILIARY DISORDERS

The liver is the largest and most complex organ in the body. In the adult, it weighs about 1500 gm and is composed primarily of specialized epithelial cells called *hepatocytes,* the major functional cells. In addition, fixed macrophages (Kupffer cells) line the sinusoids, or hollow spaces, within the liver (Fig. 13–1). Their action is phagocytic, and they remove particulate material from the circulating blood in a manner similar to that of an oil filter in an engine.

Blood comes to the liver from two distinct systems: the *arterial system* via the *hepatic artery,* and the *portal system* via the *portal vein* (Fig. 13–2). Arterial blood enters the liver at a rate of about 800 ml/min and contains the expected systemic elements. Portal blood comes from the vascular system surrounding the digestive tract and enters the liver at the rate of approximately 600 ml per minute. It contains food materials or drugs absorbed from the gastrointestinal tract. Some drugs are partly metabolized by initial passage through the liver via the portal system before entering the systemic circulation. This is referred to as the *first pass* effect. Perhaps the "purpose" of this arrangement is to detoxify harmful materials before exposing the general circulation (and thus the entire body) to them. Because of the dual blood supply to the liver, liver infarction is extremely uncommon. If a branch of one system is blocked, the other system can supply enough blood to prevent tissue damage. This is in contrast to the heart or brain, in which blockages of the single vascular system are common (myocardial and cerebral infarction).

The liver performs at least five major functions in humans.

Bile Production. The liver produces *bile salts,* which, with the liquid portion of the liver secretion, are called *bile.* Bile is secreted through canaliculi (small channels) into the common hepatic duct and collected by the gallbladder for storage (Fig. 13–3). Bile is released through the action of cholecystokinin (CCK), a hormone that controls gallbladder contraction as well as release of pancreatic juice (See Chapter 12).

Bilirubin Secretion. The liver secretes bilirubin, a compound formed from hemoglobin. When red blood cells die of old age (120 days or so) or are destroyed, hemoglobin leaks from the damaged cell and accumulates in the blood stream. The iron in hemoglobin is saved and recycled by the body so that only a small amount of new iron is needed daily in the diet. Most of the remainder of the hemoglobin molecule is converted to bilirubin, an intensely yellow

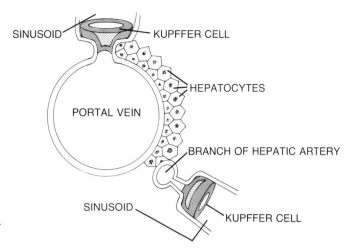

Figure 13–1. Histology of normal liver tissue.

compound. The liver conjugates (combines) bilirubin with glucuronide to form *conjugated bilirubin,* which is water-soluble and hence easily removed from the body via renal excretion. Bilirubin is excreted in the bile into the duodenum and adds a yellowish color to fecal material.

If bilirubin accumulates faster than the liver can conjugate it, the serum level increases *(hyperbilirubinemia)* and a yellow hue appears to body tissues (icterus or *jaundice*). The skin and sclera of the eye are especially affected by jaundice. Extremely high levels of bilirubin in the blood stream lead to entry into the brain, with resulting brain damage (kernicterus), especially in infants. This occurs when there is massive red blood cell destruction, as in the case with Rh factor incompatibility between mother and fetus (erythroblastosis fetalis). Liver disease or biliary obstruction can also cause jaundice. In these cases, normal amounts of bilirubin are not conjugated (liver disease) or removed (liver disease or biliary obstruction) from the body.

Detoxification. A third important activity of the liver is metabolism of drugs and other compounds for the purpose of detoxification. Were it not for this function, most drugs would stay in their original form in the body. Their effects would be exaggerated, and removal from the body might be difficult. For example, ethyl alcohol is converted to acetaldehyde and then to acetic acid largely by liver

Figure 13–2. Blood supply to liver.

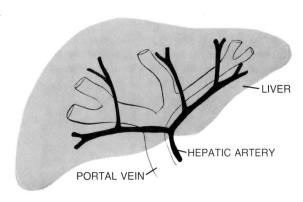

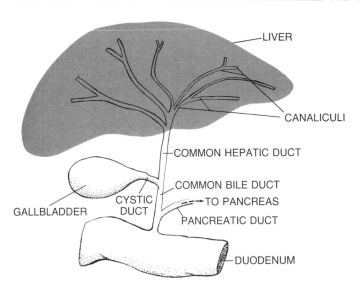

Figure 13–3. Biliary system.

action. In addition, part of the ethyl alcohol is also conjugated with glucuronide for easier removal from the body. Interestingly, some drugs are excreted to a significant degree in the bile. Examples are erythromycin estolate (Ilosone) and most tetracyclines (e.g., Achromycin). An important finding in liver disease is failure to metabolize or detoxify drugs, a process called *biotransformation.*

Protein Synthesis. By this activity, amino acids are combined to form various types of body proteins. Not only are structural proteins formed; albumins and lipoproteins are also made through liver action. In liver disease, this ability decreases and complications result. Chronic liver disease often results in *wasting,* which is due to inadequate protein synthesis and muscle atrophy. Reduced albumin level in the blood stream leads to loss of serum oncotic pressure (which holds water in the capillaries) and is partly responsible for the edema (ascites) that develops in hepatic cirrhosis (see Chapters 3 and 7). Failure to form lipoproteins, even in acute liver disease, can lead to accumulation of fat in the liver (fatty liver), since fat must be removed in the form of lipoproteins. Many blood-clotting factors are globulins, another type of protein, and require hepatic synthesis. Chronic liver disease, therefore, often leads to impaired blood coagulation and bleeding tendencies.

Conversion of Nitrogenous Waste. The liver metabolizes nitrogenous waste products (primarily ammonia) formed by protein breakdown or normal cell destruction. Ammonia is converted by the liver to *urea,* which is removed by kidney action. Failure of the liver to convert ammonia to urea results in accumulation of ammonia in the blood stream, whereas failure of the kidney to remove urea results in an increased blood urea nitrogen (BUN) level (see Chapter 11). A special problem arises in cirrhosis of the liver associated with bleeding into the digestive tract from dilated and broken down veins in the esophagus (esophageal varices). Blood is acted upon by bacteria in the colon and its proteins are metabolized, resulting in the formation of ammonia. Ammonia is absorbed through the intestinal wall and enters the blood stream. The damaged liver fails to convert all of the ammonia to urea, and the level of ammonia in the blood stream increases, leading to central nervous system malfunction.

The gallbladder functions as a storage vessel for bile so that larger amounts can be released following a large or fatty meal to aid digestion. It is an outgrowth of the common bile duct (Fig. 13–3) and is a popular site for stone formation.

The major disease processes affecting the liver and gallbladder are inflammation, infection, and neoplastic disease. Malignancy of the liver is uncommon, except as a metastatic site for other tumors. Gallbladder cancer is occasionally seen, especially in a bladder filled with gallstones, and often leads to biliary obstruction. This form of cancer has usually metastasized to the liver by the time it is diagnosed and, therefore, results of treatment are generally poor.

LIVER AND GALLBLADDER TESTS

In addition to tests of *serum albumin* and *prothrombin* levels, which indirectly measure liver synthetic functions, several other tests are used to measure hepatic function or to assess the amount of liver damage.

Total Serum Bilirubin Level. This test measures the concentration of conjugated and unconjugated bilirubin in the bloodstream. The normal value is 0.1 to 1 mg/dl, and the ratio of unconjugated to conjugated bilirubin is approximately 2:1. Jaundice develops when the liver fails to conjugate bilirubin or when red blood cells are broken down faster than the liver can conjugate the resulting formed bilirubin. The jaundice is thus caused primarily by accumulation of *unconjugated* bilirubin. Decreased *conjugated* bilirubin levels result from impaired conjugative ability as a result of liver damage or biliary tract obstruction that causes liver damage.

BSP Retention. Bromsulphalein (BSP) is primarily excreted via the biliary system and is used to measure the excretory capacity of the liver. In normal individuals, there is 0 to 5 per cent of the dye remaining in the blood stream 45 minutes after intravenous administration. *BSP retention* is increased in most types of liver disease (e.g., hepatitis, cirrhosis). Allergic reactions to BSP, unfortunately, have limited the use of the test in recent years.

Enzymes. The liver cells contain three enzymes that are normally present in the serum in small amounts but that leak out of damaged liver cells, resulting in increased serum levels. Lactic dehydrogenase (LDH), glutamic-oxaloacetic transaminase (GOT),* and glutamic-pyruvic transaminase (GPT)† normally have low levels in the serum (SLDH = 0 to 300 ImU/ml; SGOT = 0 to 15 ImU/ml; SGPT = 0 to 15 ImU/ml). The serum levels of these rise in proportion to liver cell damage and serve as a diagnostic tool for liver disease. It should be pointed out that LDH and GOT are present in other tissues, notably the heart, and high serum levels could reflect cardiac as well as hepatic damage. Glutamic-pyruvic transaminase is found primarily in the liver, and increased SGPT is thus a more specific indicator of liver damage than the other two values. In all cases, though, the enzyme changes should be correlated with other clinical findings to establish a diagnosis.

---

*Also called aspartate aminotransferase (AST).
†Also called alanine aminotransferase (ALT).

Urobilinogen. A compound formed from bilirubin, urobilinogen is excreted primarily in the stool with a small percentage excreted in the urine (normal = 0.1 to 1 Erlich unit/dl). Impaired liver function causes reduced excretion in the stool and increased urinary urobilinogen excretion. The test reflects early, minimal impairment in liver function and is therefore quite useful if other clinical findings or laboratory tests are inconclusive.

Liver Biopsy. This test is helpful in the differential diagnosis of difficult cases, permitting distinction to be made between cirrhosis of the liver and the various forms of hepatitis. It also gives information as to progress in the healing of damaged areas of the liver. A large-bore needle is inserted through the lower rib cage, after local anesthesia, and a "core sample" of liver tissue is removed for study.

X-ray Exam. The gallbladder can often be visualized on x-ray examination, especially if it contains opaque stone material. However, visualization is better if a dye is given to outline the gallbladder contents. Calcium or sodium ipodate (Oragrafin) given orally is excreted in the bile and will outline the gallbladder and its contents on x-ray film (cholecystography) and aid in the diagnosis of gallbladder disease.

Ultrasound Examination. This technique pictures the gallbladder in a manner similar to x-ray films and is also useful.

Alkaline Phosphatase. An enzyme excreted through the biliary system, alkaline phosphatase has a normal serum level of 2 to 5 Bodansky units per liter. Biliary obstruction prevents removal of the enzyme and increases the serum level. The test is useful in distinguishing obstructions of the biliary tract from primary liver disease. This is helpful, since liver damage (biliary cirrhosis) results from prolonged obstruction of the bile duct or its tributaries and can be prevented by surgical removal of the obstruction. Hepatic cirrhosis, which would give similar clinical findings but a normal serum alkaline phosphatase value, is not surgically treatable. This test would thus differentiate conditions requiring immediate surgery from those in which surgery was not indicated.

THE LIVER

HEPATITIS

Inflammation of the liver is termed hepatitis. The term does not suggest a cause for the disorder, and there are several possibilities.

Pathogenesis

The two most common causes of hepatitis are viral infection and exposure to hepatotoxic agents. A similar type of liver damage occurs in both situations. Likewise, the clinical manifestations of acute hepatitis are similar, regardless of cause, and include jaundice, enlarged liver (hepatomegaly), liver tenderness, fever, nausea, and vomiting. Hepatomegaly results from swollen hepatocytes and from the edema caused by acute inflammation of the organ (Fig. 13–4). Jaundice is caused by impaired conjugation and removal of bilirubin. Fever results from infection and/or the consequences of hepatic cell necrosis. Other findings include loss of appetite and a peculiar aversion to smoking. The cause of these symptoms is not clear but

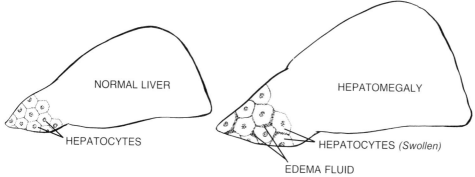

Figure 13-4. Hepatomegaly.

may be related to alteration in the sense of taste, perhaps due to accumulation of unmetabolized compounds affecting the taste buds.

Hepatitis progresses through three stages. In the *prodromal* stage, infection or cell damage is developing and clinical symptoms and signs consist of malaise, sore throat, nausea and other nonspecific findings. Mild abdominal pain may be present. Symptomatology is most noticeable during the *icteric* stage, especially jaundice and hepatomegaly. Recovery occurs during the *convalescent* stage. Occasionally, the disease increases dramatically in severity, this is called *fulminant* hepatitis. Fulminant hepatitis is difficult to treat and often leads to cirrhosis and liver failure.

At least three types of hepatitis are caused by viral infection. *Hepatitis A* ("infectious" hepatitis) and *hepatitis B* ("serum" hepatitis) are caused by different viruses and can be detected by the presence of viral antigen in the blood of an infected individual. A third distinct type (non-A, non-B) is now recognized. It is diagnosed at present by failure to find A or B antigen after testing.

Several types of hepatitis are caused by exposure to toxic drugs or chemicals. These can be termed *toxic hepatitis*. Alcohol, solvents, and certain legitimate drug products can cause liver cell injury that leads to hepatitis.

Hepatitis A

Hepatitis A is caused by a ribonucleic acid (RNA) virus. It is generally spread by oral contact, but occasionally it is transmitted via feces or transfusion of blood. Water contaminated with human fecal material is a likely source of infection, particularly in developing countries. Contact with animals is not a likely source of infection, since only marmoset monkeys and chimpanzees develop the disease. The incubation period for hepatitis A in humans is usually 30 to 40 days.

Hepatitis A is most common in children and in those living under crowded conditions. Outbreaks occur in military camps, dormitories, and other areas involving close personal contact. Chronic virus carriers do not seem to exist, and acquisition by blood transfusion is thus uncommon, since those with active disease would be excluded from blood donation. Approximately one fourth of the United States population carries antibodies to hepatitis A virus, suggesting prior exposure to the organism. In some countries in which the incidence of hepatitis A is high, 80 to 90 per cent of the population are antibody carriers. Reinfection is unlikely, since the antibody response to initial infection is excellent.

Laboratory Findings

The leukocyte count is normal or slightly lower than normal in hepatitis A. Serum levels of LDH, GOT, and GPT are elevated, reflecting necrosis of some hepatocytes; SGPT is usually greater than SGOT, in contrast to hepatic cirrhosis, in which SGOT is generally greater than SGPT. Hyperbilirubinemia is commonly seen, reflecting impaired conjugation and removal of bilirubin by the liver. Likewise, urinary urobilinogen level is also increased (hyperurobilinogenuria). Liver biopsy shows hepatocellular necrosis, with swollen hepatocytes and invasion of neutrophils to remove necrotic cells.

Diagnosis

Mononucleosis, hepatic cirrhosis, and other forms of hepatitis are the major diagnostic considerations. Mononucleosis can be detected with a special test (spot test). The other conditions can be differentiated through a combination of history and specialized laboratory tests. Influenza and drug-induced liver disease can duplicate many of the symptoms of hepatitis A.

Treatment

Bed rest, avoidance of alcohol or other drugs that affect the liver, and the use of a low-fat diet are important in providing optimal conditions for full recovery. A low-fat diet is recommended to avoid accumulation of fat in the liver, since hepatic synthesis of protein (and thus lipoprotein) may be impaired. (See the previous discussion of fat removal from the liver.) Alcohol or other drugs that could damage the liver or that require hepatic metabolism should be avoided to reduce the chance of further liver injury. Many drugs (e.g., narcotics) require liver metabolism and will produce a prolonged or exaggerated effect if metabolic functions of the liver are impaired.

Complications

Recovery from hepatitis A is usually complete in 1 to 4 months. Repeated liver enzyme, serum bilirubin, and urinary urobilinogen measurements and related studies monitor healing of liver damage. Normalization of these tests generally parallels clinical improvement, although abnormal values may occasionally be seen for 6 to 12 months. The major complications are the development of *fatty liver* (Fig. 13–5) and continuation of hepatitis in chronic form. Fatty liver often resolves with time in the absence of continuing liver injury.

Chronic active hepatitis, a complication of *acute hepatitis,* often leads eventually to hepatic cirrhosis and liver failure. It can be treated with corticosteroids (e.g., prednisone) or immunosuppressive drugs (e.g., azathioprine [Imuran]) but usually becomes progressively worse with time.

Hepatitis B

Hepatitis B is caused by a deoxyribonucleic acid (DNA) virus, sometimes referred to as a Dane particle. It is transmitted primarily by needles, including those used for blood transfusion, drug administration, tattooing, or acupuncture. Patients receiving blood products or those abusing intravenous drugs have a high incidence of hepatitis B. The virus can also be spread through oral or sexual contact or occasionally via the feces. Symptoms of hepatitis B are similar to those of hepatitis A but often develop more slowly.

The incubation period for hepatitis B is 2 to 6 months. In contrast to hepatitis A, 5 to 10 per cent of infected people become carriers and are therefore a potential source of further spread of the

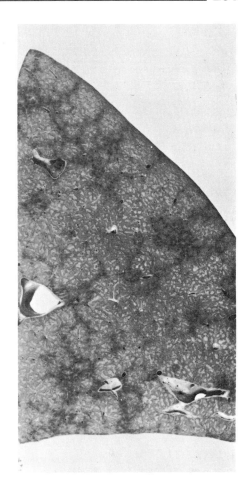

Figure 13–5. Fatty liver. (From Robbins, S. L., and Cotran, R. S.: *Pathologic Basis of Disease,* 2nd ed. Philadelphia, W. B. Saunders Company, 1979.)

disease. Hepatitis B is often a more serious infection than hepatitis A, and fulminant hepatitis or chronic hepatitis develops more frequently as a complication, sometimes leading to death. Severe chronic hepatitis may lead to kidney damage caused by toxic effects of large amounts of bilirubin excreted by the kidney (hepatorenal syndrome). The damaged kidney then fails to remove urea and uremia develops.

Laboratory Findings

Elevated SLDH, SGOT, and SGPT are seen in hepatitis B, as in hepatitis A, as are hyperbilirubinemia and hyperurobilinogenuria. The leukocyte count is normal or slightly lower than normal. As with hepatitis A, a characteristic antigen-antibody reaction identifies the type of hepatitis. The hepatitis B antigen is sometimes called *Australia antigen,* since it was originally identified in the serum of an Australian aborigine.

Diagnosis

Diagnosis is based upon the laboratory tests described, plus a history of transfusion or other potential serum to serum contact a few months before the onset of symptoms.

Treatment and Prevention

The same principles of treatment apply with hepatitis B as with hepatitis A and include bed rest, a low-fat diet, and avoidance of alcohol or other drugs affecting the liver. Unless fulminant or chronic hepatitis develops, full recovery is the rule. Recovery can be followed with the normalization of laboratory tests and improvement in symptoms.

A new vaccine (Heptavax B) is available for the prevention of hepatitis B in high-risk people. It is primarily designed for patients or personnel involved in hemodialysis, institutionalized patients, or those who have been in contact with active hepatitis B patients. The vaccine is made from human serum and given in a series of three injections. Protection is thought to last for 5 years and can be extended with booster doses. Other preventive measures include disinfection of contaminated materials, careful handwashing after contact with an infected individual, and the use of gamma globulin injections in those thought to have been exposed to the hepatitis B virus. Hepatitis B immune globulin is also available for those with heavy exposure to the virus and is effective if used within 10 days after exposure. The use of disposable syringes, needles, and other equipment has helped a great deal to avoid spread of the disease.

Hepatitis non-A, non-B

Hepatitis in which neither A nor B antigen can be detected is now recognized. Probably, there are at least two different types of non-A, non-B hepatitis (also sometimes called hepatitis C). In some studies, 90 per cent of the cases of post-transfusion hepatitis were of the non-A, non-B type. In addition, carriers of non-A, non-B have been identified. The incubation period is from 2 to 20 weeks, overlapping that of both hepatitis A and B. Clinical signs and symptoms and most laboratory findings are identical to those of hepatitis A or B. The only practical way to avoid non-A, non-B hepatitis at present is to use only blood donors who are known to be free of liver disease. It is hoped that a specific serologic test for the disease will be developed in the near future.

Alcoholic Hepatitis

Alcoholic hepatitis is a subgroup of the category of toxic hepatitis, but it occurs frequently enough to be considered a group of its own. Prolonged, heavy exposure to alcohol damages the hepatocytes, leading to inflammation and necrosis. Although complete recovery is possible, 50 per cent of cases develop permanent fibrosis associated with attempted regeneration of the liver cells. Infiltration of hyaline material into hepatocytes (alcoholic hyaline) is also common and serves as a histologic marker for the condition. Approximately 10 per cent die from acute liver failure as a complication of alcoholic hepatitis.

Approximately one third of heavy drinkers develop alcoholic hepatitis; and the incidence is greater among female than male alcoholics, for unknown reasons. Periods of 1 to 15 years of heavy drinking are usually required, and most develop the condition after about 5 years of chronic alcoholism. The acute condition often follows a recent binge, but chronic, steady consumption of smaller amounts can also cause it even if the individual does not drink enough to be obviously intoxicated. It seems that the liver, in this case, does not have the opportunity to recover from the toxic effects of chronic alcohol administration.

Alcoholic hepatitis is considered a step toward hepatic cirrhosis and often fuses into cirrhosis with continued alcohol exposure. The liver is enlarged, and the usual symptoms of hepatitis are present, often with the added features of neurologic damage associated with alcoholism. Poor diet and resulting vitamin deficiency probably play some role in promoting liver injury and may impair recovery.

Laboratory Findings   Laboratory findings are similar to those with other types of hepatitis. However, leukocytosis, thrombocytopenia, and elevated serum alkaline phosphatase levels are seen fairly often, probably reflecting more extensive hepatic necrosis than with other types of hepatitis.

Treatment and   The treatment of alcoholic hepatitis is similar to that of the
Complications   other types of hepatitis, especially emphasizing total avoidance of alcohol. Vitamin supplements, especially folic acid and thiamine (vitamin B-1), promote maximum possible recovery of damaged liver tissue.

Mild cases of alcoholic hepatitis usually resolve completely. Most cases of severe disease, however, progress inexorably toward cirrhosis, in spite of optimum treatment.

Other Toxic Forms of   Besides alcohol, a number of other drugs are occasionally
Hepatitis   associated with the development of hepatitis. Acetaminophen (Tylenol) can cause hepatitis after heavy exposure, as in a childhood overingestion. Solvents such as chloroform or carbon tetrachloride or those contained in abused chemical substances (e.g., glue sniffing) are associated with hepatitis. In these cases, the severity and duration of exposure are correlated strongly with the risk of developing the condition. Other drugs, including isoniazid (INH) and halothane (Fluothane), can cause hepatitis, but the disease is not correlated with severity or duration of exposure. The term *idiosyncrasy* (unusual reaction) describes this situation. Prior exposure to the offending drug may be necessary for sensitization, after which even small amounts trigger off disease development. With halothane, for example, only two anesthetizations, close together, may be necessary for the development of hepatitis. Still other drugs can cause a blockage of bile flow (cholestasis) by inflaming the bile canaliculi within the liver. These include erythromycin estolate (Ilosone), most phenothiazines (e.g., Thorazine), and some sulfonamides (e.g., sulfadiazine). Retention of bile within the liver for long periods of time leads to necrosis of hepatocytes and hepatitis.

Treatment and   The treatment of toxic hepatitis consists of removal of the toxic
Complications   agent and provision of conditions optimal for liver regeneration. As with other forms of hepatitis, some cases resolve completely, some become fulminant, and some become chronic with the likelihood of progression into cirrhosis.

HEPATIC CIRRHOSIS   The term cirrhosis derives from the Greek words *kirrhos* (yellow) and *sklerosis* (hardening). It describes a condition in which the liver hardens and shrinks and develops a yellowish color as a result of accumulation of fat.

Pathogenesis   The histologic picture of hepatic cirrhosis shows hepatocyte destruction with replacement of destroyed cells with regenerating liver cells and fibrous tissue. Characteristically, bands of fibrous

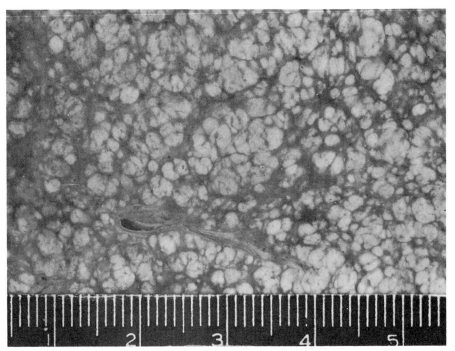

Figure 13-6. Nodule formation in hepatic cirrhosis. (From Robbins, S. L., and Cotran, R. S.: *Pathologic Basis of Disease,* 2nd ed. Philadelphia, W. B. Saunders Company, 1979.)

tissue are formed that disrupt the normal cell configuration and the regenerating cells form *nodules*. In alcohol-induced cirrhosis, the nodules are usually small (micronodules), while in cirrhosis caused by long-term infection or other injury, they are commonly large (macronodules). Often, a mixed nodular pattern is seen (Fig. 13–6).

Hepatic cirrhosis is generally the end stage of all chronic liver conditions, since it represents attempted healing of the liver under adverse conditions such as alcoholism and chronic infection. Often, the condition is multifactorial, with infection or malnutrition superimposed upon existing alcoholic liver disease. It is a common sequel to chronic hepatitis from any cause. Although alcoholism and chronic infection are common causes, rarer conditions, such as Wilson's disease (excessive deposition of copper in the liver and other body tissues) and hemochromatosis (excessive deposition of hemosiderin in the liver and other body tissues), can also cause hepatic cirrhosis. It is occasionally idiopathic as well.

Symptoms and Signs

The symptoms and signs of hepatic cirrhosis can generally be attributed to two major problems (Table 13–1). The first is the failure of the damaged liver to perform its usual functions concerning the metabolism of numerous chemical compounds or synthesis of body compounds:

1. Failure to metabolize estrogen leads to *amenorrhea* in females and *impotence* and *gynecomastia* (breast enlargement) in males, caused by the effects of increased estrogen levels. High estrogen levels are also associated with redness of the palms (palmar erythema) and breakdown of small surface blood vessels causing asterisk-shaped lesions (spider nevi).

Table 13–1. SYMPTOMS AND SIGNS OF HEPATIC CIRRHOSIS

Problems Related to Metabolic and Synthetic Failure of the Liver	Problems Related to Hardening and Shrinking of the Liver
Amenorrhea	Portal hypertension
Impotence	Esophageal varices
Gynecomastia	Hematemesis
Palmar erythema	Ascites
Spider nevi	Increased blood protein for bacterial
Reduced albumin synthesis	decomposition (caused by
Reduced clotting factor synthesis	esophageal bleeding)
Jaundice	
Increased serum ammonia level	

2. Failure of the liver to break down aldosterone is thought to be associated with the development of the edema seen in cirrhosis.

3. Reduced albumin synthesis by the damaged liver favors loss of serum water (reduced oncotic pressure) and also results in edema.

4. Reduced synthesis of clotting factors leads to increased bleeding tendencies, easy bruising, and petechial hemorrhages on body surfaces.

5. Jaundice, caused by accumulation of bilirubin, reflects failure of the liver to conjugate bilirubin with glucuronide.

6. Change in intestinal activity (constipation or diarrhea) is partly related to reduced bile secretion by the damaged liver.

7. Increased serum ammonia levels seen in late stage cirrhosis result from failure of the liver to convert ammonia to urea, which can be excreted by the kidneys.

The second problem concerns the shrinking and hardening that occur during the cirrhotic process; these events are detectable by physical examination. Shrinkage of the liver compresses veins in the portal system and causes portal obstruction and increased portal pressure (portal hypertension) (Fig. 13–7). This leads to dilation of veins in the esophagus (esophageal varices) and upper stomach (occasionally in the lower intestinal tract) that drain through the portal system. The situation is analogous to that of varicose veins in the leg. Owing to the close proximity of esophageal veins to the surface, varices frequently break down and bleed into the esophagus.

Figure 13–7. Portal hypertension.

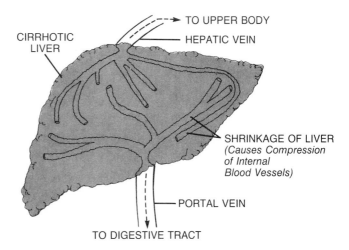

This results in *hematemesis* (vomiting of blood) and eventual decomposition of blood proteins by intestinal bacteria, forming excessive amounts of ammonia. The ammonia is absorbed into the blood stream, causing increased blood ammonia levels, as previously described. Increased portal pressure forces lymph fluid from the liver, causing *ascites* (abdominal edema). This is worsened by the associated hyperaldosteronism and hypoalbuminemia often seen in hepatic cirrhosis.

In addition to these symptoms, the individual with hepatic cirrhosis also usually suffers from weakness, malaise, loss of weight, nausea, and vomiting, possibly related to impaired digestive processes associated with liver failure. These symptoms, along with the more serious ones (hematemesis, jaundice or ascites) cause the person to seek medical attention.

Laboratory Findings   Elevated SLDH, SGOT, and SGPT reflect liver cell damage. Usually SGOT is higher than SGPT, in contrast with the findings in hepatitis. The serum bilirubin level is increased, and the albumin level is decreased (normal = 3.5 to 5.5 gm/dl). Blood-clotting ability, especially prothrombin activity, is decreased. Anemia is often seen as a result of the combined effects of esophageal bleeding, reduced clotting ability, and reduced erythrocyte formation (direct effect of alcohol). Increased BSP retention is a common finding. Liver biopsy shows histologic changes typical of cirrhosis with fibrosis, scarring, and nodule formation. Direct observation with a lighted tube inserted through the peritoneal wall (peritoneoscopy) reveals a shrunken, nodular liver.

Diagnosis   With the pertinent laboratory information plus a history of alcohol abuse or other long-term damage to the liver, the diagnosis of hepatic cirrhosis is usually not difficult. *Hepatitis* causes somewhat similar laboratory findings but is considered a potentially reversible condition. The transition from chronic hepatitis to hepatic cirrhosis is by no means clear-cut. *Biliary cirrhosis,* caused by obstruction in the biliary tract (stone, constriction, tumor) is similar to hepatic cirrhosis, but it is potentially treatable, even curable in some cases, with surgery. Cirrhosis results from the effects of bile retained by the liver as a result of the obstruction.

Treatment   Treatment of hepatic cirrhosis is multifaceted and often disappointing, since irreversible organ damage has frequently occurred prior to diagnosis. Bed rest, low-fat diet, and avoidance of alcohol, as with hepatitis, give the liver maximum help in regeneration, as do vitamin supplements. Vitamin K is helpful in promoting improved clotting factor synthesis. A low-sodium diet is prescribed if severe ascites is present, and a low-protein diet is favored if there is excessive ammonia retention. Measures to reduce esophageal bleeding include the use of vasopressin (Pitressin), which constricts blood vessels, and an expandable tube inserted into the esophagus to exert pressure on bleeding vessels. Iron supplements and/or blood transfusions are often necessary to control anemia.

Diuretics reduce the quantity of ascitic fluid, as does direct abdominal tap. Spironolactone (Aldactone) is often a diuretic of choice, since it inhibits the effect of excessive aldosterone, one cause of ascites. Other diuretics, such as furosemide (Lasix), are also useful for sodium removal. Electrolytes should be monitored frequently to chart the response to diuretic therapy.

Complications   The major complication of hepatic cirrhosis, in addition to blood loss and the respiratory difficulty caused by accumulation of ascitic fluid in the abdominal cavity, consists of absorption of ammonia formed by bacterial decomposition of protein in the intestine. Bleeding esophageal varices permit blood to enter the lower intestinal tract, where blood proteins are broken down. In the cirrhotic state, the liver is not able to convert the ammonia so formed into urea for urinary excretion and ammonia accumulates in the blood stream. High levels of ammonia cause brain malfunction (hepatic encephalopathy), including flapping tremors, aggressive behavior, and, finally, coma and death.

Attempts to lower the serum ammonia level and control hepatic encephalopathy are only partly successful. A low-protein diet and control of esophageal bleeding, if possible, will reduce the quantity of protein available for decomposition into ammonia. Sterilization of the intestinal tract with neomycin inhibits bacterial action but causes renal toxicity over long periods of treatment. A newer approach involves the use of lactulose (Cephular), a polysaccharide that breaks down under bacterial action to form nonabsorbable fragments that lower the pH in the intestine. This favors reduced ammonia absorption and a shift of ammonia from the blood stream across the intestinal membrane into the lumen. Lactulose also has a laxative effect, which removes ammonia in the feces in the form of ammonium ion (NH_4^+). Note that neomycin and lactulose should not be used together, since bacterial action is necessary for the breakdown of lactulose and its eventual effect.

Primary carcinoma of the liver is rare, but it usually occurs in a cirrhotic liver (5 per cent become malignant) and is therefore a potential complication of hepatic cirrhosis.

Prognosis   The outcome of hepatic cirrhosis depends upon the severity of the condition and whether alcohol or other hepatotoxins are strictly eliminated. In mild cases, the liver continues to function in spite of significant cellular damage. Severe cases with ascites, hematemesis, or jaundice have a 5-year survival rate of only about 35 per cent.

THE GALLBLADDER

CHOLECYSTITIS   Gallbladder inflammation (cholecystitis) can be acute or chronic. In over 90 per cent of the cases, cholelithiasis (presence of stones in gallbladder) is the cause of gallbladder inflammation, with bile duct abnormalities and pancreatitis being less common causes. Gallstones are of three types: cholesterol stones, calcium bicarbonate stones, and mixed stones containing cholesterol, calcium salts, and bile salts (Fig. 13–8).

Approximately 10 per cent of males and 20 per cent of females aged 55 to 65 in the United States have cholelithiasis, with the

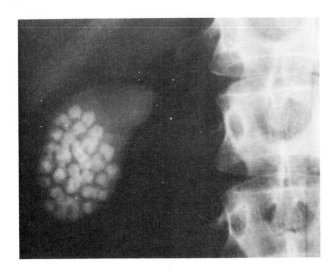

Figure 13–8. Mixed gallstones. (© 1973, Carroll H. Weiss, RBP, Camera M.D. Studios, Fort Lauderdale, Fla. Used with permission.)

highest incidence among Pima Indian women (70 per cent). Whites are more commonly affected than blacks, although blacks with sickle cell disease often develop calcium bilirubinate stones from red blood cell hemolysis. (See the discussion on sickle cell anemia in Chapter 20.)

Factors such as hypercholesterolemia, gallbladder infection, or impaired bile flow favor stone formation. Some people apparently form a bile that is deficient in bile salts necessary for solubilization of cholesterol, and cholelithiasis results. The condition favors middle-aged females who are overweight. The stools contain undigested fat, which makes them float in water and gives them a rancid odor.

Pathogenesis   Many people with cholelithiasis do not develop symptoms of cholecystitis; these people are said to have *silent gallstones*. There is argument as to whether to remove the gallbladder (cholecystectomy) in these individuals. They may never develop cholecystitis. However, their chances are greater than in those without cholelithiasis. If they do develop cholecystitis, it may be at a time when they are much older and in poorer physical condition, thus making the operation riskier. Also, there is some increased risk of gallbladder cancer if stones are retained for long periods of time. If symptoms of acute cholecystitis develop, cholecystectomy is usually warranted.

Acute cholecystitis develops when a gallstone blocks the outflow of bile from the gallbladder by impacting somewhere in the biliary system (Fig. 13–9). Continued secretion of bile into the gallbladder or inflammation behind the stone causes distention of the gallbladder and ischemia, resulting in infarction, necrosis, and infection of the organ. If the stone obstruction is in the vicinity of the sphincter of Oddi, reflux of bile into the pancreas can occur, causing secondary pancreatitis. Liver damage may result if bile is retained long enough without relief of the obstruction (biliary cirrhosis).

Acute Cholecystitis   Typical symptoms of acute cholecystitis include right upper quadrant pain (biliary colic) in the vicinity of the gallbladder, nausea and vomiting, fever, and jaundice. Fever is caused by inflammation and/or associated infection of the gallbladder. Jaundice results from

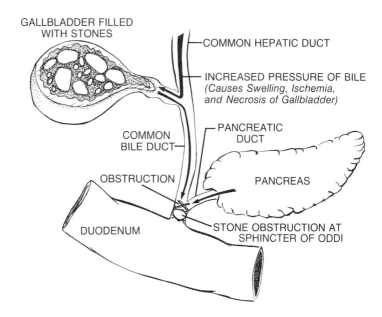

GALLBLADDER FILLED
WITH STONES

COMMON HEPATIC DUCT

INCREASED PRESSURE OF BILE
*(Causes Swelling, Ischemia,
and Necrosis of Gallbladder)*

COMMON
BILE DUCT

PANCREATIC
DUCT

OBSTRUCTION

PANCREAS

DUODENUM

STONE OBSTRUCTION AT
SPHINCTER OF ODDI

Figure 13–9. Acute cholecystitis.

impaired outflow of bile from the liver through the common bile duct. Abdominal tenderness and muscle rigidity are common clinical findings, resulting from the inflammatory reaction in the gallbladder. The distended gallbladder may be palpable during physical examination. The acute attack usually occurs after a heavy meal containing a large amount of fat, since this produces a strong demand for gallbladder contraction and results in a stone becoming dislodged into the duct system.

Laboratory Findings   Leukocytosis and hyperbilirubinemia are usually present. Elevated SGOT, SGPT, and SLDH are commonly seen, reflecting liver cell damage caused by retained bile. X-ray examination of the gallbladder area may show opacities attributable to the presence of stones. Cholesterol stones are translucent, but bile- or calcium-containing stones are more opaque to x-rays. Cholecystography, using Oragrafin, or ultrasound examination of the gallbladder is helpful in diagnosis.

Diagnosis   A number of conditions also cause upper abdominal pain and can be confused with acute cholecystitis. Pancreatitis, perforated ulcer, and hepatitis are good examples. Perforated ulcer can be detected with an upper GI series. Both pancreatitis and hepatitis cause laboratory findings that overlap with those of acute cholecystitis and are therefore hard to exclude. Good localization of pain in the right upper quadrant, along with positive cholecystography findings, strongly favors acute cholecystitis.

Treatment   A waiting period of 12 to 18 hours is usually justified, since many cases improve spontaneously without surgery. Intravenous feeding (usually glucose solution) avoids the need for digestion, which causes gallbladder contraction and worsening of symptoms. Analgesic drugs help to relieve the associated pain. Morphine and meperidine (Demerol) are contraindicated because they can cause spasm of the sphincter of Oddi and may worsen stone impaction.

Pentazocine (Talwin) is the preferred drug for pain relief. Antibiotics are often used to prevent or treat infection resulting from gallbladder ischemia and necrosis. If spontaneous improvement does not occur, especially if signs of infection or perforation develop, cholecystectomy is performed. The gallbladder is removed and the remaining cystic duct stump is ligated after removing all stones from the biliary tract. Operative mortality is less than 1 per cent.

Cholesterol stones can sometimes be dissolved with the use of oral deoxycholic acid. The process takes 1 to 2 years and must be continued indefinitely to be successful. It is a good alternative to surgery for poor-risk patients with only cholesterol stones.

Complications

Perforation with abdominal abscess or peritonitis can result, as with appendicitis, requiring intensive antibiotic treatment. Chronic cholecystitis results from repeated acute attacks.

Prognosis

Cholecystectomy is curative, and the prognosis following successful surgery is excellent. Without surgery, symptoms may return and worsen with each successive attack of acute cholecystitis.

Chronic Cholecystitis

Persistent inflammation of the gallbladder results in repeated attacks of cholecystitis and tissue changes suggestive of chronic inflammation. The gallbladder usually contains stones and is fibrotic and enlarged. Gallbladder function is impaired, and the organ may be poorly visualized by cholangiography.

Symptoms include attacks of right upper quadrant pain associated with a variety of digestive disturbances, including flatulence, belching, and intolerance to fat. Some individuals with chronic cholecystitis benefit from a low-fat diet, bile salts, and the use of antacids and anticholinergic medication. In some cases, surgery is eventually necessary to relieve symptoms.

SUMMARY

Hepatic and biliary disorders result from a variety of causes, including infection, toxicity of drugs or chemicals, and mechanical obstruction of the biliary tract. The symptoms, laboratory findings, and complications associated with the various types of acute hepatitis are similar, as is the treatment. The outcome varies, however, with some cases resolving completely and others progressing to chronic hepatitis and, eventually, to hepatic cirrhosis. Hepatic cirrhosis represents the end stage of most liver diseases, but it is not invariably fatal if progression of the liver damage can be halted. Treatment of hepatic cirrhosis involves attention to the many physiologic derangements occurring with the loss of both circulatory and metabolic functions in liver failure.

Cholecystitis usually results from cholelithiasis and is primarily an obstructive disorder of the biliary tract. Although diet and drug therapy may be helpful for treatment, surgery provides a cure for the problem.

Questions
1. Occasionally, in a newborn infant, there is failure of development of the biliary system (biliary atresia). Describe the consequences of this regarding the liver and the body in general.
2. The liver is well endowed, with a dual circulation, a bypass system for drug or chemical metabolism, and excellent regenerative capacity. Explain how this endowment was especially helpful to primitive man.
3. Explain, on a histologic basis, why acute hepatitis usually resolves completely while hepatic cirrhosis does not.
4. Compare and contrast hepatic cirrhosis and biliary cirrhosis as to cause, symptoms, laboratory findings, and treatment.
5. Hepatic diseases, cholecystitis, and pancreatitis have much in common regarding symptoms, laboratory findings and treatment. Explain how pancreatitis can be the *result* of cholecystitis and biliary cirrhosis can be the *result* of pancreatitis.

Additional Reading

Aach, R. D. and Kahn, R. A.: Post-transfusion hepatitis: Current perspectives. Ann. Intern. Med., 92:539, 1980.

Bartrum, R. J., Crow, H. C., and Foote, S. R.: Ultrasound examination of the gallbladder. J.A.M.A., 236:1147, 1976.

Lieber, C. S.: Alcohol, protein metabolism and liver injury. Gastroenterology, 79:373, 1980.

Redinger, R. N.: Cholelithiasis: Review of advances in research. Postgrad. Med., 65:56, 1979.

Seeff, L. B.: Immunoprophylaxis of viral hepatitis. Gastroenterology, 77:161, 1979.

Sherlock, S.: Chronic hepatitis. Postgrad. Med., 65:81, 1979.

Zieve, L., and Nicoloff, D. M.: Pathogenesis of hepatic coma. Ann. Rev. Med., 26:143, 1975.

CHAPTER 14

RESPIRATORY DISORDERS

The respiratory tract (Fig. 14–1) technically begins with the *nose,* whose inner mucosal layer warms air as it is inhaled. Mucus within the nasal cavity traps particulate matter and prevents it from entering the remainder of the respiratory system. An extension of the nasal cavity, the *nasopharynx,* connects the posterior portion of the nose with the *pharynx* (throat) and joins the *oral cavity,* another route for entry of air into the lungs.

Below the pharynx, the *larynx* marks the beginning of the tubular system that leads to the lungs. The larynx closes to prevent entry of foreign material into the lungs. Pressure buildup below the closed vocal cords forces them apart and expels foreign objects below the larynx. This *cough reflex* is of vital importance in clearing objects from the lungs and in removing accumulated mucus. If the cough reflex is suppressed with drugs, accumulated mucus hinders normal lung function. A special problem exists during anesthesia, when vomiting can lead to aspiration of gastric contents because of suppressed cough reflex. This may result in *aspiration pneumonia* (see Chapter 9).

Below the larynx, the respiratory tract continues as the *trachea,* a flexible tube consisting primarily of rings of cartilage. The trachea branches into the *left* and *right mainstem bronchi,* each of which leads to a lung. The mainstem bronchi, like the trachea, are composed mainly of cartilage with a lining of mucous membrane. When the bronchi enter the lungs, they branch further and their composition changes. Instead of rings of cartilage, there is now smooth muscle encircling the bronchial branches with cartilage interspersed among the muscle bundles.

Further down in the lung, the bronchial branches form *bronchioles,* which have smooth muscle but no cartilage. The bronchioles are capable of extreme constriction, owing to a lack of rigid cartilaginous framework, and this is characteristic of bronchial asthma.

The *alveoli* constitute the functional units of gas exchange in the lung. They are clustered at the ends of the terminal bronchioles like grapes, and their tremendously large surface area provides well for absorption of oxygen from the inspired air and removal of carbon dioxide via the expired air. The alveolar wall consists of a network of capillaries, a separating layer of tissue, and the alveolar epithelium. Within the alveolar epithelium is formed *pulmonary surfactant* necessary for lubrication and normal movement of the lungs. A common disease of infants, respiratory distress syndrome (RDS), occurs when too little surfactant is produced (see Chapter 22).

In addition to the effect of respiratory mucus in trapping particles (including some bacteria), additional cleansing effect is

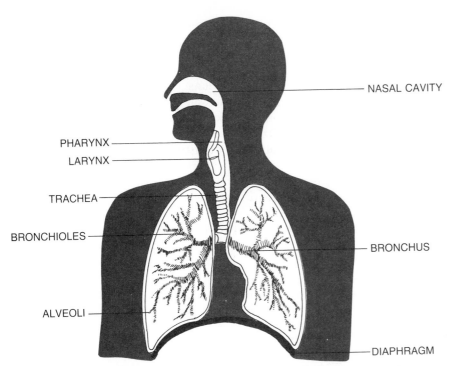

Figure 14–1. The normal respiratory tract. (From Leonard, P. C.: *Building a Medical Vocabulary.* Philadelphia, W. B. Saunders Company, 1983.)

provided by the *cilia,* hairlike projections from special cells (ciliated columnar epithelial cells) lining the bronchi and bronchioles. These move particles upward toward the trachea, eventually allowing for expectoration or swallowing of the material. Chronic inflammation of the ciliated columnar epithelial cells, as with cigarette smoke, leads to *squamous metaplasia* and loss of this specialized function (see Terms in Pathophysiology). Particles too large to be removed from the normal lung by ciliary or mucous action are trapped in alveolar macrophages and digested or propelled up the respiratory system to the pharynx. Many lung diseases (pneumonias, chronic inflammatory disorders) result from failure to remove bacteria or other particles. These conditions are much more common in those with impaired lung defense mechanisms (heavy smokers, alcoholics, those working in heavy air pollution) than in normal people.

NORMAL RESPIRATORY FUNCTION

Ventilation is defined as the process of inhalation and exhalation caused by muscular activity of the chest and diaphragm. The normal ventilatory rate is 7 to 8 liters per minute in resting adults and increases with the respiratory demands of exercise. Increased ventilatory rate and depth in a nonexercising person is called *hyperpnea* and may be the result of systemic acidosis, hysteria, or conditions that restrict air passage or gas exchange in the alveoli.

Apnea is complete failure of ventilation. It can result from complete blockage of the airway or, more commonly, from drugs that depress the medullary respiratory center (e.g., barbiturates). In the latter case, there is no spontaneous drive for respiration. Often, *respiratory depression* occurs, in which breathing does not stop altogether but ventilation is reduced to the point where hypoxia occurs. This leads to *respiratory acidosis* (see Chapter 8) because of retention of carbon dioxide (hypercarbia).

Distribution is the parceling of air into various respiratory compartments. If distribution is good, air is distributed in proportion to the vascular supply of the lung compartment, thus providing optimal gas exchange. Restricted air passage affects distribution of air within the lung and reduces gas exchange. Likewise, vascular damage prevents effective gas exchange, even though adequate air is reaching the particular area of distribution.

TESTS OF RESPIRATORY FUNCTION

Because respiratory function can be assessed with a high degree of precision, an accurate diagnosis can be made of specific respiratory disorders.

Vital Capacity (VC). This is the volume of air that can be exhaled after maximal inhalation. It is approximately 4 liters in normal adults but may be 1 liter or less in a patient with severe emphysema.

Forced Expiratory Flow (FEF). FEF is the rate of maximal air exhalation attained during vital capacity determination. Often the rate during the middle 50 per cent of air flow is measured (between 25 per cent and 75 per cent exhalation); this is called the FEF_{25-75}. It is a good indicator of disease of the small bronchioles (as in chronic bronchitis). Normal values depend upon the particular instrument employed for testing.

Total Lung Capacity (TLC). TLC is defined as the volume of air in the lung after maximal inhalation. It is normally 5 to 7 liters in adults and is increased in emphysema and other types of obstructive lung disease. The increase seen in obstructive lung disease represents vital capacity converted to unusable *residual volume* by alveolar deterioration.

Blood gas values also reflect respiratory pathophysiology, as does pH.

Arterial Oxygen Tension (Pao_2). This is normally 80 to 100 millimeters of mercury (mm Hg) pressure in adults and decreases with conditions that impair alveolar gas exchange, ventilation, or distribution of air.

Arterial Carbon Dioxide Tension ($Paco_2$). This is a useful measure of respiratory function, since impaired alveolar gas exchange, ventilation, or distribution of air increases its value almost immediately. The normal $Paco_2$ in adults is 34 to 46 mm Hg pressure. Arterial oxygen saturation is normally 94 to 100 per cent and decreases with conditions that lower Pao_2 and raise $Paco_2$. Blood pH (normal = 7.35 to 7.45) generally decreases with conditions of impaired respiratory activity (respiratory acidosis) and increases as a result of hyperventilation (respiratory alkalosis). (See Chapter 8.)

TYPES OF RESPIRATORY DISORDERS

A variety of disease processes take their toll on the respiratory tract (Table 14–1). Conditions such as cystic fibrosis and respiratory distress syndrome (RDS) in infants result partly from *faulty secretory functions* within the respiratory system.

Many respiratory disorders result from *infection*. Examples are pneumonia and acute bronchitis (Chapter 9). *Inflammatory reaction* is the major process involved in bronchial asthma, but it also plays a role in bronchitis and pneumonia.

Table 14-1. TYPES OF RESPIRATORY DISORDERS

Disease Process	Representative Disease
Faulty secretory function	Cystic fibrosis, respiratory distress syndrome in infants
Infection	Pneumonia, acute bronchitis, empyema
Inflammatory reaction	Bronchial asthma, hypersensitivity pneumonitis
Destructive lung disease	Bronchiectasis, emphysema
Neoplastic disease	Benign lung tumors, malignant lung tumors
Retention of inhaled dust	Pneumoconiosis (noninflammatory)

Destructive lung disease often results from chronic inflammation or infection. If the medium-sized *bronchi* are damaged and permanently dilated, the condition is known as *bronchiectasis.* Infection is more likely in bronchiectasis than in the normal lung, since the damaged bronchi have impaired ciliary activity. *Alveolar damage* leads to loss of surface area and reduced gas exchange associated with a loss of lung elasticity, as in emphysema.

Often the term *chronic obstructive pulmonary disease* (COPD) is used to refer to any lung condition in which there is chronic or recurrent obstruction to air flow within the lung. This general term includes chronic bronchitis, bronchial asthma, bronchiectasis (because of obstruction from the large amounts of mucus secreted), and emphysema.

Neoplastic disease represents a fifth process affecting the respiratory tract. Benign lung tumors are uncommon, but malignant tumors are, unfortunately, all too well known. (Lung cancer is discussed in detail in Chapter 21.) Other respiratory tract tumors (larynx, pharynx) are much less common than lung cancer but, like lung cancer, they also occur chiefly in smokers.

A number of lung disorders are related to the *inhalation of dust particles* in quantities that overwhelm the pulmonary defense mechanisms. Fine particles can be carried in the inhaled air deep into terminal bronchioles and alveoli, where they remain for long periods of time, sometimes permanently. These conditions are called *pneumoconioses* and result in small airway obstruction and reduced alveolar gas exchange. The problem is mainly a mechanical one, although inflammatory reaction to certain materials also occurs. Well-known examples of pneumoconiosis include *black-lung disease* (coal miners' pneumoconiosis, anthracosis), *silicosis* (seen in those who quarry rock or sandblast), and *asbestosis* (seen in those working around asbestos in any form). Asbestosis greatly increases the risk of lung cancer (90-fold in those who also smoke cigarettes) as well as the risk of mesothelioma, a normally rare pleural tumor (1000-fold).

Some pneumoconioses trigger a specific type II hypersensitivity in the victim, leading to respiratory symptoms and eventual destruction of alveolar tissue. This subgroup is sometimes called *hypersensitivity pneumonitis* and includes *farmer's lung* (sensitivity to hay mold), *bagassosis* (sensitivity to sugar cane fiber), and *bird fancier's lung* (sensitivity to proteins in bird droppings). In these cases, as in pneumoconioses in general, early removal of the offending inhalant generally reverses symptoms and prevents progressive lung damage.

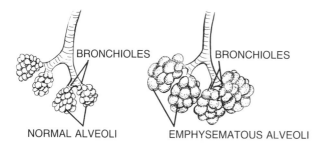

BRONCHIOLES   BRONCHIOLES

NORMAL ALVEOLI   EMPHYSEMATOUS ALVEOLI

Figure 14–2. Alveoli in normal and emphysematous lungs.

Large *foreign bodies* in the respiratory tract cause obstruction, leading to wheezing, dyspnea, and cyanosis. Examples include food items (bites of meat, peanuts, popcorn) or other objects (buttons, toothpicks). Items that pass through the larynx and trachea may obstruct smaller branches of the respiratory system. Interestingly, the majority of inhaled objects enter the right lung rather than the left, since the right mainstem bronchus is on a more direct line with the trachea. For persons with objects lodged in the bronchi, trachea, or larynx (sometimes called a "cafe coronary" because the symtoms resemble those of a heart attack), the Heimlich maneuver (sharp squeezing with pressure from below the sternum) can be life-saving.

EMPHYSEMA

Breakdown of the alveolar walls and associated capillaries causing a coalescence of alveoli into larger structures is termed emphysema (Fig. 14–2). The areas formed are called *bullae* and have greatly reduced surface area when compared with the original volume of alveoli. Also characteristic of emphysema is reduced elasticity of the alveolar tissue, leading to impaired compressibility of the lungs. As a result, the lungs are overinflated and contain trapped air that does not participate in ventilation. Exhalation, normally a passive process, becomes labored and accessory muscles of respiration are brought into play to force air from the lungs. In practice, a degree of bronchiectasis is often seen with emphysema, so that both terminal bronchioles and alveoli are permanently distended.

Pathogenesis

Emphysema generally results from chronic lung irritation, especially that caused by cigarette smoke or air pollution. It is now recognized that an inherited tendency toward the disease also exists in some people. Individuals with a deficiency of alpha-1-antitrypsin (A1AT), a protein that inactivates trypsin, are especially susceptible to emphysema. Since trypsin is a protein digestant, it is proposed that failure to inactivate it results in digestion of elastic tissue in the alveoli. Of the individuals who are homozygous for the A1AT trait, 70 to 80 per cent develop emphysema, usually before age 40. Heterozygous people also have an increased risk of emphysema, especially if they smoke or are exposed to heavy air pollution. Among white Americans, the incidence of homozygous disease is about 1 in 3500 and the incidence of heterozygous disease is about 1 in 40. Blacks carry the A1AT trait much less often than whites.

Emphysema becomes most apparent between ages 40 and 60, although autopsies of apparently healthy people often show the beginnings of the disease much earlier, even during the teenage years. Smokers show earlier changes in the lungs than nonsmokers, and progression of the disease is more rapid.

Symptoms and Signs   Dyspnea on exertion is usually the first symptom of emphysema, reflecting reduced lung capacity. Unfortunately, by the time dyspnea develops, a great portion of the lung's reserve capacity has already been lost. Cough, with expectoration of thick sputum, is also characteristic. Sputum may be clear or amber-colored, signifying coexisting infection. The affected person breathes through pursed lips to improve ventilation. Physical examination reveals an over-expanded chest, reduced diaphragm movement, and increased use of accessory muscles of respiration (especially in the neck and upper chest). Wheezing and a prolonged exhalation phase are also commonly seen.

Laboratory Findings   Chest x-ray examination is especially useful in the diagnosis of emphysema. X-rays show overinflation of the lungs, a lowered diaphragm (resulting from overinflation), and often the presence of obvious bullae in the lung fields. There is an increased TLC and residual volume. Vital capacity is often decreased, and FEF is greatly reduced; FEF is considered the most reliable indicator of emphysematous changes in the lung.

Arterial oxygen tension and arterial oxygen saturation are decreased, but $Paco_2$ is often normal or low until later in the disease because of hyperventilation occurring as a consequence of hypoxia. Some emphysema patients have a deficiency of A1AT. Long-term severely emphysematous individuals frequently show elevations of erythrocyte count, hemoglobin, and hematocrit. This is due to erythropoiesis, resulting from chronic hypoxia, and resembles the adaptation made to high altitude.

Diagnosis   Emphysema must be differentiated from bronchial asthma, chronic bronchitis, lung infection, and lung tumors. Lung infections or tumors usually produce characteristic x-ray findings. Bronchial asthma and chronic bronchitis often coexist with emphysema (COPD is the general term) with confusing clinical and laboratory findings. Exposure to irritating inhalants is a common denominator in all three lung conditions.

Treatment   There is no specific treatment for emphysema and damage already done to the lung is irreversible. Surgery is not helpful, since no repair or replacement of damaged lung tissues is currently possible. There are several useful therapeutic measures, however.

Avoiding Irritants. The disease can be slowed or halted by *cessation of smoking* or avoidance of exposure to other air pollutants.

Increased Diaphragm Movement. Breathing exercises that increase use of the diaphragm improve pulmonary ventilation, particularly exhalation. Elevation of the foot of the bed takes advantage of the weight of abdominal organs in pushing the diaphragm upward during exhalation.

Reducing Weight. Loss of weight to normal reduces the excessive demand for oxygen associated with obesity.

Drugs. Drug therapy is primarily symptomatic and includes the use of bronchodilators, antitussives, mucolytics, antibiotics, and oxygen.

Bronchodilators. Bronchodilators, such as aminophylline or isoproterenol (Isuprel), increase airway size and improve ventilation and distribution of air to some extent, especially if air passages are plugged with mucus. These drugs have considerable cardiac stimulant action and add to the workload of the heart, in addition to making the heart more vulnerable to arrhythmias. Newer drugs, such as metaproterenol (Alupent) or albuterol (Proventil), provide good bronchodilator action with less cardiac stimulation than traditional bronchodilators and are especially useful in emphysema associated with angina pectoris, hypertension, or cardiac arrhythmias.

Antitussives. Antitussive drugs, such as codeine or dextro-methorphan, control unnecessary coughing that fatigues the patient and irritates the respiratory tract. The physician must walk the narrow path of prescribing enough antitussive to suppress unnecessary coughing but also allow for productive cough. Any retention of mucus in an emphysema patient further reduces alveolar function and increases severity of symptoms.

Mucolytics. These agents, such as acetylcysteine (Mucomyst), liquefy thick mucus and promote its expectoration. Together, bronchodilators, antitussives, and mucolytics improve the accessibility of alveoli to air and make the respiratory effort more effective.

Antibiotics. Emphysema renders the lungs much more vulnerable to infection, largely because of impaired lung defense mechanisms. In addition, respiratory infection is more serious with emphysema, since respiratory function is marginal, at best, and worsens drastically with the congestion associated with infection. Respiratory infections should be treated early with antibiotics, such as ampicillin or erythromycin, that provide coverage against most common respiratory pathogens. Vaccination against influenza and types of pneumonia preventable by immunization is also a good idea and may prevent life-threatening respiratory impairment.

Oxygen. Many emphysema patients use oxygen for severe periods of dyspnea and have tanks at home or even in their cars. While oxygen therapy is extremely helpful at these times, overuse of it can depress normal respiration and lead to an increased dependence on it. Improved breathing techniques and attention to other supportive measures are better solutions to the problem in the long run.

Complications

Progressive loss of respiratory capacity is commonly seen in emphysema, in spite of optimum treatment. The individual becomes bedridden and requires more and more oxygen for survival. Even minimal exertion causes severe dyspnea. Terminal respiratory infection is common in this setting. As the disease progresses and lung capillaries are destroyed, increased capillary resistance develops. This results in an elevation of blood pressure within the pulmonary system (normally only 15 to 25 mm Hg), a condition called pulmonary hypertension or *cor pulmonale*. Cor pulmonale is not generally treatable, except by improving or halting deterioration of the respiratory condition. Eventually, symptoms of right-side heart failure develop, with dilation and loss of contractility of the right ventricle.

Prognosis   Prognosis in emphysema is usually not good. If all treatment modalities are utilized to the fullest, survival for several years is likely. Mild, early cases can often be kept from progressing rapidly by removal of causative or aggravating factors, whereas severe cases progress inexorably downhill.

BRONCHIAL ASTHMA

Bronchial asthma consists of a reversible obstruction in the bronchial tree caused by contraction of bronchial smooth muscle, associated with edema of the bronchial mucosa and production of a thick mucus (Fig. 14–3). All three changes cause reduced ventilation and/or distribution of air to the alveoli. Note that this is not an alveolar disease, as is emphysema, but results from reduced movement of air *into* and *from* the alveolar tissue.

Pathogenesis   Two major types of bronchial asthma are recognized.

Atopic Asthma. Atopic (extrinsic) asthma results from allergy to outside materials, especially inhalants. Common offenders are pollen, dust, mold spores, and tobacco smoke. Ingested materials (milk, eggs, chocolate) are less common causes of asthmatic reactions. In atopic asthma, the bronchi are the "shock tissues" of the allergic reaction. A typical type I hypersensitivity reaction, leading to mast cell rupture with resulting asthma symptoms, is seen (see Chapter 4).

Nonatopic Asthma. Nonatopic (intrinsic) asthma is apparently not related to allergy, since the individual does not have an elevation of serum IgE antibodies or a history of allergy symptoms. In these individuals, inhalation of irritating fumes or cold air, exercise, stress, or respiratory infection triggers asthma symptoms. These cases probably result from excessive parasympathetic stimulation as a reflex response to such events. Approximately equal numbers of people have each type of asthma, and many have a combination of both types. In *status asthmaticus,* the sufferer has prolonged attacks of either type. Some degree of asthma may occur all the time, and the individual is frequently resistant to many antiasthma drugs.

Bronchial asthma, since it affects such a vital function as breathing, creates considerable emotional response in the victim. The emotional stress generated often aggravates the symptoms, even with the atopic type. In addition, a psychological overlay is often seen in the asthmatic, in which the individual becomes more dependent ("Please help me to breathe") or even manipulative ("If I

Figure 14–3. Bronchi in normal and asthmatic lungs.

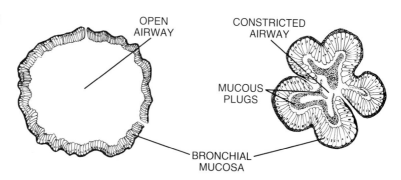

OPEN AIRWAY

CONSTRICTED AIRWAY

MUCOUS PLUGS

BRONCHIAL MUCOSA

don't get my way, I'll have an asthma attack"). In both cases, extra attention is directed toward the sufferer. It is important for the physician and family of the asthmatic individual to realize the potential for this problem and to treat the disease in a matter-of-fact manner, stressing the benefits available with appropriate treatment rather than the limitations associated with the condition.

Symptoms and Signs   Dyspnea, wheezing, and cough with production of a viscous sputum are commonly seen in bronchial asthma of any type. Wheezing can be heard with a stethoscope ("musical" rales) or often without. Exertion increases the dyspnea, and the person usually sits or lies down with the head propped up to relieve symptoms. Resistance is felt in the chest when inhaling as well as exhaling, since there is obstruction in either direction. Hard coughing often brings up a large blob of mucus (mucous plug) and relieves some of the obstruction. Individuals with atopic asthma often have other allergic disorders, such as allergic rhinitis or skin reactions (urticaria).

Laboratory Findings   Sputum examination shows a thick material containing spirals of shed epithelial tissue (Curschmann's spirals). In atopic asthma, numerous eosinophils are also seen. Sensitivity to skin tests for allergens identifies the atopic individual or the person with a combination of both types. A chest x-ray exam is not usually revealing in bronchial asthma but is helpful in ruling out emphysema, lung infection, or lung tumor, which can also produce similar symptoms. During severe attacks, decreased PaO_2, reduced arterial oxygen saturation, and increased $PaCO_2$ are seen.

Diagnosis   As with emphysema, bronchial asthma may overlap with other lung conditions in terms of etiology, symptomatology, and laboratory findings. A careful history showing a cause-and-effect relationship between exposure to allergen or other triggering factor and symptom development is extremely helpful. Negative chest x-ray findings suggest bronchial asthma rather than most other lung conditions. Foreign bodies in the respiratory tract can cause wheezing and cough, but the onset is sudden with no significant history of respiratory disease. Congestive heart failure can cause asthmalike symptoms ("cardiac asthma"), especially if acute pulmonary edema develops. (See the discussion of congestive heart failure in Chapter 10.) The cause and treatment in this case are, of course, different.

Treatment   General measures for the control of bronchial asthma include elimination or reduction of contributing factors. Avoidance of environmental allergens or hyposensitization to them reduces allergic response in atopic asthma. Avoidance of irritating fumes, cold air, or violent exercise, along with early treatment of respiratory infections, helps to prevent the nonatopic form of bronchial asthma. Reduction of stress factors may be beneficial in both types. Reassurance that bronchial asthma is seldom fatal is of great help to the sufferer.

Drug therapy is the mainstay of treatment for bronchial asthma. Mild sedative/antianxiety drugs, such as phenobarbital or diazepam (Valium), calm the person during the attack and reduce the nervousness caused by most bronchodilator drugs. Symptomatic treatment of bronchial asthma consists of using drugs for the *existing attack* or for *prevention of attacks*.

Existing Attacks. These attacks are treated primarily with *bronchodilators* and *oxygen therapy*. Epinephrine, injected subcutaneously, is very effective in terminating an attack of bronchial asthma. Aminophylline, injected intravenously in water for injection, is also effective.

Inhalers. For milder attacks, inhalers containing bronchodilators can be used. Epinephrine (Medihaler Epi), isoproterenol (Medihaler Iso), and isoetharine with phenylephrine (Bronkosol) are good examples. In severe attacks, these may not be satisfactory, since severe bronchoconstriction, edema, and mucus formation may limit their depth of penetration into the lung. A problem with all of the inhalers mentioned is that they also stimulate the heart, an effect especially undesirable during an asthma attack. Metaproterenol (Alupent), terbutaline (Brethine) and albuterol (Proventil), cause less cardiac stimulation but retain excellent bronchodilator properties, as mentioned regarding emphysema. They are especially useful in asthmatics with coexisting cardiac conditions.

Oxygen. Oxygen is useful during the acute attack. However, it should be used sparingly because it depresses the respiratory drive caused by hypoxia and may eventually create dependence on itself.

Corticosteroids. These are useful, not as bronchodilators but to suppress the inflammatory reaction leading to asthma symptoms. Intravenously administered hydrocortisone (Solu-Cortef) or methylprednisolone (Solu-Medrol) are drugs of choice. For less severe cases, orally administered prednisone or equivalent drug is often effective. These should be given in large doses initially and then tapered off or discontinued as soon as possible to reduce side effects.

Preventive Therapy. Inhalers, oral combinations, corticosteroids, and cromolyn (Intal, Aarane) are used.

Inhalers. Bronchodilator inhalers can be used for short-term preventive effect, if administered just before beginning the activity that precipitates an asthma attack. Thus, the individual can use the inhaler before shoveling snow, mowing the grass, or cleaning out the attic.

Oral Combinations. These drugs generally contain two or three bronchodilators plus a sedative to reduce nervousness caused by the other drugs and give good protection when taken three or four times per day. Representative products are Tedral and Quadrinal.

Corticosteroids. Oral corticosteroids are helpful as preventives for bronchial asthma but cause many side effects with long-term use. Corticosteroid inhalers help to avoid the long-term systemic effects of orally administered corticosteroids, since they exert most of their effect directly on the bronchial tissue with little systemic absorption. Two examples are dexamethasone inhaler (Decadron Respihaler) and beclomethasone inhaler (Vanceril Inhaler).

Cromolyn. A unique drug for the prevention of atopic bronchial asthma, cromolyn prevents mast cell breakage caused by IgE-antigen interaction (type I reaction). It is inhaled as a dry powder from a special dispensing device that punctures the capsule and delivers the powder to the lungs. Cromolyn works only as a preventive rather than a treatment for the existing attack, since mast cells have already broken with the existing attack and, like Humphty Dumpty, can't be put together again! Cromolyn often causes mild throat irritation, cough, or even slight bronchospasm as it is inhaled, since it is in powder form.

Combined Therapy. Status asthmaticus is treated primarily with aminophylline, corticosteroids, and oxygen therapy. Hospitalization, careful monitoring of fluid balance (dehydration is common), and even tracheal cannulation with respirator therapy may be required.

Complications

Bronchial asthma that is inadequately treated or resistant to treatment gets progressively worse, with hypertrophy of the bronchial musculature resulting from repeated attacks of bronchoconstriction. Often, emphysema and/or repeated respiratory infections develop as late complications. Patients on long-term corticosteroid therapy develop Cushing's syndrome, which is characterized by edema, increased fat storage and protein breakdown, and a host of other changes. Adrenal atrophy develops because the adrenal gland is no longer required to produce endogenous corticosteroids. The person finally becomes dependent upon constant steroid administration for relief of symptoms (steroid-dependent asthma). Users of bronchodilator inhalers can become both physically and psychologically habituated to the devices, so that rebound asthma attacks occur when they are not available. This is likened to the situation in which a person cannot sleep unless there is a bottle of sleeping tablets (often unused) on the nightstand.

Prognosis

Prognosis is good if every attempt is made to control contributing factors and to relieve symptoms through adequate, but conservative, drug therapy. Lack of control of contributing factors and/or poor drug therapy results in worsening of symptoms and possible eventual development of status asthmaticus.

PLEURAL EFFUSION

Accumulation of fluid in the pleural space is a *sign* of disease rather than a disease itself. A variety of conditions can result in pleural effusion, but primary pleural disease is rare. Only primary infection or tumors of the pleura are seen as primary pleural diseases. Far more commonly seen is pleural effusion related to disease of organs within the pleural cavity, especially the heart and lungs.

Pathogenesis

Pleural effusion commonly results from inflammation, infection, or neoplastic growth of organs within the pleural cavity. Another common cause is congestive heart failure, in which pulmonary edema leads to accumulation of fluid within the chest (see Chapter 10). Other conditions associated with pleural effusion are hepatic cirrhosis (causing ascites) and nephrotic syndrome. Inflammation of the lung (aspiration pneumonia), infection (pneumococcal pneumonia, empyema), or lung tumors often result in fluid accumulation in the pleural cavity. One type of effusion, a *transudate,* is formed as a result of congestive heart failure, hepatic cirrhosis, or nephrotic syndrome. The other type, an *exudate,* forms in response to inflammation, infection, or neoplastic growth. Transudates are almost pure fluid, containing little protein and few cells. Exudates contain a large number of cells, along with a protein content nearly equal to that of plasma. Exudates often contain cells formed as a result of the underlying disease process (neutrophils, pus cells, neoplastic cells).

Symptoms and Signs   Small amounts of fluid in the chest usually cause no symptoms. As the quantity of fluid increases, symptoms develop in proportion to the increase in intrathoracic pressure or interference with lung function. Dyspnea, cough, and chest pain are common symptoms. Interference with lung action causes restricted chest motion on the affected side and a decrease or change in breath sounds.

Laboratory Findings   A volume of fluid greater than 300 ml usually appears upon chest x-ray examination (Fig. 14–4). Large quantities of fluid shift the mediastinum and heart away from the effusion area, and this is visible on x-ray films.

Thoracentesis (puncture of thorax for fluid removal) permits sampling of the pleural fluid for laboratory study. Fluid can be examined for bacteria, pus cells, neutrophils produced as a result of inflammation, or neoplastic cells. In addition, cultures can be made for organisms not readily identifiable by direct smear technique.

Pleural biopsy is indicated if infection, inflammation, or neoplasia is suspected. A sample is taken from the pleural tissue (usually with a large needle) in the area of effusion, and slides are prepared. Multiple biopsies around the area of effusion can be made in this manner with very little risk to the patient.

Treatment   Since pleural effusion is a sign of disease rather than a disease itself, treatment consists of removal of the underlying cause. Antibiotic therapy of infections; surgical removal of operable tumors; and management of congestive heart failure, hepatic cirrhosis, or nephrotic syndrome will reduce the quantity of fluid formed and relieve symptoms. Removal of fluid from the chest by means of thoracentesis gives dramatic temporary relief of symptoms while treatment of the primary condition is in progress. Rapid removal of large amounts of fluid (more than 1 liter) is not recommended, since it may deplete body proteins or alter the fluid balance excessively.

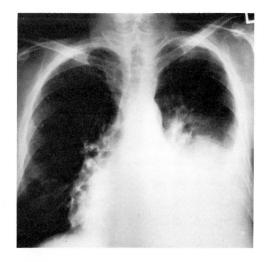

Figure 14–4. Pleural effusion. (From Griffiths, H. J., and Sarno, R. C.: *Contemporary Radiology: An Introduction to Imaging.* Philadelphia, W. B. Saunders Company, 1979.)

Prognosis   Prognosis is good if the primary disease can be cured. It is poor in intractable congestive heart failure, hepatic cirrhosis, or nephrotic syndrome or with inoperable chest tumors.

PNEUMOTHORAX   The presence of air (or, rarely, gas) in the pleural cavity is called pneumothorax. There is some superficial similarity of the condition to pleural effusion in that it is a sign of disease rather than a disease and also because symptoms are related to the mechanical effects of pressure development within the chest.

Pathogenesis   More than half of the cases of pneumothorax occur between 20 and 30 years of age and 85 per cent of this group are men. Almost all of these individuals have no significant lung disease or history of lung problem. It appears that small bullae or *blebs* form in the lungs, probably during prenatal development. Rupture of a bleb causes leakage of air into the chest cavity and partial or total lung collapse. Some individuals have repeated episodes of·pneumothorax, whereas others have only one such experience. Pneumothorax also occurs in those with existing lung disease. Cavitary tuberculosis, emphysema, or staphylococcal pneumonia is associated with bleb formation and may lead to pneumothorax. In all of the described cases, bleb rupture occurs suddenly without traumatic injury (*spontaneous pneumothorax*).

Traumatic pneumothorax occurs following an injury to the chest, most commonly as a result of a knife or gunshot wound or puncture of a lung by a fractured rib. In some cases, the chest wall also leaks air (sucking wound) and destroys the natural vacuum necessary for inflation of the lung on inspiration. Young males also have the highest incidence of traumatic pneumothorax, since they are the most likely to be shot, to be stabbed, or to suffer a broken rib.

A variation of pneumothorax occasionally occurs in which the ruptured bleb forms a one-way valve, allowing air to escape into the chest cavity but preventing re-entry into the lung. With each exhalation, air is forced into the chest cavity through the tear in the lung tissue. Inhalation closes the valve, but the pressure developed within the chest cavity prevents lung reinflation. Continued struggling to breathe results in further collapse of the lung and increased intrathoracic pressure. The mediastinum and heart are pushed toward the opposite side and the other lung is compressed. This causes severe impairment of function of the heart and other lung, in addition to the loss of function of the lung on the side of the pneumothorax. This life-threatening condition is called *tension pneumothorax* (Fig. 14–5) and must be treated immediately for survival of the patient.

Symptoms and Signs   As with pleural effusion, symptoms and signs vary considerably and depend largely upon the amount of air in the chest cavity. Common symptoms include chest pain, dyspnea, decreased breath sounds, and reduced chest motion on the affected side. Tension pneumothorax results in rapid loss of consciousness, cyanosis, shock, and death if not treated promptly.

Laboratory Findings   A chest x-ray exam is the only useful laboratory tool for the diagnosis of pneumothorax. The area of collapse can be seen on x-

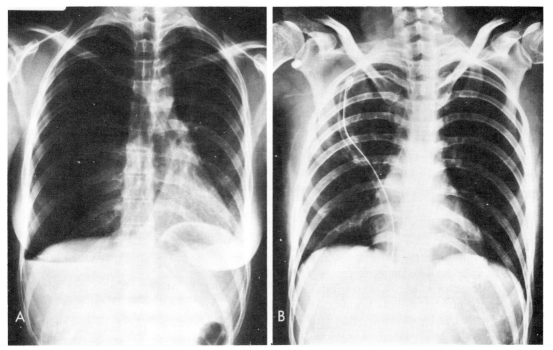

Figure 14–5. Tension pneumothorax, *(A)* before and *(B)* after insertion of chest tube. (From Griffiths, H. J., and Sarno, R. C.: *Contemporary Radiology: An Introduction to Imaging.* Philadelphia, W. B. Saunders Company, 1979.)

ray films, and shifts in the mediastinum, heart, and other lung are readily apparent (Fig. 14–5). An estimate of the degree of lung collapse can be made from the chest roentgenogram.

Diagnosis   The sudden onset of chest pain, along with dyspnea, mimics myocardial infarction or angina pectoris. However, it is not exercise-related and occurs primarily in an age group not prone to heart disease. Pulmonary embolism causes similar clinical findings, but there is often a history of a clotting problem in the immediate past (especially thrombophlebitis), hospitalization, or surgical treatment. Chest x-ray examination is the most useful way to differentiate pneumothorax from other conditions causing similar symptomatology.

Treatment   Mild cases of *spontaneous pneumothorax* resolve with little difficulty. The tear in the lung tissue heals and leakage stops. Remaining air in the chest is gradually reabsorbed. Analgesics (e.g., codeine) and antitussives (codeine, dextromethorphan) control pain and cough resulting from the lung injury. More severe cases require surgery to repair the lung tear (pneumoplasty).

Tension pneumothorax is a real medical emergency and requires immediate insertion of a chest tube (trocar) into the pleural space to relieve the excessive pressure and restore normal position and function to the lungs and heart (Fig. 14–5). Usually, the chest tube is attached to a water trap that prevents air from entering the chest through the tube. Often, a vacuum pump is also attached to gently evacuate air from the chest and provide the necessary vacuum for lung reinflation.

Sucking chest wounds (*traumatic pneumothorax*) require sealing (tape, gauze) to re-establish a vacuum within the chest. Antibiotic coverage is generally given in any situation involving penetration (accidental or surgical) of the chest wall to avoid development of lung or pleural infection. Pneumothorax associated with underlying lung disease (tuberculosis, emphysema) improves as the underlying disease is brought under control.

Prognosis   Prognosis is generally excellent with treatment, although repeated spontaneous pneumothorax episodes are fairly common. The outlook in severe cavitary lung disease is less optimistic, primarily because of the severity of the underlying condition.

SUMMARY

The respiratory tract, like other organ systems in the body, is subject to a variety of disease processes. Some problems result from impaired secretion of necessary materials (e.g., respiratory distress syndrome in infants). Others are caused by inflammatory reactions (e.g., bronchial asthma) or infection (e.g., acute bronchitis). Long-term alveolar damage leads to emphysema, a condition characterized by impaired alveolar gas exchange and loss of lung elasticity. In both pleural effusion and pneumothorax, material (fluid or air) enters the chest cavity and interferes with lung function, primarily by creating increased intrathoracic pressure. Although the symptoms are somewhat similar with the two conditions, the etiology and pathogenesis are quite different.

Treatment of respiratory disorders is directed toward removal of the underlying cause(s), if possible, combined with drug therapy to relieve symptoms and, occasionally, surgery to repair lung damage or remove fluid from the chest cavity. In general, emphysema and bronchial asthma are not treatable surgically; however, certain surgical techniques may be helpful in pleural effusion or pneumothorax.

Questions   1. Define *ventilation* and *distribution* as the terms apply to respiration. Explain how a decrease in either function leads to hypoxia.

2. Define the terms: VC, TLC (not tender loving care!), residual volume, FEF, Pa_{O_2}, Pa_{CO_2}, and arterial oxygen saturation. How is blood pH related to respiratory function?

3. Compare and contrast bronchiectasis and emphysema; pneumoconiosis (noninflammatory) and hypersensitivity pneumonitis; pleural effusion and pneumothorax.

4. Describe the typical chest x-ray findings in emphysema, bronchial asthma, pleural effusion, and pneumothorax.

5. What are the similarities and differences between atopic and nonatopic bronchial asthma regarding etiology, symptomatology, and treatment?

Additional Reading   Ballin, J. C.: Evaluation of a new aerosolized steroid for asthma therapy: Beclomethasone dipropionate (Vanceril Inhaler). J.A.M.A., 236:2891, 1976.

Leff, A. *et al.:* Pleural effusion from malignancy. Ann. Intern. Med., 88:532, 1978.

Morse, J. O.: Alpha-1-antitrypsin deficiency. N. Engl. J. Med., 299:1045, 1099, 1978.

Murray, J. F.: *The Normal Lung: The Basis for Diagnosis and Treatment of Pulmonary Disease.* Philadelphia, W. B. Saunders Company, 1976.

Snider, G. L.: The treatment of asthma. N. Engl. J. Med., 298:397, 1978.

CHAPTER 15

NEUROLOGIC DISORDERS

The central nervous system (CNS) consists of the brain and spinal cord, encased within the meninges (see Chapter 9) and bathed in cerebrospinal fluid (CSF). The brain is divided into several large areas (Fig. 15–1), including the *cerebrum, midbrain, cerebellum,* and *medulla oblongata.*

The outer shell of the cerebrum is called the *cortex* (cortex = bark). The entire cerebrum is divided into two halves, or *hemispheres,* connected by a neural bridge, the *corpus callosum.* The cortex is concerned with thinking functions and sensory perception. Emotional responses and control of body temperature, water and food intake, and sex drive have their origin in the midbrain area. The cerebellum primarily integrates muscular movements to produce smoothness in walking, talking, and other complex muscular activities. The medulla oblongata controls vital functions such as respiration, heart rate, and blood pressure, although these are modified by higher brain centers. The medulla oblongata is well protected in most animal species, demonstrating its importance in basic survival of the organism.

Within the cerebral hemispheres are four subdivisions or *lobes* (Fig. 15–2). The *frontal* lobe is located in the anterior portion of each hemisphere, in the region of the brow. The *temporal* lobe is located in the lower middle region of each hemisphere (near the temple). The *parietal* lobe is the upper, rear portion, and the *occipital* lobe is the lower, rear portion of each hemisphere.

The basal ganglia are a collection of several areas in the brain, including the *caudate nucleus, globus pallidus, putamen,* and *substantia nigra.* The function of the basal ganglia is complex, but it is thought to involve planning and programming of movement. Basal ganglia disorders are characterized by hyperkinetic movements (tremor) and hypokinetic movements (rigidity). *Parkinsonism,* a disorder involving the basal ganglia, has features of both hyperkinesis and hypokinesis.

The functional unit of all CNS tissue is the *neuron.* There are approximately 15 billion neurons in the adult cerebral cortex alone, plus additional billions in the other brain areas, contributing largely to the total weight of the adult brain, 1200 to 1400 grams. The neuron's properties of excitability and electrical transmission are shared only by muscular tissue; in addition, neurons are biochemically somewhat similar to muscle. Both possess an excitable membrane in which electrical activity is generated by ion fluxes. An important difference, however, is that neurons do not contract upon stimulation.

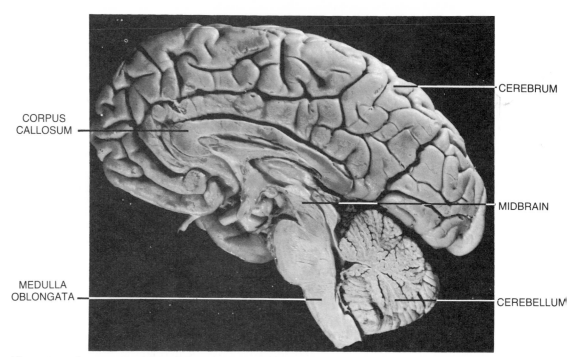

Figure 15–1. Structure of the brain. (From Gardner, E.: *Fundamentals of Neurology,* 6th ed. Philadelphia, W. B. Saunders Company, 1975.)

While it may be said that the hepatobiliary system is the most complex in the body from the standpoint of multiplicity of functions (secretory, synthetic, metabolic, circulatory), the CNS is certainly the most complex in terms of the organization and interrelationship of its various components. Integration of functions, which is well understood in the hepatobiliary system, is comprehended at only a superficial level in the CNS. The old pun that "the brain is a large gray area" certainly has some basis in fact. We make a distinction between "neurologic" disorders, in which there is generally a demonstrable pathologic change in the CNS, and "psychiatric" disorders, in which there is usually no detectable CNS pathology. This is probably a reflection of our ignorance of the subject. Our tools for measurement are crude. Interpretation of an electroencephalogram (EEG) has been likened to trying to chart the ocean floor by observing the pattern of waves a mile above. Even sophisticated x-ray studies of the brain often fail to show the cause of various neurologic disorders. We are further hampered by the fact that we cannot take a slice of living brain from a human for pathologic study. Virtually all histologic studies must be performed after death, with the exception of pathologic study of tumors surgically removed from the brain. (The thought of removing part or all of a living brain conjures up the mental image of Frankenstein and mad scientists.)

Our failure to observe histologic changes in the brains of psychotics after death does not prove that such people had normal brain activity while living. The biochemical complexity of the brain

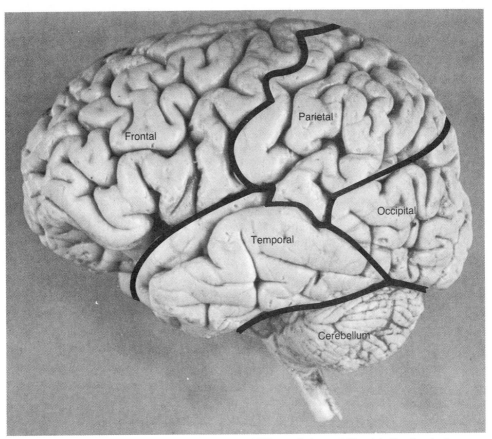

Figure 15–2. Cerebral lobes and cerebellum. (From Williams, P. L., and Warwick, R.: *Gray's Anatomy,* 36th British ed. London, W. B. Saunders Company, 1980.)

is such that subtle changes in the levels or relative proportions of various neurotransmitters can exist without our knowledge. Since we cannot assay living brain tissue for levels of norepinephrine, serotonin, or dopamine, we must rely upon assay of metabolites released into the blood stream or cerebrospinal fluid. Again, we are looking at the problem from too great a distance. There are animal models for certain neurologic disorders (e.g., epilepsy), but no such models exist for psychiatric disorders. We cannot tell whether a rat is hallucinating or experiencing paranoid feelings. Therefore, we cannot compare the neurotransmitter content of its brain with that of a normal rat, and, more importantly, we have no animal data to extrapolate to humans.

The situation is somewhat better for neurologic disorders, in which experimental brain lesions in animals often correlate well, regarding symptoms, with similar lesions in humans. A cause-and-effect relationship can thus be established, and brain areas responsible for certain CNS functions can be identified and charted. For example, selective destruction of the cerebellum in animals produces the same loss of coordination of muscular movements in animals as does cerebellar disease in humans. Destruction of areas in the basal

Table 15-1. **DISEASE PROCESSES AFFECTING THE CENTRAL NERVOUS SYSTEM**

Process	Clinical Disease or Syndrome*
Infection	Abscess, meningitis, encephalitis
Inflammation	Meningismus
Neoplasm	Glioma, meningioma
Ischemic necrosis	Stroke
Degeneration	Multiple sclerosis, amyotrophic lateral sclerosis, Huntington's chorea, Alzheimer's disease

*Representative examples.

ganglia in animals produces a disorder that mimics parkinsonism, a condition in humans that is caused by malfunction in the same brain area.

DISEASE PROCESSES AFFECTING THE CENTRAL NERVOUS SYSTEM

Like other body systems, the CNS is vulnerable to infection, inflammation, and neoplastic growth. Ischemia and degenerative disease may also affect the nervous system. Table 15-1 summarizes these processes.

Infection. Infections take the common form of abscess, meningitis (see Chapter 9), and encephalitis (generalized infection of brain matter).

Inflammation. Inflammatory processes within the CNS are poorly understood but probably account for certain degenerative disorders. Meningismus, a type of meningeal inflammation, results from nearby infections outside the CNS that cause meningeal irritation.

Neoplasia. Neoplastic growth in the CNS takes many forms, including both benign and malignant tumors. The two most common brain tumors are *gliomas* (malignant tumors that arise from connective tissue within the brain) and *meningiomas* (benign tumors arising from meningeal tissue). These, along with tumors metastasizing to the brain, comprise 85 per cent of all brain tumors.

Ischemic Necrosis. Cerebrovascular accidents (CVAs, strokes) represent episodes of brain injury and necrosis resulting from a ruptured blood vessel (cerebral hemorrhage) (Fig. 15-3) or vascular clot (cerebral thrombosis or embolism). Common sites for stroke are in the circle of Willis, a network of blood vessels at the base of the brain. Many strokes result from rupture of an existing *berry aneurysm* (Fig. 15-4) and are a common complication of hypertension (see Chapter 10).

Often there is an earlier warning of an impending stroke (in 35 per cent of cases); this is referred to as a *transient ischemic attack* (TIA). Symptoms of TIA are similar to those of a stroke and include slurring of speech, muscle weakness, dizziness, or blurred vision. However, the symptoms are milder and resolve in a day or so.

The term *stroke* derives from the early belief that it was an act of God (a stroke from heaven) and represented punishment for evildoing. Instead of muscle weakness, there is often paralysis. Loss of speech (aphonia) commonly occurs instead of slurred speech. Coma and permanent visual field loss replace dizziness and blurred vision.

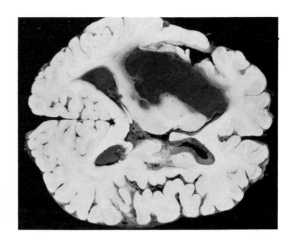

Figure 15–3. Stroke resulting from cerebral hemorrhage. (From Robbins, S. L., and Cotran, R. S.: *Pathologic Basis of Disease,* 2nd ed. Philadelphia, W. B. Saunders Company, 1979.)

Recovery from a stroke depends upon the ability of other areas in the brain to assume the functions of the damaged ones. Neural regeneration does not occur.

Nerve Degeneration. Perhaps the most interesting (and often most tragic) CNS disorders involve neural deterioration. There are more than a dozen such diseases. In some cases, an autoimmune mechanism or "slow" virus infection is suspected but not proved (see Chapters 2 and 4).

Multiple Sclerosis. This condition is associated with a loss of myelin sheath from neurons in the CNS. Symptoms include poor

Figure 15–4. Berry aneurysm in circle of Willis. (From Robbins, S. L. and Cotran, R. S.: *Pathologic Basis of Disease,* 2nd ed. Philadelphia, W. B. Saunders Company, 1979.)

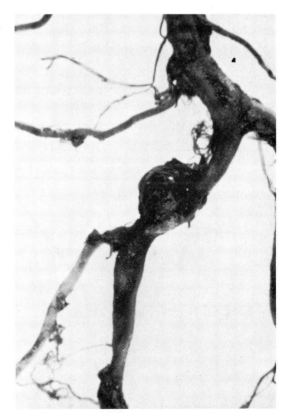

motor coordination, paralysis, and diplopia (double vision). The disease is progressive, although extremely variable in rate of progression, and there is no effective treatment at present.

Amyotrophic Lateral Sclerosis. Also called *Lou Gehrig's disease* after the famous baseball player who died from it, this disease results from degeneration of motor cells of the CNS, causing weakness and wasting of muscles of the extremities. Progressive worsening of symptoms occurs, leading to death, usually within 3 to 5 years. There is no treatment.

Huntington's Chorea. Made known to the public when it afflicted folk singer Woodie Guthrie, this disease is an inherited disorder, characterized by mental deterioration and chorea (involuntary movements). Possibly, the balance between dopamine, acetylcholine, and perhaps other neurotransmitters is abnormal in this case. Life expectancy is 10 to 15 years after onset, and there is no treatment.

Alzheimer's Disease. Also called presenile dementia, Alzheimer's disease results from atrophy of the frontal lobe of the brain associated with the formation of plaques and neural "tangles" in brain tissue. Memory loss and impaired cognitive function occur, as they do in the senile individual, but at an earlier age. On autopsy or on x-ray examination using computerized axial tomography (CAT scan), the brain is seen to be greatly decreased in size and weight. Unfortunately, there is no treatment.

COMMON CNS DISORDERS

The remainder of this chapter describes some common disorders of the central nervous system, including headache, parkinsonism, epilepsy, and organic brain syndrome.

HEADACHE
(Cephalalgia)

Headache is not a disease, but it is a common symptom of several CNS disorders, including meningitis, encephalitis, brain abscess, and brain tumor. Headache also results from hypertension, in which case the CNS is threatened by the possible complications of a stroke. Hypertensive headache often occurs upon awakening and is felt primarily in the back of the head (Fig. 15–5). The physician must consider these possible causes of headache, along with some others, in making an accurate diagnosis. Since headache is one of the most common complaints seen in patients, physicians are continually confronted with a symptom that *probably* does not result from serious disease but that *possibly* could. (This is the stuff of which gray hair—and headaches—are made!) Headaches other than those caused by these serious conditions can be categorized as *occipital, allergic, cluster,* and *migraine* (Fig. 15–5).

Occipital Headache

Pain arising from the rear portion of the skull is termed occipital or *tension* headache. The cause is usually muscle spasm in the neck area, resulting from nervous tension, fatigue, or keeping the head in one position for long periods of time (reading, studying, driving, sleeping in an awkward position). Traction of neck muscles on muscles around the skull produces the typical symptoms of pain in the back of the head or eye orbit area, or encircling the head like a

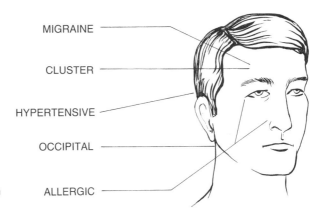

Figure 15–5. Location of pain with the common types of headache.

band (graphic demonstrations of this have been made for television commercials).

Laboratory tests are of little value in diagnosis, but a history of nervous tension, stress, or postural factors helps to pinpoint the cause of the headache.

Treatment

Treatment consists of reduction of factors that promote headache. Rest and relaxation, frequent change in position, and massage of the affected muscles, along with the application of heat to the painful areas, help to relieve symptoms. Aspirin or acetaminophen (Tylenol) relieve most occipital headaches.

For more severe cases, propoxyphene (Darvon) or combination products (e.g., Fiorinal) are helpful. Most combinations contain a sedative/antianxiety drug, such as phenobarbital, along with an analgesic agent. Phenobarbital or diazepam (Valium) is helpful if anxiety is a major cause of the problem. Narcotics should be avoided, since their powerful analgesic action is usually not needed and since they are addicting.

Allergic Headache

Allergic (sinus) headache occurs as a result of edema of nasal and sinus mucosa caused by an allergic (inflammatory) reaction. It is extremely common in allergy sufferers, especially in those with allergic rhinitis and/or sinusitis (see Chapter 18). Pain is felt in the eye orbit area or over the sinuses (especially the maxillary sinuses on each side of the nose). Nasal congestion is usually seen, and this favors poor drainage through the sinus ostia (openings) into the nasal cavity. X-ray studies of the sinuses or examination with a pencil flashlight shone through the facial tissue into the sinuses (transillumination) reveals congestion and edema of the mucosal lining.

Treatment and Complications

Treatment is directed at control of the cause. Antihistamines, such as chlorpheniramine (Chlortrimeton), are usually effective in blocking the allergic response, which is primarily related to release of histamine from mast cells. Decongestants, such as pseudoephedrine (Sudafed), administered orally, open nasal and sinus passages and improve drainage. Mild analgesics, such as aspirin, are helpful for relieving headache pain. Combinations of decongestant, antihistaminic, and/or analgesic drugs (Sinutab, Ursinus) give excellent relief of symptoms.

Nasal sprays or drops give some temporary benefit but primarily relieve only nasal congestion, since they do not penetrate well into blocked sinus passages. There is also the danger of rebound congestion induced by repeated administration of such topical decongestants (rhinitis medicamentosa).

Inadequate treatment of allergic headache may result in infection in the stagnant sinuses (see Chapter 18).

Cluster Headache

In 1939, Horton described a type of headache, later called *Horton's syndrome* or *histamine cephalalgia,* that usually affects middle-aged to older individuals. Attacks are sudden and severe, often waking the person from a sound sleep, but they are of short duration (30 to 90 minutes). Most attacks are unilateral (affecting one side of head) and occur in clusters, often 10 to 20 times per week, with headache-free periods between clusters. Nasal congestion and discharge, eye redness, lacrimation (tearing), and throbbing of blood vessels are seen on the affected side. Since these symptoms could be duplicated by injections of histamine, Horton attributed the headaches to periodic inappropriate local release of histamine. It is now thought that other compounds such as serotonin, unknown in 1939, might be involved in the pathogenesis of cluster headache. Some authorities consider cluster headache to be a variant form of migraine.

Diagnosis

Diagnosis of cluster headache is based primarily upon the pattern and types of symptoms and the exclusion of serious pathologic states. Migraine headache, its closest relative, has a slower onset and often is heralded by visual disturbances (blurring, loss of visual field).

Treatment

Horton prevented attacks with small injected doses of histamine, gradually increasing the amount, to induce desensitization to its effects. A combination of ergotamine and caffeine (Cafergot) is also used to prevent attacks. For nocturnal headaches, tablets or suppositories of Cafergot can be taken before retiring. The short duration of attacks makes treatment of an existing attack difficult because the attack may be over before the treatment takes full effect. Injections of ergotamine (Gynergen) or dihydroergotamine (DHE-45) are useful.

More recently, success has been attained with the use of methysergide (Sansert) or corticosteroids (e.g., prednisone) as preventives. Methysergide is taken three times daily for 6 months, followed by a break period of 3 to 4 weeks to minimize side effects. Corticosteroids are given in high initial doses, tapering off to withdrawal in 3 weeks. Interestingly, methysergide is a powerful serotonin antagonist.

Migraine Headache

Migraine is a peculiar form of headache in which there is a *prodromal phase,* followed by an *attack phase,* ultimately followed by a period of *edema* and *muscle contraction* in the cranial area. This form of headache is present in about 8 per cent of the population but favors women over men. It has a beginning in later childhood or during the teenage years, nearly always making its appearance by adulthood. A family history often exists with migraine, in which other members have similar attacks or variations on the same theme. Factors such as stress, premenstrual tension, or hormone changes associated with puberty or menopause may increase an existing tendency toward migraine headaches.

Many individuals with migraine are of a personality type called a "migraine personality," characterized by rigidity, shyness, perfectionism, and repressed hostility. This personality type is similar to that seen in patients with ulcer or ulcerative colitis and serves as a helpful feature in diagnosis, if present.

Pathogenesis

Migraine attacks are thought to be caused by release of a vasoconstrictor substance, followed by rebound vasodilation when the effects of the compound wear off. Both serotonin and neurokinin, a vasoactive polypeptide, have been implicated as causes of migraine attacks. During the prodromal phase, cranial and extracranial vasoconstriction is thought to cause most of the symptoms. This is followed by dilation of the same blood vessels, resulting in the attack phase. Residual edema and muscle contraction, possibly related to initial blood vessel engorgement, constitute the third phase.

Symptoms and Signs

Visual disturbances are the chief findings in the prodromal phase. These consist of blurred vision, photophobia (increased sensitivity to light), scintillating scotomas (shimmering blind spots in the visual field), and hemianopia (blindness in half the visual field). Presumably, these are caused by reduced circulation to the visual cortex and other visual structures.

The attack phase consists of throbbing and pain, usually unilateral, associated with nausea and vomiting ("sick" headache). The site for headache usually changes from side to side with each attack. Attacks require at least an hour to develop fully and last 4 to 6 hours, occasionally up to 24 to 48 hours. Residual steady pain remains after throbbing ceases, probably as a result of muscle spasm. In some individuals, "migraine equivalents," such as dizziness or gastrointestinal upset, occur without headache pain.

Diagnosis

Migraine headaches are difficult to diagnose because they occur in many forms and involve a number of organ systems besides the CNS. The pattern of headache, life history of the patient, and precise description of the attacks is often helpful in differential diagnosis. Prompt relief with ergotamine or dihydroergotamine is considered to be diagnostic evidence of migraine. Cluster headache also responds to these drugs but is thought to be a special form of migraine by many experts. The diagnosis is easier if the person has a "textbook" case (classical migraine).

Treatment

Ergotamine (Gynergen) or dihydroergotamine (DHE-45) are drugs of choice for treating existing attacks. Intramuscular injection is the preferred route of administration, but oral or sublingual tablets of Gynergen are also available, as is an inhaler. Ergotamine plus caffeine (Cafergot) is also useful as an oral tablet or as a suppository if vomiting prevents oral administration. Inhalation of 100 per cent oxygen causes reflex cranial vasoconstriction and relieves blood vessel engorgement during the attack phase. Rest in a quiet, darkened room, especially with the use of a mild sedative, will often abort an impending attack.

Successful prevention of migraine attacks has been attained with the use of methysergide (Sansert), administered as it is for cluster headache, and with propranolol (Inderal). The action of propranolol is poorly understood, but may relate to some central action involving control of vascular diameter.

Complications and
Prognosis

There are no long-term complications to migraine headache, except for side effects to drugs used for treatment or prevention of attacks. Prognosis is generally excellent.

PARKINSONISM

A constellation of symptoms including muscle rigidity, tremor, and masklike facial expression was described by Parkinson in 1817 and originally termed *paralysis agitans* because of the odd coexistence of muscle immobility and uncontrolled movement. Parkinsonism is a common disorder in people in the 50 to 60-year-old age group, but it occasionally occurs in younger individuals.

Pathogenesis

Parkinsonism is seen in a variety of settings. It occurs following brain injury, such as that caused by encephalitis (postencephalitic parkinsonism). The influenza epidemic of 1917, which resulted in many cases of encephalitis, was followed much later by a corresponding rise in the incidence of parkinsonism. The implication here is that of brain injury occurring a long time after initial insult or the persistence of "slow" virus infection in neural tissue (see Chapter 2). A similar clinical picture is seen following head injury, certain vascular disorders in the brain, or tertiary syphilis. Likewise, elderly people often have parkinsonian symptoms attributed to brain deterioration associated with aging (senile tremor). Phenothiazine tranquilizers such as chlorpromazine (Thorazine) and related drugs such as haloperidol (Haldol) and thiothixene (Taractan) cause parkinsonian symptoms as a side effect. This is especially troublesome to psychotic patients who require large doses of these drugs for control.

The common denominator in all of these situations is reduced effect of the neurotransmitter *dopamine* in the basal ganglia region of the brain. Phenothiazines and other similar drugs block the effect of dopamine and result in the pharmacologic equivalent of dopamine depletion. In the other conditions, depletion of dopamine occurs when cells in the basal ganglia are damaged and they fail to produce normal quantities of it. Autopsies of individuals suffering from parkinsonism show depigmentation of basal ganglia tissue and the presence of hyaline structures (Lewy bodies) within some of the remaining pigmented basal ganglia cells (Fig. 15–6). One theory of the pathogenesis of parkinsonism states that there must be a balance between the effective quantities of dopamine and acetylcholine for optimum muscle control (Fig. 15–7). Too little dopamine activity compared with acetylcholine activity results in parkinsonism; too much dopamine activity compared with acetylcholine activity causes a type of spastic muscle activity.

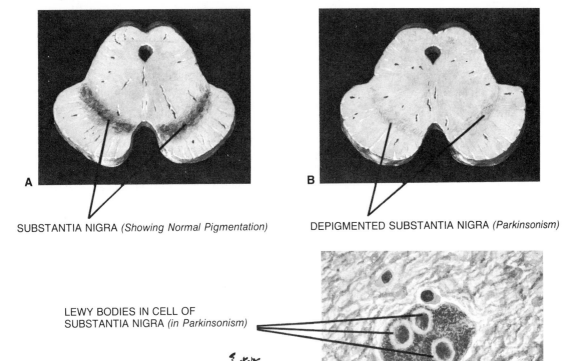

A — SUBSTANTIA NIGRA *(Showing Normal Pigmentation)*

B — DEPIGMENTED SUBSTANTIA NIGRA *(Parkinsonism)*

LEWY BODIES IN CELL OF SUBSTANTIA NIGRA *(in Parkinsonism)*

C

Figure 15–6. *(A–C)* Histologic appearance of substantia nigra in parkinsonism. (From Clinical Symposium on Parkinsonism, Vol. 28, No. 1, p. 21. © Copyright 1976, CIBA Pharmaceutical Company, Division of CIBA-GEIGY Corporation. Reprinted with permission from Clinical Symposia, illustrated by Frank H. Netter, M.D. All rights reserved. Legends adapted.)

Symptoms and Signs   Muscle rigidity, tremor, and masklike facial expression are the major symptoms of parkinsonism. Muscle rigidity gives the movements a plastic appearance (lead-pipe rigidity) or a robotlike motion (cogwheel rigidity). The term "poverty of movement" is used to describe the lack of all but essential muscle activity. Tremor results

Figure 15–7. Balance of neurotransmitters in basal ganglia (proposed relationship to motor function). DA-Dopamine; ACH-acetylcholine.

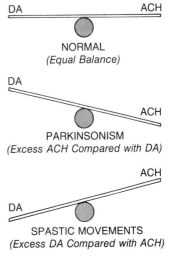

DA ——————————————— ACH
NORMAL
(Equal Balance)

DA ——————————————— ACH
PARKINSONISM
(Excess ACH Compared with DA)

ACH ——————————————— DA
SPASTIC MOVEMENTS
(Excess DA Compared with ACH)

in a rapid, involuntary movement of the hands at rest ("pill-rolling" movement) that improves if the muscles are occupied with some activity. Handwriting is often small and irregular, and some cases are diagnosed by bankers who note a gradual deterioration in its appearance. Fortunately, the biochemical process responsible for parkinsonism does not spread from the basal ganglia and intellectual and vital functions remain intact.

Diagnosis   Parkinsonism is diagnosed primarily from observation of symptoms, coupled with pertinent history. Catatonic states (characterized by muscle rigidity or paralysis) and arthritic conditions can mimic some of the clinical findings of parkinsonism. However, the combination of tremor and rigidity is relatively specific for the condition. Intention tremor (tremor during use of the muscle rather than during rest) usually signifies cerebellar disease rather than disease of the basal ganglia.

Treatment   Exercise and reassurance that general brain deterioration will not occur are helpful to all parkinsonism patients. Attempts should be made to use muscles as much as possible to prevent atrophy.

Surgery. Surgical treatments, in which specific areas of the basal ganglia are destroyed by freezing or ultrasound vibration, have been largely replaced by modern drug therapy. Surgical treatment of parkinsonism is often dramatically effective but is reserved for selected cases that have responded poorly to drug therapy.

Drugs. Drug therapy began with the use of *anticholinergic agents,* such as atropine or scopolamine. These drugs block the effect of acetylcholine in the basal ganglia when given in high doses but cause many side effects in areas outside the brain. More specific anticholinergic agents, which enter the brain more readily, were developed later. These include benztropine (Cogentin) and trihexyphenidyl (Artane). The effect of these is to better balance the dopamine *versus* acetylcholine ratio.

Amantadine (Symmetrel) was first used in the 1960s as an antiviral drug for type A_2 influenza (Asian "flu"). Elderly people and those with debilitating illness were selectively given the drug to prevent or treat the disease, since they would suffer the most severe consequences from it. It was noticed that among elderly people with parkinsonism, symptoms improved greatly after administration of amantadine. The agent is now used as a treatment for parkinsonism in all types of individuals and is thought to act by causing release of dopamine in certain brain areas, including the basal ganglia.

Levodopa (Dopar) is also currently used to increase levels of dopamine in the basal ganglia. The drug is converted to dopamine after entering the brain. Dopamine itself is not useful as an antiparkinsonism agent, since it does not enter the brain in any quantity. Its effects are only on the peripheral areas of the body, and it is employed primarily as a cardiac stimulant. Although levodopa is effective in the treatment of parkinsonism, unfortunately a large amount of it is converted to dopamine before reaching the brain by an enzyme called *dopa decarboxylase.* This means that large amounts of levodopa are needed for treatment and that numerous peripheral effects, related to dopamine activity, occur. The currently used combination of levodopa plus carbidopa (a dopa decarboxylase inhibitor) gives much better results, since it prevents peripheral conversion of levodopa to dopamine and results in higher brain levels of dopamine with lower doses of drug. The commercial combination is called Sinemet.

Complications and Prognosis

Gradual worsening of the condition is usually seen, often associated with mental depression or anxiety. Intellectual function is generally not affected. Overtreatment with levodopa or Sinemet causes spastic movements resulting from an excessive ratio of dopamine activity to acetylcholine activity. This can be corrected by a reduction in drug dosage. Vitamin preparations containing pyridoxine (vitamin B-6) should be avoided while on therapy with levodopa or Sinemet because pyridoxine destroys the effect of levodopa.

EPILEPSY

The general term *seizure* (fit) is used to describe involuntary bursts of brain activity that result in convulsions, loss of consciousness, changes in behavior, and other symptoms. *Seizure* is not synonymous with *epileptic attack,* although all epileptic attacks are forms of seizure. That is, epilepsy represents only one group of seizures.

A great many conditions can result in seizure activity, including traumatic brain injury, stroke, brain tumor, infections (meningitis), hyperthermia (febrile seizures), hypoglycemia (low blood sugar), uremia (often associated with renal failure), and overhydration. In epilepsy, there is generally a repetitive pattern of seizure activity with predictable symptoms and signs. It is considered a syndrome, rather than a disease, since it has multiple etiology.

Epilepsy has an interesting, if bizarre, history. The Greeks called it "falling sickness," since loss of motor control is the most obvious feature of some forms of it. It was also attributed to divine control of the individual or, conversely, to possession by the devil. The unfortunate victim, therefore, suffered much at the hands of the ignorant or, rarely, was exhalted for this anomaly. In the 1800s, epilepsy was recognized as a medical disorder and was treated with diet and, later, with drugs.

Pathogenesis

Epilepsy may result from some of the previously mentioned conditions, notably head injury leading to brain damage and scarring, stroke, and brain tumor. However, most cases are idiopathic. There is often a family history of epilepsy and a personal history of lapses of consciousness or other symptoms in the affected individual. Idiopathic epilepsy usually surfaces before age 30, whereas epileptic seizures caused by organic brain disease (tumor, stroke) are most often seen in those over 30. A history of febrile seizures in an infant often correlates with later development of epileptic (nonfebrile) seizures. It appears here that fever, which increases seizure tendency in all individuals, brings the epileptic individual to the threshold for seizures but usually fails to cause seizures in the normal individual. In other words, fever does not cause the person to become epileptic but brings out a natural tendency toward the condition.

In general, epileptic seizures result from uncontrolled bursts of electrical activity that spread across areas of the brain and produce symptoms that correlate with known functions of the specific areas affected. For example, electrical discharge in the motor area of the cortex results in convulsive muscular activity and temporal lobe discharges result in behavioral disturbances. Often, by observing the behavior of the individual during an attack, the location of the abnormal discharge can be estimated.

The international classification of epileptic seizures includes four major groups of seizure types: partial, generalized, unilateral, and unclassified. The commonly seen partial seizures include *temporal lobe* (psychomotor) seizures and *jacksonian* seizures. Generalized seizures take two common clinical forms: *tonic-clonic* (grand mal) and *absence* (petit mal). Unilateral and unclassified seizures are relatively rare.

Tonic-Clonic (Grand Mal) Epilepsy

The term "tonic-clonic" is now used in place of the older term "grand mal" (big malady) to describe a type of epilepsy characterized by stiffening of limb muscles (tonus) followed by symmetric twitching movements of the limbs (clonus). Other symptoms may include loss of consciousness, urinary and fecal incontinence, frothing at the mouth, and dyspnea. Dyspnea results from interference with respiratory muscle activity and often leads to temporary cyanosis.

Quite frequently (60 per cent of the time) the convulsive phase of tonic-clonic epilepsy is preceded by an "aura," which takes the form of a peculiar odor or taste (usually unpleasant), flashes of light, or sounds. Sometimes a complete visual scene is perceived or a tune is heard. Minor muscle movements in the head and face may occur and serve as an additional warning of an impending attack. The aura is usually specific for the individual; that is, the person has the same aura each time and can thus predict the onset of an impending attack.

After the seizure has subsided, unconsciousness may persist. Upon awakening, the individual is drowsy, confused, and disoriented for a period of time, and may then sleep deeply for several hours after the attack. It seems as if the CNS requires a rest period after such violent electrical discharge and must "recharge its batteries," as it were.

Tongue biting is often seen in tonic-clonic attacks and may cause injury to the organ. Swallowing of the tongue is uncommon but should be watched for during the acute attack.

Tonic-clonic attacks are the most common type of epilepsy in adults and also occur frequently in children and adolescents.

The major helpful laboratory test in epilepsy is the EEG, the technique for which was developed in the late 1920s. An EEG is made by attaching 20 or more electrodes to areas of the scalp with special conducting paste and amplifying the brain-wave activity more than 100,000 times. A graphic record of brain-wave activity is then made by the instrument. The normal wave frequency in the alert, resting individual is 8 to 14 per second. During tonic-clonic attacks, rapid spiking of waves is seen, especially over motor areas of the brain, corresponding to muscle contractions occurring at that time. Between attacks, the EEG may be completely normal in the epileptic individual.

The test is made more sensitive by flashing a strobe light in the eyes of the subject and varying the frequency of flashing (photic stimulation). Photic stimulation often causes abnormal EEG patterns suggestive of tonic-clonic seizures to occur in the epileptic person, but it does not usually affect the normal person. Not surprisingly, some epileptics have seizures while watching a flickering television set or when driving down a highway at dusk, with fence pickets or trees cutting the sunlight to produce a strobe effect.

Other laboratory tests are generally normal in idiopathic epilepsy. However, the numerous organic causes of seizure can be identified with a variety of laboratory tests, including skull x-ray studies or CAT scans, cerebral angiography, spinal tap, and others.

Absence (Petit Mal) Epilepsy

The term *"absence"* is used to describe a type of epilepsy formerly called "petit mal" (little malady), characterized by brief loss of consciousness (blank spells), loss of body motion (akinetic seizures), and slight muscle movements in the limbs, eyes, or mouth (myoclonic jerks) without falling or tonic-clonic convulsions. The three characteristic symptoms are called the *petit mal triad*. The current name absence refers to the absence of awareness and lack of participation in activity during the attack. Absence epilepsy is the most common form of epilepsy in childhood and adolescence. The victim has a blank facial expression during the attack and is unaware of conversation. It is as if a switch were flipped during the attack and the person's CNS were shut off temporarily. Children with absence epilepsy are often thought to be mentally retarded, autistic, or simply uncooperative before being diagnosed correctly. They frequently do poorly in school, since they miss important points of discussion or questions from the teacher. Some individuals have as many as a hundred attacks per day, which seriously interfere with normal functioning. Attacks last for a period of a few seconds to a minute or two.

An EEG taken during the attack shows characteristic 3-per-second (extremely slow) wave activity in several brain areas. This resembles the pattern during sleep somewhat and correlates with the clinical features previously described. Attacks can often be precipitated by hyperventilation, usually by voluntary rapid breathing on a count given by the examiner. Hyperventilation causes respiratory alkalosis and increases the susceptibility of the CNS to seizure discharge (see Chapter 8).

Temporal Lobe (Psychomotor) Epilepsy

Temporal lobe epilepsy represents a type of partial seizure associated with clouding of consciousness, amnesia, and peculiar body movements. Movements are purposeful but not appropriate at the time of the seizure (tying and untying shoes, buttoning and unbuttoning clothing). Robotlike stereotyped activities (automatisms) are common. These include smacking of the lips; movements of the head, eyes, and extremities; and muttering (often swearing). The term "psychomotor" refers to this odd combination of behavioral and motor activities. Although temporal lobe epileptics generally mean no harm, their actions are often misinterpreted by others, even to the point of arrest or assault. The attack usually terminates in 30 seconds to 2 minutes, leaving the person in a dazed condition with little memory of the attack itself.

Temporal lobe epileptics show spike activity in the temporal areas of the cortex. Attacks often occur during sleep, and it is desirable to obtain a portion of the EEG during sleep. This is accomplished by awakening the individual early on the day of the test, then placing him on a comfortable bed in a dark, quiet room during the test period, often late in the afternoon when the individual is tired.

Some interesting legal defenses have been mounted on the basis that temporal lobe epileptics are unaware of their actions during attacks and may, therefore, not be legally responsible for them. In the most famous of these cases, Jack Ruby was charged with the lethal shooting of Lee Harvey Oswald, who had been arrested following the assassination of President John F. Kennedy. On the basis of a temporal lobe variant pattern in Ruby's EEG, his defense counsel attempted to prove that Ruby was not aware of his actions during the shooting. However, the defense was unsuccessful, since Ruby was adjudged to be one of the 10 per cent of the population who are not epileptic but have a slightly abnormal EEG. Ironically, Ruby later died of cancer while in prison.

Jacksonian Epilepsy

An interesting, if somewhat bizarre, form of partial epileptic seizure is jacksonian epilepsy, named after the father of modern concepts of epilepsy, John Hughlings Jackson. Jacksonian seizures generally start on one side of the body with twitching of the thumb. Twitching progresses from thumb to hand to wrist to arm to shoulder to leg on the affected side (jacksonian march). Consciousness is not lost, and general tonic-clonic seizures do not occur in classical jacksonian epilepsy; however, the attack can trigger off a tonic-clonic seizure in one so afflicted. The progression of muscular twitching results from spread of the electrical discharge across the motor cortex, stimulating adjacent areas for motor control. Adjacent motor areas generally control body areas that are anatomically connected. That is, the motor area controlling thumb movement is adjacent to the area controlling movements of other parts of the same hand. The motor area for the wrist is adjacent to the area for the forearm, and so forth. Mapping of brain motor areas to show the body areas controlled results in a diagram of an odd figure called a *homunculus* (Fig. 15–8).

Jacksonian epilepsy shows EEG patterns of spike activity in the motor area of the cortex, with progression along the motor area corresponding to the jacksonian march seen during the attack.

Diagnosis of Epileptic Seizures

Diagnosis of a particular type of epilepsy is made from the characteristic EEG tracing. This is often obtained with the help of photic stimulation, hyperventilation, or sleep. Occasionally, mixed seizures that combine elements of more than one type are seen. Not all types fit neatly into the categories described. As mentioned, approximately 10 per cent of the normal (nonepileptic) population have some abnormality in the EEG pattern. If such an individual also has seizure activity from some other cause (e.g., organic brain disease), an erroneous diagnosis of idiopathic epilepsy may be made.

Apparent "epilepsy" can be caused by fainting, hysteria, or *narcolepsy,* a curious affliction in which the victim has attacks of

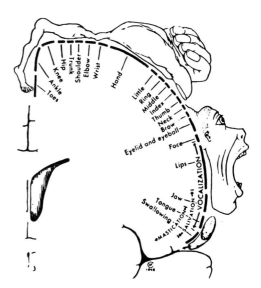

Figure 15–8. Motor homunculus. (Adapted from Penfield, W. and Rasmussen, J.,: *The Cerebral Cortex of Man: A Clinical Study of Localization of Function.* New York, Macmillan, 1950.)

falling asleep. Fainting and narcolepsy are not associated with convulsive muscular activity, and the pattern of muscle movement (or lack of it) and other symptoms in hysteria is often bizarre and related to an underlying psychiatric disorder. Careful history, observation of the attack if possible, and positive EEG evidence are needed for an accurate diagnosis of true epilepsy.

Treatment

General measures include adequate rest and avoidance of fatigue, abstinence from alcohol (which may cause seizures as the CNS rebounds from its depressive effects), and a nutritious, well-balanced diet. Any controllable causative or contributory factors should be eliminated. In past times, a "ketogenic" diet was often used as a treatment for epilepsy. The high-fat content of such a diet resulted in ketosis and systemic acidosis, which made the CNS less sensitive to seizure (see Chapter 8). This treatment has been almost entirely supplanted by drug therapy. Driving a vehicle, swimming, or operating hazardous machinery should be curtailed until seizures are completely controlled for many months and should be avoided if complete control is not attainable. Appropriate attention should be paid to the psychological and emotional aspects of the condition, since trauma in these areas will likely worsen seizure activity.

Surgical treatment of epilepsy is limited to removal of operable scar tissue in those with brain damage. Often, such scar tissue is not accessible without causing further brain injury. An experimental approach to severe, intractable tonic-clonic epilepsy involves severing the corpus callosum connecting the two hemispheres of the brain. For reasons poorly understood, this usually stops seizures; however, the procedure creates an individual with "two brains inside the same skull," since most of the intercommunication between hemispheres has been lost. By using special techniques, it can be shown that at certain times one side of the brain literally does not know what the other side is doing. (For example, if one hemisphere is "asked"— by presenting a visual question only to *its* visual field—something that the other hemisphere has just been "told"—by presenting only

Table 15–2. DRUG TREATMENT IN EPILEPSY

Type	Drugs of Choice*
Tonic-clonic	Phenytoin (Dilantin) Phenobarbital (Luminal) Primidone (Mysoline) Mephobarbital (Mebaral) Carbamazepine (Tegretol)
Absence	Ethosuximide (Zarontin) Valproic acid (Depakene) Clonazepam (Clonopin)
Temporal lobe	Phenytoin (Dilantin) Methsuximide (Celontin) Carbamazepine (Tegretol)
Jacksonian	Phenytoin (Dilantin) Phenobarbital (Luminal)
Status epilepticus	Phenytoin (Dilantin) intravenously Diazepam (Valium) intravenously Phenobarbital (Luminal) intravenously

*Orally administered unless specified otherwise.

to *its* visual field—the first hemisphere will not know the answer. It will then make up an answer to save face!) Obviously, this type of surgery is not for everyone with epilepsy.

Drug therapy is the mainstay for control of epileptic seizures. The current drugs of choice for the common types of epilepsy are listed in Table 15–2. In general, phenytoin (Dilantin) and phenobarbital (Luminal) are first-line drugs for tonic-clonic seizures, and ethosuximide (Zarontin) and valproic acid (Depakene) are first choices for absence seizures. Phenytoin and methsuximide (Celontin) are drugs of choice for temporal lobe epilepsy, and phenytoin and phenobarbital are recommended for jacksonian epilepsy. Phenobarbital often aggravates temporal lobe seizures and should be avoided in those cases. Because phenytoin and related hydantoin drugs often aggravate absence seizures and trimethadione (Tridione) and related oxazolidone drugs may aggravate tonic-clonic seizures, drug therapy is difficult in mixed forms of epilepsy. Combinations of drugs are often required to obtain satisfactory control, and abrupt withdrawal of any drug should be avoided because withdrawal may precipitate an attack.

All drugs should be taken strictly according to dosage schedule, and adjustments in dosage should be made gradually. Changing from one drug to another should be done slowly, making sure that the patient increases the dose of the new drug as the old drug is being tapered off. Most antiepileptic drugs are now given according to blood level monitoring to assure administration of doses that will provide adequate seizure protection. Periodic repeated blood level determinations are necessary to make sure that the correct level is maintained.

Certain diuretics, such as acetazolamide (Diamox), are often used as adjunctive therapy in all types of epilepsy. These *carbonic anhydrase inhibitors* cause a metabolic acidosis and render the individual less susceptible to seizures (see Chapter 8). Generally, these are not potent enough to be used as the sole treatment agent, but they may allow the major antiepileptic drug(s) to be used in smaller doses.

Amphetamines are sometimes used in small doses as adjunctive therapy for epilepsy, primarily to combat the drowsiness caused by most antiepileptic drugs. Small doses do not affect seizure tendency one way or the other, but large doses will increase the likelihood of seizure and should be avoided.

It is helpful for epileptics to carry a card indicating that they are prone to seizures. In this way, much time, effort, and embarrassment are saved should a seizure occur while away from home.

Complications

Approximately one third of patients with absence epilepsy develop tonic-clonic epilepsy later in life, although many outgrow the problem. Abrupt withdrawal of medication often precipitates *status epilepticus,* the epileptic counterpart of status asthmaticus. Status epilepticus consists of repetitive or continuous seizures, leading to exhaustion, hyperthermia, and death if not interrupted. Abrupt withdrawal of medication often occurs when the individual runs out of drug on the weekend, forgets to take a dose or two, or if a new drug is introduced too quickly (without allowing time for an adequate blood level to be developed before stopping the existing drug). Drugs of choice for treatment of status epilepticus are phenytoin, diazepam (Valium), or phenobarbital, injected *intravenously,* followed by re-establishment of the oral medication for long-term control.

Prognosis

Prognosis depends upon the nature of the underlying condition and the success in treating it. In idiopathic epilepsy, prognosis is generally good and improvement, if not complete freedom from seizures, can be attained through careful use of drugs in the vast majority of cases.

ORGANIC BRAIN SYNDROME

Organic brain syndrome (OBS) is a nonspecific alteration in brain function in which there is an organic basis for the malfunction. The term *organic* distinguishes the condition from psychosis, which is considered a *functional,* rather than an organic, problem. This distinction may be a result of our failure to find existing organic causes for psychosis.

Pathogenesis

Common causes of OBS include head injury (brain concussion or hemorrhage), infection (e.g., encephalitis), effects of drugs, or impaired circulation to the brain (stroke, generalized cerebrovascular disease). Less common causes include degenerative diseases (Alzheimer's disease, Huntington's chorea), endocrine disorders (e.g., Cushing's syndrome), or brain tumor.

Drug-induced OBS may result from drug intoxication (alcohol, sedative/hypnotics, atropine) or drug withdrawal (alcohol, sedative/hypnotics). Long-term alcohol abuse causes damage to cortical brain areas (Korsakoff's "psychosis"). Tertiary syphilis was a common cause of OBS in earlier times and was often responsive to "fever therapy" (see Chapter 9). Brain tumors can cause OBS symptoms, presumably as a result of pressure and resulting damage to brain tissue (pressure atrophy), along with destruction of normal brain tissue as the tumor replaces it.

Elderly people tend to have some degree of brain degeneration associated with aging. They may also have impaired circulation to the brain as a result of cerebrovascular disease.

Symptoms and Signs   Symptoms of OBS are extremely variable and run the gamut from mild confusion and disorientation to hallucinations, delusions, and severe distortion of reality. In between these extremes, common clinical findings are loss of recent memory, confabulation (making up information to fill in gaps of memory), and clouding of thinking processes. Hallucinations, if they occur, are usually visual (snakes, insects, Martians) and are often a source of great terror to the sufferer. Acute OBS caused by drug intoxication or withdrawal, acute brain injury, or short-term brain infection may resolve completely when the cause is removed. Chronic OBS caused by gradual brain deterioration and/or impaired circulation is usually irreversible, although it may improve somewhat at certain times.

Diagnosis   Organic brain syndrome must be distinguished from psychosis, in which no obvious organic brain condition exists. The EEG is usually abnormal in OBS but is normal in psychosis. Psychotics generally have auditory hallucinations (commonly voices) and have normal memory and orientation. It must be remembered that organic factors can exacerbate existing or latent psychosis.

Treatment and Prognosis   Acute OBS responds well to removal of the cause (e.g., infection, drug effect). Chronic OBS is largely irreversible but may be improved with the use of vasodilators, such as isoxsuprine (Vasodilan) or nylidrin (Arlidin). Anticonvulsive drugs, such as phenytoin, are helpful in improving brain-wave patterns, even though the individual does not convulse. This often relieves symptoms to some extent. Antipsychotic drugs, such as chlorpromazine (Thorazine) or thioridazine (Mellaril), frequently lessen hallucinations and reduce delusional thinking. This is not too surprising, since there is at least a superficial resemblance between OBS and psychosis.

Supportive care is often as helpful as drug therapy. The individual is often elderly and is coping with failing health, dying friends, loss of usefulness and, sometimes, a neglectful family. New interests and activities, tasks that are useful but within the person's capabilities, and attention to existing physical problems will do much to improve the overall functioning of the older individual with chronic OBS.

SUMMARY

The complexity of the central nervous system exceeds that of the most sophisticated computer. We are just beginning to scratch the surface regarding brain function and at present lack the techniques necessary to probe to a depth necessary for an understanding of the biochemistry of psychosis.

Certain neurologic disorders are understood as to etiology and pathogenesis. Many of these represent degenerative processes that cannot be reversed at present, such as Alzheimer's disease and Huntington's chorea. With other neurologic problems, however, great progress has been made toward treatment or control of the underlying disease process. Parkinsonism is often successfully controlled with drugs or, occasionally, surgery. Epilepsy can be controlled both by removal of existing causes and by the use of drugs that suppress abnormal brain-wave activity. Headache can be accurately diagnosed, with the use of sophisticated x-ray techniques, cerebral angiograms, and other modern laboratory tests. Most types of functional headache can be controlled with appropriate drug therapy. Acute organic brain syndrome can be cured if the cause is removable, as with drug intoxication or withdrawal, infection, or concussion. Even chronic organic brain syndrome can often be improved with drug therapy and with attention to psychological and social factors in the person's environment.

Questions

1. The human brain is protected from the effects of many drugs and chemical compounds by the blood-brain barrier. No such protection is afforded the liver. Comment on this difference as it relates to the fact that liver tissue is capable of regeneration, whereas brain tissue is not.
2. Why does rupture of a blood vessel most often occur in the brain, rather than in other body organs or tissues?
3. Explain why dopamine itself is not an effective drug for the treatment of parkinsonism.
4. Compare and contrast tonic-clonic epilepsy with temporal lobe epilepsy; jacksonian epilepsy with absence epilepsy.
5. Assuming that chronic OBS is related to impaired cerebrovascular circulation, give some reasons why drug therapy with vasodilators might not be effective, even though the drugs cause vasodilation in cerebral arteries of normal individuals and animal preparations.

Additional Reading

Bergman, H. D.: Convulsive disorders. Southern Pharmacy Journal, 69:11, 1977. (*Good general coverage of the various types of convulsions.*)

Parkinsonism. *CIBA Clinical Symposium,* Vol. 28, No. 1, 1976. (*Good overview.*)

Ferguson, G. G.: Common types of headache and their treatment. Southern Pharmacy Journal, 70:14, 1977. (*Discussion of headaches and drug therapy.*)

Gazzaniga, M. S.: *The Bisected Brain.* New York, Appleton-Century-Crofts, 1970.

Jarvik, L. F., Ruth, V., and Matsuyama, S. S.: Organic brain syndrome and aging. Archives of General Psychiatry, 240:382, 1980.

Toole, J. F. *et al.*: Transient ischemic attacks: A study of 225 patients. Neurology, 28:746, 1978.

CHAPTER 16

ENDOCRINE DISORDERS

The term *endocrine* is reserved for those glands that secrete their products directly into the blood stream; the term *exocrine* refers to glands secreting through a duct into an area other than the blood stream. Thus, the adrenals, gonads, and thyroid are endocrine glands, whereas the sweat glands, salivary glands, and acid-secreting glands of the stomach are exocrine glands. A *hormone* is defined as a chemical compound that travels through the blood stream to another part of the body and exerts a regulatory function. Hormones, therefore, are produced by endocrine, rather than exocrine, glands. Some organs have both endocrine and exocrine functions. The pancreas, for example, produces insulin and glucagon, which are secreted into the blood stream (endocrine), and pancreatic juice, which is secreted into the duodenum through the pancreatic duct (exocrine).

Traditional thinking regarding the endocrine system has placed the pituitary gland at the center of operations. It seems now, however, that the hypothalamus has a number of regulatory controls over the pituitary and perhaps should more rightly be called the "control center" of the body. Recent discoveries of releasing factors produced by the hypothalamus clearly show that most pituitary functions are regulated by hypothalamic activity (Table 16–1).

With the development of improved techniques for assay of hormones in the blood stream, it has become clear that a cause-and-effect relationship exists among the various types of regulatory hormones. Release of most pituitary hormones is controlled by secretion of corresponding *releasing factors* from the hypothalamus. Hypothalamic releasing factors trigger pituitary release of *tropic hormones,* which travel through the blood stream to the appropriate *target gland* (or tissue) and exert a stimulating effect. *Target hormones,* which exert effects on various body systems and tissues, are produced as a result of this stimulation. In the case of somatotropic (growth) hormone (STH), the tropic hormone exerts a direct effect upon body tissues, resulting in body growth.

As the level of target hormone in the blood stream increases, the higher level is detected by receptors in the hypothalamus that monitor circulating blood. This results in suppression of the secretion of releasing factor, leading to reduced tropic hormone secretion by the anterior pituitary gland. Target gland stimulation decreases and the blood level of hormone declines. Lowered blood level results in less hypothalamic suppression and increased production of releasing factor, tropic hormone, and target hormone. This interaction, called a *negative feedback system,* enables the body to maintain target hormone levels at the correct point, compensating for loss of

Table 16–1. RELEASING FACTORS, TROPIC HORMONES, AND TARGET HORMONES

Hypothalamic Releasing Factor	Tropic Hormone	Target Hormone (or Response)
TRF (TRH)*	TSH (Thyrotropin)	T_4 and T_3
CRF	ACTH (Corticotropin)	Corticosteroids
Gn-RH (LRF, FRF)	LH FSH	Progesterone Estrogen
GHRF (SRF)†	GH (STH)	Body growth

Abbreviations: TRF = Thyrotropin releasing factor; TRH = thyrotropin releasing hormone; CRF = corticotropin releasing factor; Gn-RH = gonadotropin-releasing hormone; LRF = luteinizing hormone releasing factor; FRF = follicle-stimulating hormone releasing factor; GHRF = growth hormone releasing factor; SRF = somatotropin releasing factor; TSH = thyroid-stimulating hormone; ACTH = adrenocorticotropic hormone; LH = luteinizing hormone; FSH = follicle-stimulating hormone; GH = growth hormone; STH = somatotropic hormone; T_4 = thyroxine; T_3 = tri-iodothyronine.
†Proposed.

hormone through metabolism or increase through exogenous administration of it (Fig. 16–1). For most target hormones (e.g., thyroid hormone, adrenal corticosteroids, androgens), the level is maintained relatively constant with only slight *diurnal variation* (fluctuations during the day and night). Estrogen and progesterone levels, however, fluctuate widely during a monthly period, forming the basis for the *menstrual cycle*. Negative feedback occurs here, too, but control is less tightly maintained and takes place over a longer time period. Were it not for these wide fluctuations, the changes in reproductive organs needed to ensure fertility, and thus survival, could not occur.

Hormones from the posterior pituitary (oxytocin and antidiuretic hormone [vasopressin, ADH]) do not appear to function in quite the same way as those from the anterior pituitary. These hormones are formed by neurons in the hypothalamus and travel down the pituitary stalk to the posterior pituitary gland. Release of these hormones results in contraction of the pregnant uterus plus other effects (oxytocin) and in an antidiuretic effect (ADH). These effects are exerted directly on the tissues, namely, the musculature of the uterus or collecting duct of kidney, without an intermediate tropic hormone.

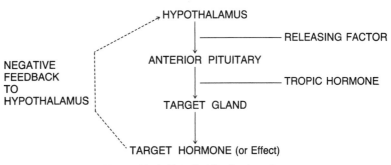

Figure 16–1. Negative feedback system.

DISEASE PROCESSES AFFECTING THE ENDOCRINE SYSTEM

Glands and tissues of the endocrine system are vulnerable to the same disease processes as are those of other body systems, namely, infection, inflammation, and neoplastic growth.

Infection

Infection is not a common cause of endocrine disorders, but it is seen occasionally. Some cases of diabetes mellitus are thought to be caused by prior viral infection in the pancreas, damaging the insulin-secreting beta cells. Widespread tuberculosis, histoplasmosis, or blastomycosis sometimes involves the adrenal gland, producing damage and resulting in *Addison's disease,* characterized by greatly reduced gland function.

Inflammation

Inflammation may result from infection in these cases and contributes to damage and loss of glandular function. In addition, inflammation resulting from an autoimmune reaction is thought to be the cause of thyroid damage in *Hashimoto's thyroiditis.* In this condition, specific antithyroid antibodies are formed. These attack the thyroid gland, causing pain, swelling, and loss of function (see Chapter 4).

Neoplasia

Neoplastic growth occasionally occurs in endocrine tissue. Both benign and malignant tumors occur. Malignant tumors are somewhat less common than benign tumors in general, and they are often detected by a loss of gland function. For example, malignant thyroid tumors trap less radioactive iodine following a test dose and show less radioactivity on thyroid scan than does the surrounding normal tissue. The malignant area is therefore identified as a "cold" area on the scan. Loss of function results from replacement of normal specialized glandular tissue with primitive, nonfunctional tumor tissue (see Chapter 6). Rarely, malignant tumors are hormone-secreting and are detected by physiologic responses to the excess hormone activity. Some examples of malignant and benign hormone-secreting tumors follow.

Oat Cell Carcinoma of the Lung. This primitive and highly malignant tumor may secrete ADH and cause excessive water retention, leading to edema (inappropriate ADH secretion).

Benign Tumors of Endocrine Tissue. These are often hormone-secreting, since they resemble the parent tissue closely and therefore retain its basic functions.

Thyroid Adenomas. These cause hypersecretion of thyroid hormones, leading to clinical hyperthyroidism.

Adrenal Cortical Adenomas. These tumors produce excessive amounts of corticosteroids, resulting in Cushing's syndrome. This disorder, which can also be caused by over-administration of corticosteroids or adrenocorticotropic hormone (ACTH) has complex symptomatology. Major symptoms are edema, hypertension, obesity, increased blood glucose level, and a tendency to store fat below the neck (buffalo hump) (Fig. 16–2). Facial edema causes a round, full face (moon face) to develop. Other common symptoms are stretch marks on the abdomen (abdominal striae) resulting from edema, osteoporosis (loss of bone calcium due to effects of corticosteroids), and changes in personality (occasionally psychosis). If

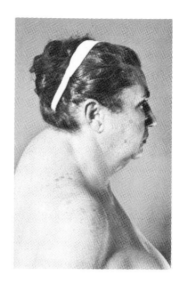

Figure 16–2. Cushing's syndrome, showing "buffalo hump," facial edema, and obesity.

aldosterone is the major hormone hypersecreted, a complex of hypertension, sodium retention, and potassium loss occurs (Conn's syndrome).

Islet Cell Adenomas of the Pancreas. These cause excessive insulin secretion and result in hypoglycemia, giving symptoms of faintness, difficulty in concentrating, diplopia (double vision), and loss of consciousness.

Pheochromocytomas. These tumors of the adrenal medulla may be benign or malignant but are usually benign. They hypersecrete epinephrine, norepinephrine, and other compounds, resulting in increased blood pressure, tachycardia, and palpitations (see Chapter 10). In nearly all cases, the tumors can be removed surgically, resulting in reduced gland secretion and reversal of clinical symptoms.

Other Disease Processes

Many endocrine disorders are caused by *hypersecretion* or *hyposecretion* of a particular gland. There is no tumor, but the gland tissue undergoes hyperplasia or atrophy for some reason. Sometimes decreased glandular function results from exogenous drug administration. Thus, in patients taking large doses of corticosteroids for extended periods of time, the adrenal cortex atrophies. The continued hypothalamic feedback suppression resulting from sustained high levels of corticosteroids prevents release of tropic hormone (ACTH) and normal simulation of the adrenal cortex. This problem can be prevented by using the tropic hormone (ACTH) rather than the target hormone (corticosteroid), thus stimulating the body's own adrenal cortex tissue to produce corticosteroids rather than supplying them from outside. Hyperplasia of the adrenal cortex occurs occasionally, usually for unknown reasons. The end result is the same as with a cortical adenoma; i.e., Cushing's syndrome.

Pituitary hypersecretion results in excessive growth of children, leading to *giantism*. Adult-onset hyperpituitarism cannot increase the height of the individual, since the long bones can no longer respond to growth hormone. However, the hands, feet, and skull enlarge, giving them a massive appearance, and the person complains

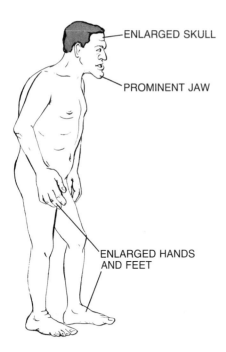

ENLARGED SKULL

PROMINENT JAW

ENLARGED HANDS
AND FEET

Figure 16–3. Acromegaly.

that hats and shoes keep getting too small. The condition is called *acromegaly* (Fig. 16–3).

Panhypopituitarism (Simmond's disease) causes the undeveloped child to become a midget and the adult to suffer a variety of symptoms caused by target organ hyposecretion (e.g., hypothyroidism, hypogonadism). This is, of course, caused by reduced secretion of tropic hormones by the hypofunctioning pituitary.

Hypofunction of the adrenal cortex results in *Addison's disease,* which is characterized by loss of sodium and retention of potassium, dehydration, low blood pressure, and weakness. It is essentially the opposite side of the coin from Cushing's syndrome. If only the posterior portion of the pituitary fails to secrete adequate amounts of hormones, the major result is *diabetes insipidus,* caused by reduced ADH activity. Oxytocin deficiency is not as obvious and may be undetected in males. The chief symptom of diabetes insipidus is the production of a large volume of dilute (insipid) urine (polyuria). In severe cases, 15 to 20 liters per day of urine are lost, resulting in rapid dehydration if intake does not equal loss.

Occasionally, a mistake is made in the biochemistry of hormone synthesis and one hormone is produced at a low level while another is overproduced. In the *adrenogenital syndrome,* the individual fails to produce adequate amounts of cortisone (an anti-inflammatory corticosteroid) because of deficiency of certain enzymes necessary for its synthesis. Thus there is deficient feedback suppression of ACTH, and increased secretion of ACTH results. Since cortisone synthesis is hampered by the enzyme deficiency, increased quantities of *androgenic* corticosteroids are formed and masculinization results. Boys with this condition mature at an early age (4 to 8 years) and show excessive muscular development resulting from androgenic stimulation ("little Atlas," "little Hercules"). Girls develop male sexual characteristics, such as growth of facial hair, muscular development, and enlargement of the clitoris.

With increased understanding of the complex interaction of hormones along with the ability to determine their levels in the blood stream with accuracy, great strides have been made in the diagnosis and treatment of endocrine disorders. Surgery is often effective for the removal of glandular tumors and usually results in permanent cure of the condition. Drug therapy, directed at controlling the hormone imbalance through supplementation of deficient hormones, is usually successful and has resulted in dramatic improvement in Addison's disease, hypothyroidism, hypopituitarism, and other deficiency states. Drugs are also used to control gland hypersecretion or its results in hyperthyroidism, Conn's syndrome, adrenogenital syndrome, and other conditions.

The rest of this chapter describes some common endocrine disorders.

THE PARATHYROID GLAND

HYPOPARA-THYROIDISM

Reduced secretion of parathormone (parathyroid hormone) from the parathyroid glands results from destruction of the glands owing to infection or to inflammatory process or following their surgical removal. The glands are tiny (30 mg each in weight) and are surrounded by thyroid tissue. In early days of thyroid surgery, the parathyroids were often accidentally removed with the thyroid tissue, resulting in a sudden drastic drop in parathormone level. Since parathormone causes mobilization of calcium from bones and renal secretion of phosphate ion, low blood levels of parathormone resulted in hypocalcemia and hyperphosphatemia.

The chief symptoms of hypoparathyroidism are muscle spasm (calcium tetany) and peripheral nerve malfunction (tingling and numbness). In severe cases, laryngeal tetany and dyspnea result (see Chapter 7).

Treatment is accomplished with the use of parathormone injections along with intravenous calcium compounds to raise the blood calcium level.

HYPERPARA-THYROIDISM

Increased parathormone secretion results in hypercalcemia and hypophosphatemia. The condition can be either *primary* or *secondary*. Eighty percent of the cases of primary hyperparathyroidism are caused by parathyroid adenoma. Secondary hyperparathyroidism generally results from chronic renal failure (see Chapter 11). Loss of calcium and failure to secrete phosphate ion by the failing kidney results in hypocalcemia and hyperphosphatemia, leading to increased secretion of parathormone. This causes bone deterioration and various skeletal deformities to occur and also results in hyperplasia of the parathyroid gland.

Treatment

Treatment is usually surgical. Parathyroid adenomas can be removed, leading to normalization of gland function. Hyperplastic parathyroid tissue formed as a result of chronic renal failure can be surgically removed but will reoccur unless the renal problem can be brought under control. The best solution is a renal transplant, although careful dialysis treatment that maintains physiologic levels of electrolytes may prevent the development of secondary hyperparathyroidism.

THE THYROID GLAND

HYPOTHYROIDISM
(Gull's Disease)

In 1874, Gull described the adult form of hypothyroidism, adding to the description of the childhood form given by Fagge three years earlier. It was seen that the conditions were identical but that the age of onset was important in determining the extent of clinical manifestations in the afflicted individual.

Pathogenesis

Hypothyroidism is the most common disorder affecting the thyroid gland. There are multiple etiologic factors, and the condition is more properly called a syndrome than a disease. In children, the condition often results from defective development of the gland, producing a rudimentary, poorly functioning gland, or, occasionally, no gland at all. Maternal hypothyroidism may be a cause of congenital hypothyroidism in the newborn. Older children and adults develop the condition for several additional reasons.

Deficiency of iodine in the diet is a common cause of the condition in many parts of the world but is now uncommon in the United States since the introduction of iodized salt. Prior to the widespread use of iodized salt, the Great Lakes area was known for its high incidence of hypothyroidism and resulting enlargement of the gland (goiter). In the *goiter belt* (as this area was called), the soil contained almost no iodine and very little seafood (a good source of iodine) was consumed, leading to iodine deficiency. In the face of deficient iodine intake, the thyroid gland failed to synthesize normal amounts of thyroxine (T_4) and tri-iodothyronine (T_3). This resulted in reduced feedback suppression of thyrotropin-releasing factor (TRF) and thyroid-stimulating hormone (TSH), and excessive gland stimulation resulted, causing gland hyperplasia (Table 16–1). With the introduction of iodized salt, the problem virtually disappeared.

Certain vegetables also cause inhibition of thyroid function when eaten to excess. Cabbage, rutabagas, and turnips contain a compound called *progoitrin,* which is converted into *goitrin* in the intestinal tract (or within the vegetable itself if eaten raw).

Chronic inflammation of the gland also leads to damage and reduced function. Some cases probably result from autoimmune reaction, since antithyroid antibodies are occasionally found in the blood of the hypothyroid individual. Other causes include surgical removal of thyroid tissue or gland damage because of radiation exposure (to x-ray or radioactive iodine). Many cases are termed idiopathic, since no cause can be found.

Symptoms and Signs

In the adult form of hypothyroidism, the symptoms include lethargy, easy fatigue, intolerance to cold, and dryness of the skin. The fingernails are brittle, and the skin has a puffy, edematous look, caused by deposition of mucopolysaccharide. This edema is called *myxedema,* and the term is often used to describe adult hypothyroidism in general. Reflexes are depressed and the speech is slow and monotonous. Heart rate and body temperature are decreased, and there is a tendency toward weight gain. (Most cases of obesity do not result from hypothyroidism, however.)

Severe hypothyroidism can lead to psychiatric symptoms. In one case, an elderly man wandered into a large metropolitan hospital muttering and acting in a bizarre manner. The initial impression was that of senile dementia, but after the observation that he wore three sweaters on a warm day, hypothyroidism was suspected. When this was confirmed and corrected, the patient became completely lucid.

Hypothyroidism has a more devastating effect in children than in adults and leads to retarded physical and mental development, along with the other symptoms just mentioned. The condition is called *cretinism.* The affected person is abnormally short, with a potbelly and an umbilical hernia, mental retardation, and delayed sexual maturation. Neonatal thyroid function testing is now done at most hospitals to detect cretinism at a stage when it can be completely reversed.

The wide variety of symptoms seen in hypothyroidism is a reflection of the fact that thyroid hormones affect virtually every metabolic process in the body. Since thyroid hormone is required for the breakdown of cholesterol to bile acids, for example, the reduced breakdown seen in hypothyroidism causes an increased cholesterol level and the possibility of increased atherosclerosis. Many other such examples exist.

Laboratory Findings

The chief laboratory findings in hypothyroidism are reduced serum levels of thyroxine (normal = 4 to 11 μg/dl) and triiodothyronine (normal = 25 to 35 percent uptake using a radioactive isotope). A composite of T_3 and T_4 (T_7) is often used as a single figure that represents both values. This is determined indirectly from T_3 and T_4 values (normal = 1 to 3.8). Serum TSH is usually elevated, since there is reduced feedback suppression of its release. The normal value for TSH is up to 10 microunits/ml. The cholesterol level is often increased, as previously mentioned, as a result of reduced metabolism. In cretinism, delayed bone and tooth development, which is visible on x-ray films, is also seen in addition to the findings described.

Diagnosis

Hypothyroidism can result from hypopituitarism, along with other types of gland hypofunction. In this case, TSH level is decreased instead of increased and hypothyroidism results from insufficient pituitary stimulation of the thyroid gland. Down's syndrome in infants superficially resembles cretinism, but it is caused by the presence of an additional chromosome (47 instead of the normal 46). Unfortunately, this condition is not treatable and mental retardation and other defects persist. Fatigue and lethargy, similar to that seen in hypothyroidism, can result from mental depression or hidden infection, such as tuberculosis. Laboratory tests of thyroid function are of great benefit in the differential diagnosis of these conditions.

Treatment   Hypothyroidism in the child or adult is easily treated by oral replacement of thyroid hormones in quantities dictated by serum hormone assays. Whole-gland preparations (thyroid extract), purified thyroglobulin (Proloid), and individual T_4 (Synthroid) and T_3 (Cytomel) are available. The doses of the pure T_4 or T_3 products are, of course, smaller than those of the whole-gland or thyroglobulin products, since the latter contain inert material extracted along with the active hormones. An interesting product called liotrix (Thyrolar, Euthroid) is synthetic but combines T_4 and T_3 in a physiologic ratio to give a balanced action. Liotrix is given in tablets equivalent in strength to the older whole-gland preparations. In general, any thyroid preparation will effectively treat most cases of hypothyroidism. Treatment is usually required for life, since spontaneous return of thyroid activity is rare.

Complications   Too-rapid administration of thyroid hormones can cause excessive cardiac stimulation, leading to arrhythmias, angina symptoms, or heart failure (high-output failure) (see Chapter 10). The dose should be brought up step by step to the correct level. Severe hypothyroidism can lead to *myxedema coma,* in which hypothermia, cardiac and respiratory depression, and death are common consequences. Intravenous injection of T_4, along with expert supportive treatment, is necessary for patient survival. Hypothyroid individuals are exceedingly sensitive to narcotic drugs and can die from usual doses of them. Narcotic drugs should be withheld completely or used in much lower doses, if needed, in hypothyroidism. Chronic administration of T_4 or T_3 in doses larger than those needed for replacement results in excessive feedback suppression and eventual atrophy of the thyroid gland. This is similar to the situation that occurs in the adrenal cortex with prolonged administration of large doses of corticosteroids.

Prognosis   The prognosis in hypothyroidism is generally good. Early treatment in children prevents the ravages of cretinism, and treatment of adults reverses their symptoms. Periodic re-evaluation is necessary to ensure maintenance of the correct level of hormone intake for adequate treatment of the condition.

HYPERTHYROIDISM
(Thyrotoxicosis)   Overactivity of the thyroid gland occurs primarily in women in the 20- to 40-year-old age group. The ratio of women to men affected is about 6:1. Parry reported in 1825 an association between enlarged thyroid, cardiac effects, and ophthalmic changes and defined the condition as we know it today. Later, Graves and Basedow refined the definition to include particular ocular changes (exophthalmos) and goiter (exophthalmic goiter) in some hyperthyroid individuals. This subgroup is said to have *Graves' disease.*

Pathogenesis   Most people with hyperthyroidism have Graves' disease. In 90 percent of these individuals, a thyroid antibody—thyroid-stimulating immunoglobulin (TSI)—is formed, presumably the result of an autoimmune reaction. TSI binds to TSH receptors in the gland and causes thyroid hyperfunction. The exact nature of TSI is not known. Since TSI operates outside the feedback system, it is not inhibited by the hypothalamic-pituitary suppression that occurs as a result of hyperthyroidism, and the increased production of T_4 and T_3 continues unabated. In addition, for poorly understood reasons, there is also deposition of mucopolysaccharide in the eye orbits, along with orbital edema. The eyes are forced outward, and the individual has a staring, surprised look with impaired eyelid function (exophthalmos) (Fig. 16–4). A fraction of TSI that causes exophthalmos without causing thyroid stimulation has been identified; this is called exophthalmos-producing factor (EPF).

The reasons for the autoimmune reaction leading to the production of TSI and EPF are not clear. Women in the 20- to 40-year-old age group are prone to a number of other autoimmune disorders, including rheumatoid arthritis and lupus erythematosus. Perhaps this represents an immune system abnormality in these people. There is a hereditary tendency toward Graves' disease, and this supports the concept of an inherited immune system abnormality.

The other major form of hyperthyroidism is *Plummer's disease,* caused by thyroid adenoma. This is not associated with exophthalmos and is not considered to be an autoimmune disorder, since TSI and EPF are not found in the blood stream.

Symptoms and Signs The symptomatology in hyperthyroidism is almost exactly the reverse of that in hypothyroidism. The individual is energetic, nervous, has difficulty in sleeping, suffers greatly from the heat because of increased body metabolism and heat production, and has an elevated body temperature. Excessive sweating is common. Heart rate is increased, and arrhythmias (especially atrial fibrillation) are common. The appetite is voracious, but loss of weight occurs because of increased metabolic rate. Hyperreflexia and a fine tremor of the hands are usually seen. Speech is rapid, and flow of thoughts is fast, often to the point of difficulty in concentrating. Exophthalmos (Fig. 16–4) is frequently present, with eye redness, irritation, or even infection resulting from impaired eyelid function and reduced tear flow over the eyeball. The thyroid gland is often enlarged or nodular, reflecting the hyperactivity and the effects of excessive gland stimulation.

Laboratory Findings The T_3, T_4, and T_7 levels are elevated in hyperthyroidism. The TSH level is depressed because of feedback inhibition, and the

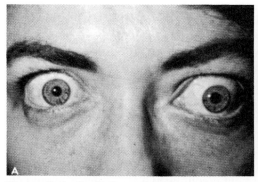 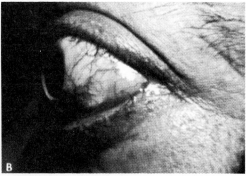

Figure 16–4. *(A, B)* Graves' disease, showing exophthalmos. (From Scheie, H. G., and Albert, D. M.: *Textbook of Ophthalmology,* 9th ed. Philadelphia, W. B. Saunders Company, 1977.)

serum cholesterol level is usually below normal because of an increased breakdown to bile acids. In Graves' disease, TSI is present; in Plummer's disease, it is absent. The electrocardiogram shows tachycardia and often atrial fibrillation.

Diagnosis   Anxiety neurosis causes many of the symptoms of hyperthyroidism. However, thyroid tests are normal. Pheochromocytoma gives many of the clinical findings of hyperthyroidism, but, again, serum thyroid tests are normal. In addition, the urinary vanillylmandelic acid (VMA) level is increased (see Chapter 10). In Hashimoto's thyroiditis, the gland is painful and obviously inflamed.

Treatment   Three different forms of treatment are available for hyperthyroidism, depending upon the circumstances of the case.

Surgery. Removal of the majority of the gland (subtotal thyroidectomy) is relatively safe and curative. It is preferred for young, healthy patients who are willing to undergo operation. Before surgery, the gland must be prepared with drugs so that good results can be attained. In the hyperthyroid state, the gland is hyperplastic, hypervascular, and loaded with T_4 and T_3. An attempt at surgery under these conditions may result in excessive bleeding and release of large amounts of thyroid hormones into the blood stream, leading to hyperthermia and cardiac arrhythmias *(thyroid storm)*. Pretreatment with propylthiouracil or methimazole (Tapazole) for 2 to 3 weeks before surgery inhibits production of thyroid hormones. These are then depleted from the gland as the body uses them, preventing the possibility of thyroid storm. Treatment with large doses of iodine or iodide ion (usually Lugol's solution) for 1 to 2 weeks before surgery causes gland involution and loss of vascularity. This prevents excessive bleeding during thyroid surgery. Iodine-iodide administration is often continued for a week or so after surgery to promote quicker tissue healing with less bleeding.

Long-Term Thyroid Inhibitor Therapy. Propylthiouracil or methimazole in lower doses gives chronic thyroid suppression. The treatment period is usually 6 to 18 months. Sometimes thyroid activity eventually returns to normal and the drug can be withdrawn with no further treatment. The possibility of blood disorders (especially agranulocytosis) prevents unlimited duration of treatment, however.

Radioactive Iodine. Given by intravenous injection or orally ("^{131}I cocktail"), this is a third approach to hyperthyroidism. Since the gland concentrates iodine from the blood stream, it will accumulate enough ^{131}I from doses harmless to other body areas to cause gland destruction. If the dose of ^{131}I is correct, enough selective gland damage occurs so that the hyperthyroidism is corrected. This form of treatment is ideal for older patients, especially those with conditions that preclude surgery. There is a slightly increased risk of thyroid cancer when this treatment is given to young people, presumably because of their longer life expectancy and the long-term effects of ^{131}I on the gland. However, the risk is no greater than in those who are treated surgically. Another complication to this form of treatment is continued gland damage, eventually making the person severely *hypothyroid* and requiring thyroid replacement therapy.

Complications   Exophthalmos that does not respond to treatment of hyperthyroidism (progressive exophthalmos) is occasionally seen in the individual with Graves' disease. Eye infection, severe damage, and blindness can result. In these cases, surgery to reseat the eyeball in the orbit can be done. Fatal arrhythmias sometimes occur in hyperthyroidism. Drugs such as propranolol (Inderal) can be given while the condition is being brought under control to protect the heart from excessive stimulation. Existing cardiac conditions (angina, congestive heart failure) are worsened by hyperthyroidism and are often refractory to conventional therapy until the thyroid condition is controlled.

Prognosis   Long-term outlook is good in hyperthyroidism, since the disease can usually be controlled. Complete remission, with normal thyroid tests in the absence of drug therapy, occasionally occurs.

THE PANCREAS

DIABETES MELLITUS   The term diabetes mellitus derives from words meaning *siphon* and *sweet* and describes a condition characterized by the production of a large volume of urine (siphon action) containing sugar (sweet). The only common feature of diabetes insipidus, previously mentioned, and diabetes mellitus is that a large urine volume (polyuria) is produced. The causes, symptomatology, and treatments of the two conditions are otherwise different. Diabetes mellitus is a complex disorder, consisting of much more than polyuria and sugar excretion.

The incidence of diabetes mellitus is approximately 2 percent in the United States population, with about equal male and female prevalence. It favors American Indians over other Americans, especially the Pimas, who have an incidence of about 35 percent. Among world populations, the Polynesians and Australian aborigines have an unusually high incidence as well.

Types of
Diabetes Mellitus   Most authorities recognize two general types of diabetes mellitus, based upon requirements for treatment.

Insulin-Dependent Diabetes Mellitus (IDDM). Individuals with this type require insulin for treatment. Most of these patients were formerly classified as *juvenile* (brittle) diabetics, although this form also occasionally occurs in adults. Insulin production is virtually absent, and pancreatic beta cells are unresponsive to drugs that stimulate insulin production from normal beta cells (oral antidiabetic agents).

Non–insulin-dependent Diabetes Mellitus (NIDDM). This type is primarily an adult disorder but is occasionally seen in juveniles. Insulin is not usually required for treatment, since beta cells are functional and are sensitive to oral antidiabetic drugs. This form of abetes mellitus is milder and produces fewer complications than IDDM. Two subgroups of NIDDM exist. In one, the individual is not obese and has a somewhat reduced insulin production. This type was formerly called *mature onset* diabetes mellitus. In the other, insulin level is normal or even elevated, but resistance to insulin is present. The most common situation here is obesity, with the presence of enlarged adipocytes (fat cells), usually caused by overeating for a long period of time. An increase in the amount of stored body fat increases insulin resistance. Certain endocrine disorders, notably Cushing's syndrome, cause an elevated blood glucose level (hyperglycemia) with a normal insulin level. The problem in these cases is not with the pancreas but with too great a demand for insulin.

In addition to those with established diabetes mellitus, there are individuals who may later develop clinical or overt diabetes. These are said to have *prediabetes*. Those with no symptoms but with an abnormal tolerance for glucose are said to have *chemical diabetes*. These categories are important, since the natural progression is from prediabetes to chemical diabetes to overt diabetes.

Pathogenesis   Volumes have been written concerning possible causes of diabetes mellitus. Many diabetics seem to have an *inherited tendency* toward the condition, and it is assumed that a genetic predisposition exists. Indeed, abnormalities in certain genes of diabetic individuals have been noted. In addition, strong concordance (both have the condition) is seen in identical twins. This approaches 100 percent in NIDDM. Close relatives of diabetics are more prone to the condition than relatives of nondiabetics. However, the situation is not clear-cut and diabetes mellitus is sometimes called a "geneticist's nightmare."

Viral infection is thought to be important in some cases of diabetes mellitus. The condition sometimes develops following infection with mumps virus or coxsackievirus and its overall incidence parallels the seasonal variation in viral infections. Virus particles can be seen in pancreatic tissue from some diabetics, and the condition can be duplicated in mice by intentional viral inoculation.

Chronic pancreatitis is occasionally followed by the development of diabetes mellitus. This is presumably due to beta cell destruction caused by chronic inflammation.

Autoimmune reactions seem important in the etiology of some cases of diabetes mellitus. Pancreatic tissue from individuals dying during an acute diabetic episode show heavy infiltration of lymphocytes, monocytes, and other cells in the islets of Langerhans, where beta cells are located. This supports the idea of an immune response. In addition, anti-islet cell antibodies are seen in 75 percent of those with IDDM but in only about 1 percent of the normal population.

"Overwork" of the pancreas, caused by a lifetime of heavy carbohydrate ingestion, may be important in some cases of NIDDM.

Insulin resistance may not only be related to obesity but may be seen in body tissues other than adipocytes. This might explain the unusually large doses of insulin needed by some diabetics.

An interesting hypothesis, proposed by Neel, is that a mild diabetic tendency is actually beneficial, in that it promotes fat storage and slower metabolism of glucose. The individual with this "thrifty gene" for mild diabetes survives periods of famine better than the nondiabetic. Populations with a high incidence of diabetes mellitus today have a history of famine periods. The American Indians and the Australian aborigines, in earlier days, were nomadic people who often faced severe food shortage. The Polynesians are thought to have migrated from the coast of South America across the Pacific

Ocean in balsa wood rafts and undergone starvation on the way. Survivors of these three groups, according to Neel, would likely carry the "thrifty gene." Intermarriage within the surviving population group would strengthen the diabetic tendency and result in a high incidence of diabetes mellitus later on.

It is likely that diabetes mellitus is not caused by a single entity but by several factors working together to cause pancreatic damage or malfunction. Possibly, a genetic tendency, coupled with viral infection, an autoimmune reaction, or both represent "partners in crime" in the development of the clinical condition (Fig. 16–5).

Symptoms and Signs

Symptoms and signs of acute diabetes mellitus vary greatly. Common findings are loss of energy and easy fatigue, polyuria, thirst, and a large volume of fluid intake (polydipsia). In IDDM, increased food consumption (polyphagia), often associated with weight loss, is seen. This is not as pronounced in NIDDM, since there is some insulin activity and partial utilization of glucose as a source of calories. Thirst and dehydration result primarily from the osmotic effects of glucose excretion in the urine, as do dryness of the skin and itching. Fatigue and wasting result from impaired utilization of glucose, since the normal effect of insulin in promoting uptake of glucose into body cells is diminished or absent. This causes the body to break down its own tissues for energy, a relatively inefficient process.

Diabetics are more prone to all types of infection, particularly those involving the lower extremities and the vagina. This is due in part to impaired protein synthesis and also to the higher glucose content of body tissues. Reduced circulation is probably a contributory factor in infections of the lower extremities. Early visual symptoms, such as blurring and change in refractive power of the

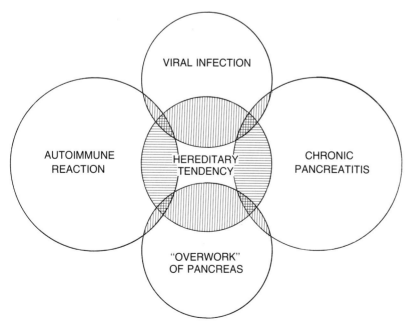

Figure 16–5. Interaction of etiologic factors in diabetes mellitus.

eyes, are common and many cases of diabetes mellitus are diagnosed by ophthalmologists or optometrists before other symptoms are apparent. A particular type of retinal vascular pattern is seen on ophthalmic examination, often very early in the course of the condition.

Diabetic symptoms are generally more severe in IDDM than in NIDDM. This gives rise to interesting speculations regarding their etiology.

Laboratory Findings   The primary manifestations of diabetes mellius are *hypergly-cemia, glycosuria,* and an *abnormal glucose tolerance.*

The normal fasting blood sugar (FBS) level, obtained after an overnight fast, is 60 to 110 mg/dl. Values over 110 mg/dl are suggestive of diabetes mellitus. The FBS level can be determined by assay of a blood sample or with the use of a test strip (Dextrostix) impregnated with glucose oxidase, an enzyme that oxidizes glucose and triggers a color reaction. The color change can be read from a chart on the bottle or with an instrument that accurately measures the intensity of color (reflectance meter). Such instruments are now sold for home use.

Glycosuria results from the passage of nonabsorbed glucose into the urine. Glycosuria usually appears at a blood glucose level of about 170 mg/dl. The large quantity of glucose filtered by the glomeruli at that blood glucose level exceeds the reabsorptive capacity of the tubular transport system and passes through into the urine (sugar spill). Therefore, the appearance of glycosuria usually means that the blood glucose level is at least 170 mg/dl. Urine glucose can be detected with Clinitest tablets, which utilize a nonspecific oxidation-reduction reaction, or with Testape, a glucose oxidase-impregnated test strip that reacts only to glucose. Both tests can be rendered inaccurate if the individual is excreting large amounts of reducing agent (vitamin C, for example) at the time of the test.

Ketosis, seen with IDDM but not with NIDDM, results from breakdown of fatty acids for energy, with the accumulation of nonmetabolizable residues (ketone bodies) left over when the fatty acid chain is metabolized. The condition is indicated by an increased level of ketone bodies (acetone, beta-hydroxybutyric acid, aceto-acetic acid) in the blood stream. This results in *metabolic acidosis,* partly from accumulation of acidic compounds and partly through electrolyte imbalance (see Chapters 7 and 8). *Ketonuria* occurs as ketone bodies are excreted in the urine. It can be detected with Acetest tablets or Ketostix. Ketosis and the resulting acidosis and ketonuria signify a more severe diabetic state, since they occur only when glucose utilization is minimal or absent.

A *glucose tolerance test* is given to diabetics to test their ability to metabolize a specific amount of glucose given quickly. An FBS is done first, then 100 gm of glucose is given as a drink (Glucola). The blood glucose level is determined at hourly intervals for 3 or 5 hours after administration of glucose. The diabetic individual has a higher FBS and reaches higher blood glucose values at the hourly points than does a nondiabetic person (Fig. 16–6). Insulin levels are lower in IDDM and in nonobese NIDDM but are normal or even elevated

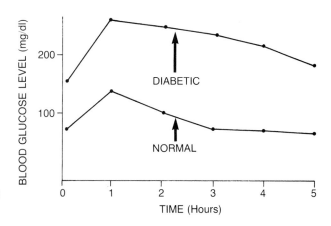

Figure 16–6. Glucose tolerance curve (normal versus diabetic).

in obese NIDDM, reflecting the insulin resistance characteristic of this type. Cholesterol and triglyceride levels are often elevated in diabetics of all types.

Diagnosis   Several nondiabetic conditions result in the appearance of sugar in the urine. *Renal glycosuria* is a disorder in which normal amounts of glucose fail to be reabsorbed at the renal tubule. Thus, sugar spill occurs at normal blood glucose levels. The individual is not diabetic and has a normal glucose tolerance but appears diabetic if only a urine test is performed. No treatment is required.

Cushing's syndrome causes hyperglycemia and glycosuria because of increased gluconeogenesis (synthesis of glucose). The treatment is to remove or control the cause of the condition. Rarely, other sugars (fructose, galactose) are excreted in the urine, giving a positive Clinitest reaction. However, testing with Testape reveals no *glucose* in the urine and points to the existence of a different metabolic disorder.

Treatment   *General measures* helpful for the diabetic include moderate exercise, avoidance of smoking, and early control of infections to prevent complications. Exercise tends to lower the blood glucose level, even in those with IDDM. Smoking increases the atherosclerotic tendency already present in the diabetic person. Early control of infection is vitally important, since the diabetic individual has subnormal defenses against minor, routine infections, for a variety of reasons. A stubbed toe easily becomes infected and then gangrenous if neglected.

A good mental attitude is essential for optimal health and happiness. While there are certain limitations placed on the individual by the condition, a full life is possible if these are dealt with in a matter-of-fact manner. Regularity of eating habits, exercise, and drug administration are critical for good control of the diabetic state.

Specific treatment for diabetes mellitus revolves around diet, insulin, and oral antidiabetic drugs.

Diet. The diet currently recommended by the American Diabetes Association consists of 35 percent of dietary calories obtained from fat (primarily unsaturated fat), reduced cholesterol intake, up to 50 percent of dietary calories from starches (eliminating concentrated sources of sugar), and liberal protein intake. This diet is considered healthier for the diabetic than the diet formerly recommended (before 1976), which stressed a higher fat intake and reduced starch intake. Since the diabetic person risks increased atherosclerosis, the current diet is more prudent but does not sacrifice good diabetic control. Virtually all diabetics should use this diet, even if they also take insulin or use oral antidiabetic drugs.

Insulin. Insulin is available in several forms:

1. Regular insulin (crystalline zinc insulin—CZI) is short-acting and has a rapid onset of action. It can be given intravenously in an emergency, as well as subcutaneously, since it is a clear solution.

2. Neutral protamine Hagedorn (NPH) insulin is intermediate in duration and onset of action and is given by subcutaneous injection.

3. Protamine zinc insulin (PZI) has a long duration and slow onset of action. It is also given by subcutaneous injection.

4. In addition, various forms of Lente insulin (regular, semi-, ultra-) are available. These roughly correspond to the three types just described.

Many diabetics mix insulins to get a quick onset but a prolonged effect. A commonly used combination is CZI plus NPH.

Oral Antidiabetic Drugs. These act by increasing the release of insulin from pancreatic beta cells. There are four products currently on the market: Tolbutamide (Orinase) has a short duration of action; tolazamide (Tolinase) and acetohexamide (Dymelor) are intermediate in action; and chlorpropamide (Diabinese) has a long duration of action. These work only if the pancreatic beta cells are functional and therefore are not effective for IDDM.

The choice of treatments for diabetes mellitus depends upon the type of condition (Table 16–2). Diet and insulin treatment can be used for all types, but diet and oral antidiabetic drugs are recommended for nonobese NIDDM. Obese NIDDM is best treated with weight reduction to decrease insulin resistance.

Complications   There are complications both to diabetes mellitus itself and to insulin therapy for it.

Reactions to Insulin. Chronic administration of insulin can cause damage to fatty tissue beneath the skin, resulting in dimpling (lipodystrophy). This problem is less common now than in the past, since newer insulin preparations are purer and closer to normal body pH. If it is a problem, the injection sites can be rotated to minimize the effect.

Some people are allergic to foreign proteins contained in insulin preparations. Commercial insulin is obtained from beef or pork

Table 16–2. TREATMENT OF DIABETES MELLITUS

Type	Treatment
IDDM*	Diet, insulin
NIDDM (Nonobese)	Diet, oral antidiabetic drugs
NIDDM (Obese)	Diet to promote weight loss

Abbreviations: IDDM = Insulin-dependent diabetes mellitus; NIDDM = non–insulin-dependent diabetes mellitus.

pancreas. Allergy to beef or pork protein often causes reactions to the preparation. There is also reaction to the insulin molecule, which is slightly different from human insulin, in these preparations. The problem can usually be overcome by switching to a form that does not promote allergy. For those allergic to foreign proteins in the insulin preparations rather than the insulin molecule itself, the newer *single-peak* or *single-component* insulins (highly purified preparations) are often a solution.

Insulin shock results when the blood glucose level drops to an abnormally low point (hypoglycemia), usually below 50 mg/dl. Early symptoms are weakness, headache, diplopia, irritability, and mental confusion. Later, unconsciousness, convulsions, coma, and even death can result. Symptoms occur because the brain effectively uses only glucose for fuel and malfunctions when the blood glucose level falls too low. Treatment consists of oral administration of sugar (candy, sweet drink, packet of sugar) if the person is conscious and the intravenous administration of glucose if unconscious.

Complications of Diabetes Mellitus. Complications of diabetes mellitus itself include diabetic ketoacidosis, large vascular disease, small vascular disease, and diabetic neuropathy.

Diabetic Ketoacidosis. This condition results from loss of control of the condition, often in an individual who discontinues insulin, drastically alters the diet, or both. Severe hyperglycemia, glycosuria, ketosis, and metabolic acidosis develop over a period of days; hypokalemia, polyuria, dehydration, and central nervous system depression result, often progressing to coma. Respiration is rapid and deep (Kussmaul respiration) with an acetone breath odor. Treatment consists of hydration, administration of potassium, and re-establishment of insulin control, usually with intravenous administration of CZI.

Vascular Complications. Diabetics suffer from both large and small blood vessel disease (Fig. 16–7). *Large vessel disease* (occlusive vascular disease) is primarily an atherosclerotic process, affecting the arteries of the legs and feet, heart, and cerebral system. Consequently, the affected individual is more likely to develop impaired circulation to the legs and feet, myocardial infarction, or stroke. Reduced circulation to the lower extremities increases the susceptibility to infection, ulceration, and gangrene of the feet.

Small vessel disease affects the blood vessels of the retina

Figure 16–7. Diabetic vascular disease in large and small vessels.

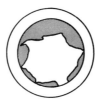

NORMAL

LARGE VESSEL
DISEASE
(Atherosclerotic
Deposits
in Lumen)

SMALL VESSEL
DISEASE
(Glycoprotein
Deposits in
Basement
Membrane)

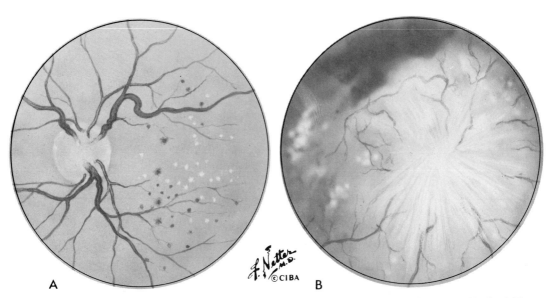

Figure 16–8. Diabetic retinopathy. *(A)* Venous dilatation, microaneurysms, minute hemorrhages, and (yellowish) spots in the ocular fundus. *(B)* Retinitis proliferans and massive hemorrhage. (From CIBA, Plate Number 23, Vol. 4, Section V. © Copyright 1965, CIBA Pharmaceutical Company, Division of CIBA-GEIGY Corporation. Reprinted with permission from the CIBA Collection of Medical Illustrations, illustrated by Frank H. Netter, M.D. All rights reserved.)

(retinopathy) and kidney *(nephropathy)*. It is characterized by deposition of glycoprotein in the basement membrane of the affected vessel, leading to reduced vessel size. In the kidney, this results in progressive loss of renal tissue and the eventual development of chronic renal failure. In the retina, microaneurysms and tiny hemorrhages develop. Diabetic retinopathy is of two types (Fig. 16–8): *background,* the type just described, and *proliferative,* a progressive form characterized by overgrowth of new vascular tissue (neovascularization) in the retina. Proliferative retinopathy causes obliteration of the retinal nerve cell layer (rods and cones) and leads to blindness. Detached retina is also common, as is cataract.

The vascular complications of diabetes mellitus are currently the subject of debate. One line of thought is that they are primarily due to the wide fluctuations in blood glucose level seen in diabetics. The other point of view is that blood glucose level is not a factor in the development of vascular complications. The debate cannot be settled at present because it is not possible to completely control blood glucose levels in diabetics to see whether or not this would prevent vascular complications. In the future, this question may be answered because it may be possible to control blood glucose levels effectively with an infusion pump that releases the required quantity of insulin automatically.

Diabetic Neuropathy. This condition is thought to result from impaired blood supply to peripheral or autonomic nerve fibers but it is poorly understood. Reduced autonomic activity, loss of peripheral sensation, and other symptoms are frequently seen in long-term diabetics. A variety of drugs are employed for treatment, but none is particularly effective.

Complications of diabetes mellitus are more severe in IDDM than in NIDDM, since IDDM is a more severe form of the condition and has an earlier onset in most cases. The best possible control of the diabetic state should be sought. This will reduce, but not eliminate, complications.

Prognosis   Prognosis in IDDM is not as good as in NIDDM for reasons already stated. There is great variation in long-term prognosis of diabetes mellitus because of the variability of the disorder among individuals. In general, the life expectancy is about 7 to 9 years less than for nondiabetics. The major causes of death are myocardial infarction, renal failure, and stroke, Some individuals, however, especially those with firm control of the condition, live 40 years or more after the onset of IDDM with minimal complications.

Future Development   Three important avenues of research are being explored today
in Treatment of   to aid in treatment of the diabetic individual.
Diabetes Mellitus   *Insulin pumps,* originally used in the late 1970s, provide a steady release of insulin into subcutaneous tissues, usually by means of an abdominal needle, and give much better control than traditional insulin injections. The rate can be increased manually at mealtime. A future improvement would be a pump that constantly monitors blood glucose level and releases the correct amount of insulin as needed, as does the normal pancreas.

Recombinant DNA research with *Escherichia coli* bacteria has produced a strain that manufactures human insulin, now marketed as Humulin. This insulin can be used in those who react adversely to beef or pork insulin or in those who develop antibody resistance to those products.

Successful transplant of islet cells has been accomplished in animals. The transplanted islet cells, which contain beta cells, grow and secrete insulin. This has not been accomplished in humans because of tissue incompatibility but may eventually be possible. The future has never looked brighter for the diabetic.

SUMMARY

Endocrine hormone activity is maintained through a complex system of feedback control involving the hypothalamus, anterior pituitary, and target gland. For most hormones, a relatively constant level is maintained in the blood stream. Estrogen and progesterone, however, undergo wide swings in level, giving support to reproductive tissues that is necessary for normal fertility.

Endocrine glands are affected by the same disease processes that affect other body tissues: infection, inflammation, and neoplasia. In addition, clinical disorders result from hypersecretion or hyposecretion of glands and from perverted synthesis of particular hormones. Hypothyroidism and hyperthyroidism are examples of disorders caused by secretion of incorrect amounts of thyroid hormones. Likewise, hypoparathyroidism and hyperparathyroidism result from inadequate or excessive secretion of parathormone. The adrenogenital syndrome is an example of a condition caused by perversion of synthesis (androgenic corticosteroids instead of anti-inflammatory corticosteroids).

Diabetes mellitus is a complex disorder, primarily related to a lack of insulin secretion or the development of resistance to it. Many etiologic factors seem important in its development, including heredity, viral infection, obesity, and autoimmune reaction. Although it cannot be cured, good control can usually be obtained with a combination of dietary, insulin, and oral antidiabetic therapy. Insulin and oral antidiabetic drugs are not used together in the same patient but each can be used in conjunction with diet. There is much argument about the causes of complications with diabetes mellitus. However, most agree that tight control of the condition will help to avoid or minimize long-term complications.

Questions

1. Speculate on ways by which the negative feedback system could allow wide swings in estrogen and progesterone to occur but would maintain relatively constant levels of androgen.
2. Compare and contrast the effects of a thyroid adenoma with those of a thyroid carcinoma in terms of histology, symptomatology, and treatment.
3. How do cretinism and myxedema differ? Is the treatment the same?
4. Compare and contrast Graves' disease and Plummer's disease.
5. Explain the rationale for treatment of IDDM with insulin, obese NIDDM with a weight-reducing diet, and nonobese NIDDM with oral antidiabetic drugs.

Additional Reading

Brown, J. *et al.:* Autoimmune thyroid diseases—Graves' and Hashimoto's. Ann. Intern. Med., 88:379, 1978.

Diabetes Mellitus. Indianapolis, Eli Lilly and Co., 1980. *(Excellent detailed and well-illustrated monograph.)*

Gilliland, P. F.: Myxedema: Recognition and treatment. Postgrad. Med., 57:61, 1975.

Krieger, D. T.: Endocrine disease and ills influenced by hormones. Pharmacy Times, 43:79, 1977. *(Brief overview of endocrinology.)*

Neel, J. V.: Diabetes mellitus: A "thrifty" genotype rendered detrimental by "progress"? Am. J. Human Genetics, 14:353, 1962. *(Fascinating theory of the etiology of diabetes mellitus.)*

Riesenberg, L. B.: Recombinant DNA—The containment debate. Chemistry, 50:13, 1977. *(Concise, well-illustrated treatment of gene splicing.)*

CHAPTER 17 INFLAMMATORY DISORDERS

The term *inflammatory disorder* is, admittedly, a vague one, since most diseases are associated with, if not caused by, inflammation. It is a nonspecific response to tissue injury. However, some conditions have symptomatology directly related to tissue or organ inflammation. Complications develop as a result of chronic inflammation and the major thrust of therapy is suppression of inflammation. It is obvious that in these conditions, inflammation is the central theme. These rightly deserve the dubious honor of being called inflammatory disorders.

The concepts of *acute* and *chronic inflammation* have been discussed in detail in Chapter 3. Pain, edema, warmth, redness, and loss of function are the major features of acute inflammation. Chronic inflammation often results from unresolved acute inflammation and takes the form of abscess development (suppurative) or granuloma formation (granulomatous). Inherent in the concept of chronic inflammation are the consequences of fibrosis and attempted repair of tissue damage which often result in structural and functional alteration in the affected tissue. An understanding of both acute and chronic inflammation is necessary for clarification of the symptoms, signs, laboratory findings, treatment, and complications of inflammatory disorders.

A process tightly intertwined with the etiology and pathogenesis of many inflammatory disorders is *autoimmune reaction* (see Chapter 4). The body's immune system is directed against certain tissues, cells, or chemical compounds, yielding an inflammatory reaction. Possible causes for such a reaction are numerous. Slight alteration in a body component, resulting from damage or attachment to an external element, could cause body surveillance systems to perceive it as a foreign component. Antigenic substances sequestered within cells could become accessible to immune surveillance when the cells were damaged. The immune system itself could be altered, so that it would "read" normal components as being abnormal. Examples of diseases associated with these abnormalities are given in Chapter 4. In many cases, there is evidence for the existence of an autoimmune reaction but the exact cause is lacking. Antibodies to various body components are found in the blood stream, but the mechanism for autoimmune reaction is not known.

Autoimmune disorders vary greatly in the type and extent of inflammation seen. With *Hashimoto's thyroiditis,* for example, only the thyroid gland is affected. *Myasthenia gravis* is characterized by selective autoimmune damage to receptors for acetylcholine at the somatic neuroeffector (myoneural) junction. *Pernicious anemia* is caused by specific damage to the gastric mucosa. Other autoimmune

269

disorders are more generalized. Interestingly, there is often a similar pattern of organ and tissue involvement in the systemic autoimmune conditions. The *joints, skin,* and *kidneys* are most often affected by the circulating immune complexes. This causes considerable overlap of symptoms among the various disorders and wide variability in symptoms within a particular disorder. Diagnosis is often difficult for these reasons.

Well-known systemic diseases thought to be caused by autoimmune reaction include rheumatoid arthritis, systemic lupus erythematosus, dermatomyositis, and scleroderma (now also called progressive systemic sclerosis). Of the four disorders, rheumatoid arthritis and lupus erythematosus are the most common.

RHEUMATOID ARTHRITIS

Rheumatoid arthritis is a chronic, systemic inflammatory disorder, primarily affecting the joints. The condition favors females over males in the ratio of 3:1, with a general incidence in the mixed population of about 2 per cent. Females in the 20- to 40-year-old age group are especially affected. This is interesting, since this group is also prone to other allegedly autoimmune disorders, such as lupus erythematosus. In addition to the joints, the heart, small blood vessels, pleural cavity, and eyes are frequently involved in the disease process. However, symptomatology generated by lesions in these areas is generally overshadowed by that of the joints.

The designation *rheumatoid* (oid = like) derives from the observation that the joint inflammation is identical to that of rheumatic fever (see Chapter 10). Various forms of the condition exist. If the vertebral column is the major site, it is called *ankylosing spondylitis.* If enlargement of the spleen (splenomegaly) and leg ulcers occur in conjuction with arthritis, it is known as *Felty's syndrome. Juvenile rheumatoid arthritis* is, by definition, a form having an onset before age 16. This form is similar to, but not exactly the same as, the adult form. All forms of the condition are characterized by exacerbations and remissions (waxing and waning) of symptoms over periods of days, weeks, or months.

Pathogenesis

There appears to be an inherited tendency toward rheumatoid arthritis. The condition usually surfaces in adult life, and its onset may follow severe emotional trauma (divorce, death of loved one, injury, surgery). In these cases, the traumatic event appears to be the "last straw" for disease development.

The characteristic lesion in rheumatoid arthritis is destruction of collagen tissue. Sometimes, the disorder is classified as a collagen disease, along with other autoimmune disorders. Lesions develop not only in the joints but also in other body tissues. Subcutaneous nodules (a type of granuloma) are seen in about 20 per cent of those with rheumatoid arthritis and nodules are often seen in the sclera of the eye. Joint involvement begins as inflammation of the synovial membrane (Fig. 17–1). Later, proliferation of connective tissue, associated with infiltration of lymphocytes and plasma cells, occurs. Granulation tissue forms in the inflamed area and is called *pannus.* Eventually, the cartilage covering the bone ends is destroyed and fibrosis occurs as a result of chronic inflammation. This causes immobility of the joint (fibrous ankylosis). In severe cases, the bony tissues unite, causing a permanently frozen joint (bony ankylosis).

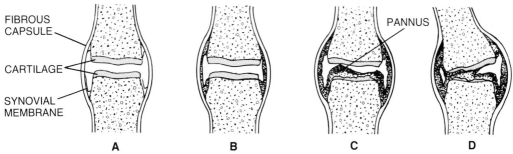

FIBROUS CAPSULE

CARTILAGE

SYNOVIAL MEMBRANE

PANNUS

A   B   C   D

Figure 17–1. Stages in rheumatoid arthritis. *(A)* Normal joint. *(B)* Synovial inflammation. *(C)* Pannus formation. *(D)* Subluxation.

Symptoms and Signs   The chief symptoms in rheumatoid arthritis are pain, stiffness, and warmth in the affected joints, especially on awakening and after heavy exercise. Joint involvement is usually symmetric and especially affects the fingers, wrists, knees, and ankles. In ankylosing spondylitis, the spine is severely affected but other joints have only minimal involvement. Fever, lethargy, loss of appetite, and weakness are also common findings. Some patients have subcutaneous nodules, as mentioned, usually over pressure points (bone edges, bursae), which are a useful diagnostic sign. Long-standing cases show joint ankylosis and disuse atrophy of muscles around affected joints. Arthritic joints are reddish-colored and swollen, the swelling accentuated by surrounding muscular atrophy. Frequently, the articulating bones of a joint are shifted out of alignment by fibrosis and pannus development, producing *subluxation* of the joint (Fig. 17–1).

Laboratory Findings   Leukocytosis and elevated erythrocyte sedimentation rate (ESR) are commonly seen during symptomatic periods. If the disease is in a remission period, these findings may be normal. Hypochromic (pale erythrocyte color) anemia is often seen and is thought to be caused by blood leaking into the inflamed joints or by reduced erythropoiesis.

The most characteristic laboratory finding in rheumatoid arthritis is a macroglobulin called *rheumatoid factor* (RF), found in the serum of at least 75 per cent of rheumatoid arthritis patients. This is an antibody primarily directed against IgG, but it also attacks other immunoglobulins in some cases. Complexes of RF-IgG are thought to circulate through the blood stream to joints and other areas, where they initiate an inflammatory response. This is similar to the situation with the arthritis seen in rheumatic fever. Because some arthritics, especially those with juvenile rheumatoid arthritis, do not have RF in the serum, this proposed mechanism must remain only speculative at this point.

Diagnosis   Rheumatoid arthritis must be differentiated from other arthritic conditions. Rheumatic fever produces identical joint symptoms, but there is no rheumatoid factor in the serum. In addition, elevated antistreptolysin O (ASO) titer and heart murmur are frequent clinical findings (see Chapter 10).

Osteoarthritis (also called degenerative joint disease) is primarily a "wear and tear" phenomenon, affecting weight-bearing joints and those subject to misuse or overuse, such as the shoulder in baseball pitchers. Osteoarthritis can produce somewhat similar symptoms to rheumatoid arthritis, but it is strictly a local joint disease with no systemic involvement and no serum findings.

Gouty arthritis (to be discussed) is associated with asymmetric joint inflammation and an elevated serum uric acid level.

Infectious (pyogenic) arthritis appears as a secondary complication to other infection (e.g., gonorrhea), especially when there is invasion of the blood stream by the infecting organism. Usually, the primary infection can be identified and treated.

Treatment   Probably no disease has ever been fought with such a wide variety of weapons as has rheumatoid arthritis. People suffering from chronic, relentless pain will try anything to obtain relief. Therapy has ranged from Chinese herbal teas, to copper bracelets, to snake oil, to brake fluid. (Snake oil and brake fluid are applied externally!) *Special diets* emphasizing vitamins C and E, alfalfa, and zinc have been recommended. It appears that some patients may actually be deficient in zinc. Most of these and many other remedies wither and die in the light of a controlled clinical trial. The variable nature of rheumatoid arthritis makes some remedies appear to work at first. They are generally used when the disease is at its worst, just before a remission period begins. Thus, the electromagnetic device placed around an inflamed joint and sold by the arthritis huckster (there actually was such a device) provides "relief." The only relief is that the victim is relieved of a lot of money!

Dimethyl sulfoxide *(DMSO)* is still controversial and not yet approved for use in treating human arthritis. The drug seems to have some benefit as an anti-inflammatory agent and, in addition, acts as a vehicle to carry other drugs (e.g., corticosteroids) into the joints. However, its long-term safety in humans has not been established.

Conventional treatment of rheumatoid arthritis revolves around the use of *aspirin* or aspirin substitutes, corticosteroids, and assorted other anti-inflammatory drugs. Aspirin is the mainstay of treatment for those who tolerate the large amounts needed for control of rheumatoid arthritis. For those who experience gastric irritation, bleeding tendencies, allergy or tinnitus (ringing in the ears) from aspirin, several substitutes are available. Aspirin-type side effects are reduced, but not always eliminated, with these drugs. Examples of currently used products are ibuprofen (Motrin), naproxen (Naprosyn), sulindac (Clinoril), and meclofenamate (Meclomen).

Corticosteroid therapy is reserved for those individuals who fail to obtain adequate relief from aspirin or aspirin substitutes. In addition to prednisone, a wide variety of other drugs are available, including dexamethasone (Decadron), triamcinolone (Aristocort), and methylprednisolone (Medrol). These drugs give excellent relief of symptoms by suppressing the inflammatory response, but they cause Cushing's syndrome and adrenal atrophy with long-term use. Intra-articular (into the joint) injections and alternate-day therapy help to reduce toxicity. Still, the drugs must be used sparingly and only during acute inflammatory episodes if toxic effects are to be avoided.

A number of other drugs used for rheumatoid arthritis have an *anti-inflammatory action* that relieves symptoms. Indomethacin (Indocin) and gold compounds are examples. As with other drugs, toxicity or undesirable side effects reduce their suitability as treatment modalities.

In addition to drug therapy, certain *surgical procedures* are used in some arthrics. These include joint replacement and repair (arthroplasty). The need for surgery is often avoided today because of the more definitive drug therapy available.

Arthritics should get adequate rest, but also exercise enough to prevent stiffness of the joints. This is often a narrow path to walk. Emotional stress should be avoided, since this definitely causes worsening of arthritic symptoms. Heat (warm baths, heating pads, melted paraffin applied to joint) often relieves symptoms, although some arthritics obtain more relief from cold materials applied to the affected joints. Mild irritants (e.g., Deep Heet Rub) increase circulation and often lessen symptoms in mild cases.

The diet should be well balanced but no different than for a nonarthritic. The low-fat diet currently employed is healthful but has not proved effective for the relief of arthritic symptoms.

Complications and Prognosis
Complications and prognosis are closely interrelated, since the most common complication — progressive joint deformity — affects long-term prognosis by causing crippling. However, fewer than half of the arthritis patients suffer severe limitation of activities. In some individuals, the disease progresses very slowly, never restricting activities. A few spontaneously recover and no longer require therapy of any type. An uncommon complication to rheumatoid arthritis is the development of deposits of amyloid material in various body organs and tissues (amyloidosis), presumably because of chronic inflammation. The liver, kidneys, and spleen are commonly affected, as are the adrenal glands. Symptoms are quite variable and are referable to the particular organs and tissues affected. Aside from the complication of amyloidosis, rheumatoid arthritis does not generally shorten the life expectancy.

LUPUS ERYTHEMATOSUS
Lupus erythematosus is the second most common of the allegedly autoimmune disorders. The disease exists in two forms: *chronic discoid lupus erythematosus* and *systemic lupus erythematosus* (SLE). The discoid form affects only the skin and produces erythematous (red) scaly lesions that scar upon healing. If the scalp is affected, alopecia (hair loss) occurs in addition. This condition only rarely progresses to SLE. Systemic lupus erythematosus affects a wide variety of organs and tissues, in addition to the skin, producing variable symptoms. The incidence of SLE is about 1:2000, women outnumbering men 9:1. Women in the 20- to 40-year-old age group are especially affected. Blacks are more prone to SLE than are other individuals. A hereditary tendency seems to exist, as with other autoimmune diseases, but, again, clinical disease usually develops in adult life.

Pathogenesis
The onset of SLE often follows *exposure to ultraviolet light (sunlight or sun lamp) or ingestion of certain drugs.* Hydralazine (Apresoline), a drug used to treat hypertension (see Chapter 10)

causes the greatest frequency of lupus reactions. Procainamide (Pronestyl), phenothiazines (e.g., chlorpromazine), and sulfonamides (e.g., sulfisoxazole) are also occasionally associated with the onset of SLE. Possibly, both ultraviolet light and certain drugs act as "partners in crime" in disease development. It is of interest that most of these drugs can also cause photosensitization of the skin (sensitivity to ultraviolet light) without causing SLE. Drug-induced SLE is usually reversible when the drug is discontinued.

Viral infection has also been proposed as a cause of SLE. Increased antibody titer to common viral diseases (measles, rubella) is seen in many SLE patients. Virus-related particles have been found in SLE lesions, and a similar disease, caused by a virus, is seen in mice and minks. However, there is no direct proof that viruses cause human SLE. Viruses may move into tissues already damaged by the inflammatory process.

The basic problem in SLE is the formation of antibodies to a variety of body components. The typical SLE patient has serum antibodies to erythrocytes, leukocytes, thrombocytes, cell nuclei, and deoxyribonucleic acid (DNA). Complexes formed between DNA and anti-DNA antibody are deposited in small capillaries, causing vascular obstruction. In addition, the three "shock areas" for autoimmune disorders (joints, skin and kidneys) frequently react to the circulating immune complexes. Antinuclear antibody (ANA) acts on the nuclei of damaged leukocytes, causing swelling of the nuclei and ejection of them from within the cell. The ejected nuclei, called *LE bodies,* are then engulfed by other leukocytes and the resulting cells are termed *LE cells.* These can be detected in the serum of the SLE patient. It is thought that reduced formation of T lymphocytes may alter body surveillance so that normal components are misread as being foreign and thus are antigenic. This immune defect could easily be hereditary.

Symptoms and Signs

Those with a textbook case of SLE demonstrate a "butterfly" rash across the bridge of the nose, alopecia, arthritis, weakness, fever, and vague nerve and muscle aches ("neuralgia," "myalgia"). Raynaud's phenomenon (see Chapter 10) occurs in about 20 per cent of SLE patients. Lung disease (pneumonia, pneumonitis) is also common. Kidney involvement (as an "innocent bystander") occurs frequently, as do anemia and oral ulceration. Symptoms vary tremendously, however, and some SLE patients present with only arthritis, some with skin eruptions, and others with Raynaud's phenomenon as the only discernible finding.

Laboratory Findings

Nonspecific findings of increased ESR and anemia are usually seen. In addition, leukopenia and thrombocytopenia are often seen; ANA is present in 95 per cent of SLE patients, LE cells are found in about 65 per cent, and specific anti-DNA antibodies are present in 90 per cent of SLE patients. Not all findings occur in each patient, and all do not necessarily occur at the same time in those who show all of the common laboratory findings; LE cells and ANA are seen in patients with other autoimmune diseases. Both Veneral Disease Research Laboratory (VDRL) and fluorescent treponemal antibody-absorption (FTA-ABS) tests, which are used in the diagnosis of syphilis (see Chapter 9), often give false-positive results in SLE. This is apparently due to reaction of the test antigens with some of the many antibodies circulating in the blood stream of the SLE patient.

Other laboratory tests reflect organ damage caused by autoimmune reaction. The kidney is especially affected, but hepatitis and endocarditis also occur.

Diagnosis   Systemic lupus erythematosus can mimic the other autoimmune disorders quite well. Rheumatoid arthritis, scleroderma, and dermatomyositis must be differentiated from SLE on the basis of history, symptoms, and laboratory tests. Syphilis (especially tertiary stage) produces a similar type of hypersensitivity reaction involving multiple organs and tissues. The exclusion of syphilis is made more difficult by the false-positive serologic tests for syphilis that are frequently seen.

Treatment   Patients with systemic or discoid lupus erythematosus should avoid ultraviolet light. All drugs under suspicion should be withdrawn to remove causes of the disease. *Aspirin* is effective for the arthritic component of SLE. Rest and avoidance of emotional stress will help to reduce the severity of symptoms.

Systemic corticosteroids are useful for certain complications, such as glomerulonephritis or lung involvement, but are not generally used as a primary treatment. Topically applied corticosteroids are very helpful for skin reactions and produce little systemic toxicity, since they are poorly absorbed.

Immunosuppressive drugs (e.g., azathioprine [Imuran]) and *anticancer agents* (e.g., cyclophosphamide [Cytoxan]) are good backup drugs for severe glomerulonephritis, since they suppress the immune response that leads to kidney damage. However, they are quite toxic.

Complications and   Prognosis depends upon the extent of organ damage. Renal
Prognosis   failure is the most common cause of death, but lung and heart damage is also common. Some patients experience spontaneous remission with normalization of laboratory findings. Many complications develop from too-vigorous drug therapy, such as bone marrow damage with reduced blood count, Cushing's syndrome, and alopecia. This points up the wisdom of conservative treatment ("first do no harm"). An overall 10-year survival rate of over 90 per cent is now seen with SLE, much better than in previous times.

GOUT   Gout is a disease with a colorful history. Such notables as Benjamin Franklin and Samuel Johnson suffered from it. The typical gout sufferer in early days was depicted as a middle-aged male, usually of the aristocracy, and given to excess in eating and drinking. It was felt that gout was the price to pay for living the good life. English peasants were glad to see noblemen suffer from a disease seldom encountered by the poorer classes. There were two major reasons for the high incidence of gout among the English nobility: they could afford a diet rich in purines (red meat, seafood), and they intermarried to preserve the royal bloodline, thus strengthening any tendency toward the disease.

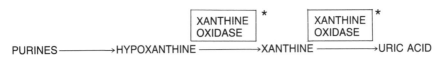

*Site of action of allopurinol (Zyloprim).

Figure 17–2. Pathway for uric acid synthesis. Overproduction of uric acid is the most common cause of gout.

Gout can be considered a metabolic disorder, since the common form is caused by a metabolic defect. It is also an inflammatory disorder, consisting chiefly of arthritis, and can be considered along with the other forms of arthritis. Since some forms of gout are not related to metabolic defect, they fall into the second category.

Males over 30 years of age make up 95 per cent of the gout victims. Afflicted females are almost always past menopause. It is thought that estrogen gives some protection from gout in the premenopausal female. A hereditary tendency toward gout is often seen.

Pathogenesis   *Primary gout* usually results from hereditary overproduction of uric acid (Fig. 17–2). Purine compounds are metabolized to uric acid to such an extent that the serum uric acid level is increased above the normal range (hyperuricemia). Some primary gout sufferers have *reduced renal excretion* of uric acid (not related to kidney damage) or a combination of both conditions.

Secondary gout results from renal disease (causing reduced uric acid excretion), treatment of neoplastic disease, or the use of drugs that raise the serum uric acid level (e.g., chlorothiazide). *Drug-induced gout* is uncommon, except in those with a predisposition toward the disease. Renal failure is a common cause of secondary gout. Gout associated with malignancy (especially leukemia) and its drug therapy is caused by massive cell destruction, which releases large quantities of purine compounds into the blood stream. These are converted to uric acid, causing marked hyperuricemia. An interesting irony exists in that renal failure causes gout and the hyperuricemia associated with gout leads to renal damage *(gouty nephropathy)*. A vicious cycle, once generated, can therefore be maintained and augmented.

Diet is not considered extremely important in gout development today, as it once was. However, in the individual predisposed to gout, massive ingestion of purines can trigger an acute gout attack. Such attacks occur following crab festivals on the east coast and shrimp and crawfish festivals in southern Louisiana.

The characteristic lesion in gout is called a *tophus*, caused by deposition of uric acid in joints, bursae, or soft tissues. Tophi represent uric acid that has precipitated from body fluids and accumulated to form nodules. Such nodules are found most often around joints of the big toes, fingers, elbows, or in the rims of the ear (Fig. 17–3). Precipitation of uric acid from the urine gives rise

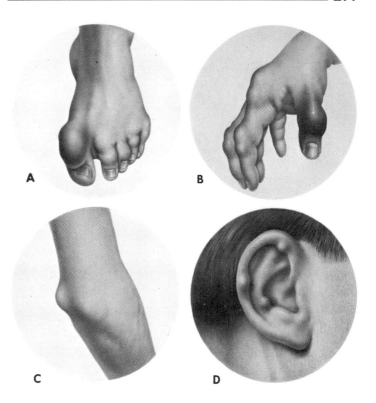

Figure 17–3. Common sites for tophi in gout. *(A)* Big toe. *(B)* Thumb (and other joints of the hand). *(C)* Bursa of elbow. *(D)* Rim of ear. (Reproduced by permission of Merck Sharp & Dohme, Division of Merck & Co., Inc.)

to renal deposits (Fig. 17–4). Inflammation results from tissue irritation caused by the sharp, needle-shaped crystals. In chronic gout, tophaceous deposits within the joint lead to impaired joint function and, eventually, to joint deterioration.

Symptoms and Signs

The typical gout attack occurs in the big toe and is asymmetric; that is, gout affects the big toe on only one foot. Typical signs of acute inflammation develop, with excruciating pain. Constitutional

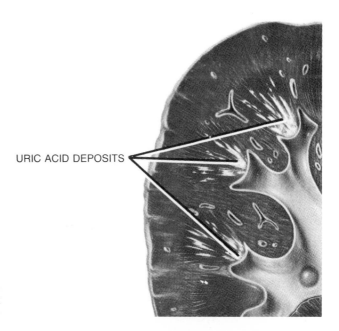

URIC ACID DEPOSITS

Figure 17–4. Renal deposits of uric acid in gout. (Reproduced by permission of Merck Sharp & Dohme, Division of Merck & Co., Inc.)

symptoms of headache, fever, and weakness are also common as a result of the inflammation. Within a few days, symptoms subside and itching and peeling of the skin over the affected joint develop, as they do with sunburn. The pattern of inflammation and recovery is similar with other joints.

Laboratory Findings   The most important finding in gout is hyperuricemia (normal = 2 to 7.5 mg/dl). It should be pointed out, however, that whereas hyperuricemia is necessary for gout, four out of five individuals with hyperuricemia never develop an acute gout attack. They are said to have *asymptomatic hyperuricemia.* Nonspecific findings include elevated ESR and leukocytosis during an acute attack. Examination of fluid from the affected joint shows crystals of uric acid. X-ray studies show tophaceous deposits in various body areas in long-standing cases but may not show abnormalities in the first acute attack. Later, x-ray findings suggestive of decreased bone density in the affected area are seen.

Diagnosis   Gout must be differentiated from *pseudogout,* in which deposits of calcium pyrophosphate are found in fluid from affected joints. Crystals of calcium pyrophosphate have a different appearance from uric acid crystals and the serum uric acid level is normal in pseudogout. Other forms of arthritis can also be confusing. However, the demonstration of uric acid crystals in fluid from arthritic joints along with asymmetric joint involvement and hyperuricemia strongly suggests gout.

Treatment   Gout therapy consists of two general approaches. If attacks occur infrequently, *symptomatic treatment* of each attack is indicated. The drugs of choice are colchicine, indomethacin (Indocin), phenylbutazone (Butazolidin), and oxyphenbutazone (Tandearil). All have anti-inflammatory action, but colchicine is specifically effective for gout without being effective for other inflammatory disorders. It is occasionally used as a diagnostic agent for gout, since it brings relief of symptoms only in gouty arthritis, not in rheumatoid or other forms of arthritis. Colchicine is usually effective within 12 hours. The other drugs are given for 3 to 5 days.

Preventive gout therapy is employed if attacks are frequent or if there is evidence of progressively increasing uric acid deposition. Drugs that increase uric acid excretion, such as probenecid (Benemid) and sulfinpyrazone (Anturane), are used to treat chronic gout. These are called *uricosurics.* They deplete uric acid and lower the serum level but increase the risk of gouty nephropathy because the urine concentration of uric acid increases. An alternative approach is to use allopurinol (Zyloprim), a drug that prevents uric acid synthesis by blocking xanthine oxidase (Fig. 17–2). This lowers both the serum level and the urinary level of uric acid.

Diet restriction is not particularly helpful in gout. However, moderation in the intake of high-purine foods and mineral water ingestion (to prevent precipitation of uric acid in the urine) are recommended.

Complications and   Gouty nephropathy, leading to renal failure, is the major risk
Prognosis in chronic gout. Permanent joint deformity results from prolonged
gout, especially if inadequately treated. The modern treatments
available can prevent most complications of gout and ensure a
normal life span, with reduction or elimination of symptoms.

SUMMARY

Inflammation is a disease process central to most clinical conditions, either as cause or effect. With the diseases classified as
inflammatory disorders, however, there is a pattern of involvement
of body areas particularly vulnerable to the effects of circulating
immune complexes or inflammatory compounds. The joints and
kidneys are frequently affected. In the subgroup called autoimmune
inflammatory disorders, the skin is also a common site for inflammation caused by contact with immune complexes.

Rheumatoid arthritis and systemic lupus erythematosus are the
most common of the so-called autoimmune disorders. They have
much in common regarding etiology, symptomatology, laboratory
findings, and treatment. Gout is somewhat different, since it is
caused by a chemical agent (uric acid) that deposits in and around
joints, causing inflammation. However, the arthritic component of
all three conditions is often similar.

Questions   1. Discuss various ways in which the body could begin reacting to its own
tissues.
2. Compare and contrast rheumatic fever and rheumatoid arthritis; gout
and osteoarthritis (degenerative joint disease).
3. Discuss the problems encountered in trying to prove a viral etiology for
autoimmune disorders.
4. Give the common causes for gout, and explain the reason for the
hyperuricemia in each case.
5. How do Felty's syndrome and ankylosing spondylitis, two forms of
rheumatoid arthritis, differ?

Additional Reading   Baum, J.: Modern concepts in the treatment of gout. Drug Therapy, 8:76, 1978.
Calin, A.: Rheumatoid arthritis. American Family Physician, 18:89, 1978.
Decker, J. L. et al.: Systemic lupus erythematosus: Evolving concepts. Ann. Intern.
Med., 91:587, 1979.
Healey, L. A.: Gout and hyperuricemia are different, but readily managed. Pharmacy
Times, 44:60, 1978.
Ridolfo, A. S.: Nonsteroidal anti-inflammatory agents in arthritis. American Family
Physician, 17:131, 1978.

CHAPTER 18 EYE, EAR, NOSE, AND THROAT DISORDERS

Diseases of the eye, ear, nose, and throat are often considered together because of the proximity of these structures in the body. In earlier times, physicians specialized in diseases of all four areas, but with the rapid development of technology in the fields, a need developed for a separation into two distinct areas of specialty. Now, the medical specialty of eye disorders and treatment (ophthalmology) is distinct from that of ear, nose, and throat (ENT) disorders (otorhinolaryngology). In addition, there is considerable subspecialization within each area, with some practitioners performing only eye surgery and others only ear surgery, for example. Allergy is a common disease process involving the eyes, ears, nose, or throat. The field of allergy treatment is a subspecialty of internal medicine, and allergists represent a third group of practitioners frequently called upon to treat diseases of these areas. While ENT disorders are usually primary and self-limited, eye disorders fairly often reflect systemic diseases. We have discussed retinopathies associated with hypertension and diabetes mellitus and ocular manifestations of systemic autoimmune diseases. There are also other conditions the eye specialist must look for in performing a routine eye examination so that correct treatment can be started and ocular and systemic complications can be avoided.

The disease processes most commonly encountered in eye and ENT disorders are *inflammation* and *infection. Anatomic factors* are also important and contribute toward glaucoma, otitis media, sinusitis, and other diseases. *Allergy,* itself a cause of inflammation, is often a cause of or a contributing factor toward diseases in these areas. *Environmental factors* figure into these diseases as well, since exposure to smoke or air pollution is a common cause of eye, nose, or throat irritation.

The principles of treatment of these disorders are similar to those of other diseases previously discussed. Inflammation and infection can be eliminated or controlled, as can allergic reactions. Anatomic defects are often surgically correctable. Irritating materials in the environment can be removed or the individual protected from their effects. Early treatment of an acute disorder often prevents tissue damage and the development of complications. Although complications to these disorders are not generally life-threatening, serious problems such as brain abscess resulting from extension of sinusitis occasionally occur.

THE EYE

CONJUNCTIVITIS

Inflammation of the conjunctiva (outer covering of the eyeball and inner lining of the eyelid) is the most common eye disease in the United States. A highly contagious form of infectious conjunctivitis called *pink eye* is especially common in the spring and fall.

Pathogenesis

The causes of conjunctivitis are numerous. Infection with bacteria, such as *Staphylococcus aureus* and pneumococci, or adenoviruses (cold or "flu" viruses) is extremely common. Less common causes of infectious conjunctivitis include *Neisseria gonorrhoeae* (see Chapter 9) and chlamydiae. Chlamydial conjunctivitis closely resembles gonococcal conjunctivitis, both in symptomatology and in methods of spread. Rarely, fungi or parasites cause infectious conjunctivitis. The infectious organisms contact the eye from air or droplet spread or from another part of the infected person's body (nose, throat). Rubbing the eye with contaminated fingers is also a common method of contact.

Allergic reactions are an important cause of conjunctivitis. Ocular allergy usually occurs in those with other allergic manifestations (allergic rhinitis). Irritation resulting from contact with tobacco smoke, air pollution, or irritating fluids (e.g., chlorinated swimming pool water) is extremely common. Overuse of the eyes in reading, studying, or watching television also results in eye irritation. Ultraviolet light (sunlight, sun lamp, arc welder) can also cause eye irritation.

Symptoms and Signs

The symptoms of conjunctivitis of any cause include redness of the eye, with itching, lacrimation (tearing), and dilated blood vessels ("bloodshot" eye). The eye discharge can be watery, stringy (especially in allergy), or purulent (in infection). Chemosis (edema of the conjunctiva around the cornea) is also common, especially if allergy is the cause of conjunctivitis. Pain is usually absent or minimal and vision is not directly affected, since only the exterior eye membrane is involved.

Diagnosis

Severe eye conditions, such as acute glaucoma, corneal injury, or iritis (inflammation of the iris) can mimic some of the symptoms of conjunctivitis. These usually require the expertise of the ophthalmologist for examination, diagnosis, and treatment.

Treatment

The treatment of conjunctivitis varies with its cause. Infectious conjunctivitis caused by most bacteria can be treated with eye drops or ointments containing neomycin, tetracycline, or sulfonamide. Chlamydial infection requires topical tetracycline often plus oral tetracycline administration for cure.

Only a few antiviral drugs are available, such as idoxuridine (Stoxil), and these are used only for corneal infection with *Herpes simplex*. There is no effective antiviral therapy for the common adenovirus infections.

Fungal conjunctivitis is treated with drops containing amphotericin B (Fungizone) or mycostatin (Nystatin). Parasitic infection requires specialized treatment, which depends upon the causative organism. Note that penicillin is not generally recommended for eye infections, since it often causes sensitization when applied topically. Allergic conjunctivitis responds well to anti-inflammatory corticosteroids applied to the conjunctiva in drop form. Dexamethasone (Decadron) is a representative product. Good symptomatic relief is also obtained with commercial eye drops (Murine or Visine) or with boric acid solution.

It is important to avoid contamination of the eye with the fingers, dust, smoke, or pollen to allow the inflammation to subside and to prevent further irritation. Often, these factors are contributory to other causes of conjunctivitis. Any other factors (eyestrain, ultraviolet light, irritating fluids) that cause or contribute toward the condition should be eliminated.

CATARACT
Cataracts represent cloudy or opacified areas in the lens. The lens has no blood supply and is vulnerable to outside influences, possibly because of its lack of circulation and the reparative processes to go with it.

Pathogenesis
Usually, the condition develops slowly, often taking years before the vision is severely impaired. Cataracts are often bilateral and may occur at birth. More often, however, they develop in later life. Some degree of opacity is seen in individuals in the 60- to 80-year-old age range (senile cataract), but the degree may be relatively slight. Eye trauma and radiation exposure also frequently cause cataract. Causes of secondary cataract include diabetes mellitus and uveitis (inflammation of the iris, ciliary body, and choroid). Prolonged high-dose corticosteroid administration is also associated with cataract formation. This is often the treatment employed for uveitis, as well as for other inflammatory diseases.

Diagnosis
The lens cloudiness associated with cataract formation can be seen with an ophthalmoscope, an instrument used to examine the eye, or often with the naked eye (Fig. 18–1). As the opacity worsens, the retina becomes less and less visible until, finally, it cannot be seen. During this time, vision in the affected eye worsens progressively.

Treatment
There is no treatment that will remove the cloudiness and return the lens to normal. However, surgical lens removal is routinely done and is quite safe even in elderly or debilitated people. The diseased

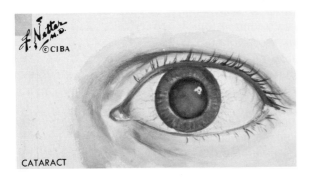

CATARACT

Figure 18–1. Cataract. Note cloudiness of pupil. (©Copyright 1965, CIBA Pharmaceutical Company, Division of CIBA-GEIGY Corporation. Reprinted with permission from the CIBA Collection of Medical Illustrations, illustrated by Frank H. Netter, M.D. All rights reserved.)

lens can be removed using a special instrument that nibbles it away and draws out the lens material through a tiny tube at the same time. The traditional procedure has been to remove the entire lens at once through a surgical incision, and this is still done in many cases. Corrective glasses or contact lenses are then needed to compensate for the loss of refractive power formerly provided by the lens. Lens implants are now being made on selected cataract patients with some success. When all of the technical problems associated with this procedure are controlled, the technique will probably become widely used.

GLAUCOMA

Glaucoma refers to the presence of increased intraocular pressure. Approximately 1 per cent of the United States population have glaucoma, although at least 25 per cent of the cases are undetected. Most cases occur in individuals over 40, but congenital glaucoma is also fairly common.

In the normally functioning eye, there is a balance between the *formation* and *removal* of fluid in the anterior chamber (aqueous humor). Fluid is manufactured by the *iris, ciliary body,* and *cornea* and is removed through the *canal of Schlemm* and its tributaries, the *trabecular network.* Accordingly, intraocular pressure remains in the normal range (10 to 25 mm Hg). In glaucoma, this balance is upset, so that aqueous humor is removed too slowly compared with its rate of formation, resulting in increased intraocular pressure.

Types of Glaucoma

Glaucoma can be *primary* or *secondary.* Secondary glaucoma results from conditions that lead to reduced outflow of aqueous humor, especially eye trauma, tumors, uveitis, or advanced cataracts. In these cases, there is mechanical obstruction (tumor cells, cell debris, swelling) of the trabecular network. Secondary glaucoma is usually unilateral, since the disease processes that cause it do not generally affect both eyes to an equal degree.

Primary glaucoma is often bilateral and is of two general types: *narrow-angle* and *open-angle.*

Narrow-Angle Glaucoma. This condition occurs when the angle between the base of the iris and the cornea is too shallow (less than 20 degrees) (Fig. 18–2). Narrow-angle glaucoma is seen most often in women in the 40- to 60-year-old age group who have an anatomically shallow anterior chamber. Narrow-angle glaucoma is prone to develop into *angle-closure glaucoma* (Fig. 18–2). Anything that results in further narrowing of the angle can completely obstruct the trabecular network, causing a dramatic increase in intraocular pressure, severe eye pain (to the point of causing vomiting), and threatened vision. Common causes of angle closure are excitement, which causes release of epinephrine, and the use of anticholinergic medications (e.g., atropine). In both cases, the pupil dilates widely, thickening the base of the iris musculature and completely blocking aqueous outflow.

Open-Angle Glaucoma. This type of glaucoma (Fig. 18–2) affects 90 per cent of cases and can occur as a congenital defect, usually in association with other eye defects or other systemic abnormalities (as in rubella). These cases are caused by alteration of the trabecular network, reducing the rate of removal of aqueous

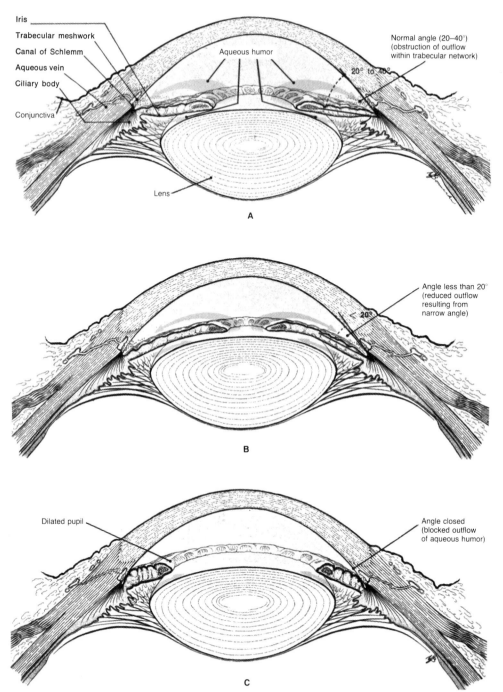

Iris
Trabecular meshwork
Canal of Schlemm
Aqueous vein
Ciliary body
Conjunctiva

Aqueous humor

Normal angle (20–40°)
(obstruction of outflow
within trabecular network)

20° to 40°

Lens

A

Angle less than 20°
(reduced outflow
resulting from
narrow angle)

< 20°

B

Dilated pupil

Angle closed
(blocked outflow
of aqueous humor)

C

Figure 18–2. Anatomic features of glaucoma. *(A)* Open-angle glaucoma. *(B)* Narrow-angle glaucoma. *(C)* Angle-closure glaucoma. (From Soll, D. B.: Glaucoma. Am. Fam. Physician, 9:126, 1974.)

humor. Similarly, in open-angle glaucoma developing in adults, there is outflow obstruction, presumably as a result of an inherited tendency that surfaces later in life. In both cases, the angle is over 20 degrees and obstruction is apparently within the trabecular network itself, rather than at the angle.

Symptoms in glaucoma vary from none, in most cases of chronic open-angle disease, to the severe symptoms seen in angle-closure glaucoma. A progressive loss of visual field (particularly peripheral vision) is seen in all types of glaucoma, giving it the nickname "the thief of vision," since this loss is not noticed in the early stages. Very high intraocular pressure results in eye pain, a "halo" around lights and objects, and rapid visual field loss. Loss of visual field is due to impaired circulation in the retina as a result of the high intraocular pressure. Retinal blood vessels are squeezed by the high pressure, and the impaired circulation causes permanent damage to the rods and cones.

Diagnosis   Glaucoma is diagnosed primarily by measuring the intraocular pressure (*tonometry*), either directly, with an instrument applied externally to the eye surface after local anesthesia, or indirectly, with an instrument that shoots a puff of air at the eye and measures flexing of the eyeball surface. Flexing is inversely related to intraocular pressure. The air-puff test requires no local anesthetic. Cupping of the optic disc occurs when intraocular pressure is high and can be used as a rough indicator of glaucoma when examining the eye, although tonometry is much more accurate. *Perimetry* measures and charts the visual field and detects areas of visual loss (scotomas).

Treatment   Surgical treatment is used primarily for angle-closure glaucoma, congenital glaucoma, and correction of cataract and certain other causes of secondary glaucoma. An operation called an *iridectomy* is used to relieve pressure in angle-closure glaucoma or to prevent development of angle-closure glaucoma in a person with narrow-angle glaucoma.

Drug therapy is the mainstay for most cases of glaucoma and is usually the sole treatment for adult, open-angle glaucoma. Most drugs act by reducing the rate of formation of aqueous humor, thus improving the balance between its formation and removal and reducing intraocular pressure. Carbonic anhydrase inhibitors, such as acetazolamide (Diamox) (see Chapter 8) are used orally, and timolol (Timoptic) and epinephrine are applied topically to the eye. Epinephrine is effective in open-angle glaucoma, even though it dilates the pupil (mydriasis). Its beneficial action here is not well understood. It is specifically contraindicated in narrow-angle glaucoma, since it may precipitate angle-closure glaucoma. Pilocarpine (Pilocel) acts by causing pupil constriction (miosis), thus thinning the base of the iris musculature and improving drainage through the trabecular network. In addition to eye drops, which have been used for decades, there is also now a delivery device for pilocarpine that is placed in the conjunctival sac. The device (Ocusert) gives a steady release of pilocarpine for 7 days, instead of the short-term benefit (4 to 6 hours) provided by eye drops. In addition, the drug effect is more uniform from hour to hour, avoiding the rebound increase in intraocular pressure seen when the effect of the drops wears off. After a week, the dispensing device is discarded and a new one is inserted.

Glaucoma patients should avoid excessive excitement or stress and should watch for anticholinergic effects, such as dryness of the mouth or constipation, in drugs they take. Nonprescription drugs having anticholinergic side effects, such as antihistamines, are usually labeled for the benefit of the consumer who has glaucoma. If drugs with anticholinergic effects or side effects must be taken by an individual with open-angle glaucoma, the effects can usually be canceled out by using larger amounts of antiglaucoma drugs at that time. However, those with narrow-angle glaucoma should avoid such drugs entirely if possible.

The biggest risk in glaucoma is severe visual field loss, leading to blindness or very limited sight ("gun-barrel" vision). Visual loss can occur quickly in angle-closure glaucoma or gradually in open-angle glaucoma. Most visual field loss can be prevented through early diagnosis and treatment. Routine tonometry is recommended for those over 40 to spot early glaucoma and for others with eye disorders that could cause secondary glaucoma.

THE EAR

EXTERNAL OTITIS

Inflammation of the external auditory canal is a common clinical finding (Fig. 18–3). It results from infection, allergy, or irritation of the canal and can be part of a more general surface inflammation (e.g., seborrheic dermatitis). A large number of cases are caused by swimming in fresh water or poorly chlorinated swimming pools (swimmer's ear). In these cases, microbial contaminants enter the ear canal and infection develops. Common infecting bacteria in external otitis are staphylococci and coliforms. Fungi, such as Aspergillus, Mucor, and others, also infect the ear canal or secondarily infect a canal with existing bacterial infection. Infection is facilitated by retaining moisture in the ear after swimming or bathing. Attempts to clean the ear canal with hairpins or other rough objects scratch the surface layer of tissue and promote inflammation, infection, or

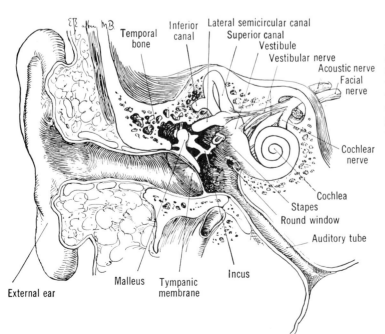

Figure 18–3. Semischematic drawing of the ear. Note the ossicles extending across the middle ear cavity. The greater part of the course of the facial nerve through the ear has been omitted. (From Gardner, E.: *Fundamentals of Neurology: A Psychophysiological Approach,* 6th ed. Philadelphia, W. B. Saunders Company, 1975.)

both. (The old advice to "use nothing in your ear smaller than your elbow" is certainly well taken.) Allergy to metal in earrings, especially nickel, and irritation caused by hearing aid earpieces also cause external otitis. Often, in these cases, the auricle (external ear) is inflamed as well.

Symptoms and Signs　　Symptoms associated with external otitis include pain, itching, and discharge from the ear canal. The discharge can be purulent or watery, depending upon the cause of the condition. Excessive wax accumulation is also common, resulting from overactivity of ceruminous (wax-producing) glands in response to inflammation. There is usually some degree of hearing loss, often severe, as the canal becomes occluded by a combination of discharge, wax, scaly material sloughed from the inflamed tissue, and edema. In severe cases of infectious external otitis, fever and enlarged lymph nodes near the affected ear are seen.

Diagnosis　　The major conditions to rule out in the diagnosis of external otitis are otitis media (middle ear infection), boil (furuncle) of the ear canal, and the presence of a foreign body in the canal. Otitis media, to be discussed shortly, mimics the symptoms of pain, fever, and hearing loss. In addition, if the eardrum is perforated, pus can drain from the middle ear to the outside. Furuncles of the ear canal can cause pain and local inflammation, even though they may be no larger than a pinhead. Children are famous for putting objects into the ear canal (beans, buttons, small toys), and these can cause or duplicate the symptoms of external otitis. In all of these cases, examination of the ear with a lighted magnifying instrument (otoscope) is necessary for accurate diagnosis.

Treatment　　External otitis caused by infection is treatable with anti-infective drops placed in the ear canal and secured with a cotton wick. Bacitracin, neomycin, and polymyxin are drugs of choice. Several excellent combination products (e.g., Neosporin) are available. Some products combine anti-inflammatory corticosteroids with anti-infective agents (e.g., Cortisporin). Antifungal agents, such as natamycin (Natacyn), combat the common fungal causes of external otitis. Burow's (aluminum acetate) solution is helpful when applied to the ear canal with a moistened wick. The preparation dries secretions and reduces itching. It can also be applied to the auricle as well. Irrigation of the ear canal with diluted Burow's solution, 3 per cent hydrogen peroxide solution, or warm water removes scales and crusts from the inflamed mucosa. Hydrogen peroxide and carbamide peroxide in glycerin (Debrox) have a foaming action on contact with body tissues and float material from the ear canal. Severe infectious external otitis may require systemic antibiotic therapy.

Complications　　There are few complications to external otitis. In severely debilitated patients, especially elderly diabetics, penetration of the mucosa and nearby bone tissue occasionally occurs, eventually spreading to the brain. This is called *malignant external otitis*. It is usually caused by *Pseudomonas aeruginosa* and is a life-threatening condition, requiring vigorous antibiotic and supportive treatment.

OTITIS MEDIA   Inflammation of the ear in the area between the tympanic membrane (eardrum) and the cochlea (Fig. 18–3) is termed otitis media. The condition is almost always caused by bacterial infection, resulting from passage of infected material from the nasopharynx through the eustachian (auditory) tube into the middle ear. Most often there has been previous infection, such as pharyngitis, sinusitis, or tonsillitis, but occasionally resident bacteria in the area migrate into the middle ear.

Children between 6 months and 2 years of age and between 4 and 6 years of age are the most vulnerable to otitis media, with boys slightly favored over girls. In children, the eustachian tubes are almost horizontal, on a level with the nasopharynx and middle ear. This makes it easy for bacteria to enter the middle ear from the nasopharynx. The eustachian tubes in adults dip slightly from middle ear to nasopharynx, causing natural drainge of middle ear fluid and making bacterial migration into the middle ear more difficult. Accordingly, adults are less often affected than children. However, infection is still possible, especially if the nose is blown vigorously, forcing bacteria up the eustachian tubes.

Symptoms and Signs   When otitis media occurs, the typical changes associated with acute inflammation are seen. The tissue lining the middle ear becomes edematous, and fluid and cellular exudates are formed. The opening of the eustachian tube is blocked by edema, and the only avenue for fluid removal is lost. Further fluid accumulation causes pressure to develop, with pain and a sense of fullness in the ear. Hearing loss is common because of the dampening effect of accumulated fluid on normal vibratory action of the eardrum and auditory ossicles (incus, malleus, and stapes). Continued pressure buildup causes bulging and thinning of the eardrum and the danger of rupture. Otoscopic examination shows the drum bulged toward the outer ear, along with hyperemia and dilation of the blood vessels of the eardrum.

Laboratory Findings   The most common pathogenic organisms in otitis media are
and Diagnosis   pneumococci, staphylococci, beta-hemolytic streptococci, and *Haemophilus influenzae*. *H. influenzae* is becoming a more prevalent pathogen than in previous years and is often resistant to conventional drug therapy. However, it can be eradicated with appropriate antibiotics, sulfonamides, or both. In practice, routine culture of the middle ear contents is not done, since it requires puncture of the eardrum to obtain a sample. It can be performed in refractory cases, however, to establish the identity of the causative organism.

The leukocyte count is usually elevated in otitis media, reflecting systemic response to the localized infection. Other laboratory tests are not helpful. Diagnosis is based upon this finding, plus otoscopic findings and a history of a recent upper respiratory tract infection. It should be pointed out that colds, although caused by a virus, can promote otitis media by causing eustachian tube obstruction and impairing drainage from the middle ear into the upper throat. The same problem occurs with enlarged adenoids or allergy.

Several conditions can be confused with otitis media. *External otitis* causes overlapping symptomatology, as previously mentioned.

Myringitis bullosa, caused by a virus, consists of eardrum inflammation with bullae (blebs) on the eardrum. Although antibiotic treatment is often given, it is mainly to prevent secondary bacterial infection. Toothache or impaction of an upper third molar ("wisdom" tooth) causes pain that may seem to come from the middle ear. Arthritis of the joint between the mandible (jawbone) and temporal bone (temporomandibular joint disease—TMJ) also causes pain suggestive of otitis media. This condition is most often caused by malocclusion of the teeth. In both situations, otoscopy and hearing are normal.

Treatment

Topically applied antibiotics are ineffective for the treatment of otitis media, in contrast to external otitis, since the infection is behind the eardrum and inaccessible from the outside. However, analgesic drops (e.g., Tympagesic) will give some relief of eardrum pain while the infection is being treated. Drugs of choice for *systemic* administration include penicillin, ampicillin (Polycillin), and amoxacillin (Amoxil). Erythromycin (Erythrocin) is useful if penicillin allergy, which involves all three drugs, is present. Cephalosporins and co-trimoxazole (Bactrim, Septra) are also effective against most organisms. For staphylococcal infection, a cephalosporin such as cefaclor (Ceclor) or a penicillinase-resistant penicillin such as oxacillin (Prostaphlin) is recommended. Resistant forms of *H. influenzae* can be treated with a combination of erythromycin and a sulfonamide, such as sulfisoxazole (Gantrisin). It is important that anti-infective treatment of otitis media be continued for 7 to 10 days to completely eradicate the infection.

The only commonly employed surgical treatment for otitis media is *myringotomy,* in which the eardrum is deliberately punctured, under local anesthesia, with a special knife. This relieves pressure and promotes drainage and healing of the infection. Spontaneous rupture of the eardrum, which occurs in severe infections if myringotomy is not done, often results in scarring and hearing loss upon healing, whereas intentional, clean incisions heal with little or no scarring. If drug treatment of otitis media is started soon enough, myrinogtomy is usually not necessary.

Complications

Today, otitis media almost always resolves completely with appropriate treatment. In the past, however, *chronic otitis media* frequently developed because drugs that could cure the infection were not yet available. Chronic otitis media is characterized by persistent middle ear infection, with the development of perforation of the eardrum and constant drainage through the perforation into the ear canal (tubal ear). A dreaded result of this is extension of infection into the mastoid bone around the middle ear area. Mastoiditis requires intensive antibiotic therapy, and often surgery to remove necrotic tissue, for cure.

The same conditions that favor otitis media also favor *serous otitis media.* Here, there is no infection, but the middle ear fills with serous or mucoid fluid, giving symptoms similar to those of infectious otitis media. Pain and fever, however, are absent. Infection often occurs under these conditions of impaired drainage from the middle ear area. Treatment of serous otitis media often requires tonsillectomy and adenoidectomy (T and A), plus the insertion of ventilation tubes through the eardrums for cure. If allergy is a contributing factor, antihistamines and decongestants may be of great benefit in reducing eustachian tube blockage.

THE NOSE

ALLERGIC RHINITIS

Inflammation of the nasal mucosa that is due to allergic reaction is called allergic rhinitis (hay fever). It affects about 10 per cent of the population and often coexists with other manifestations of allergy, such as sinusitis, bronchial asthma, or allergic dermatitis. The tendency toward allergy is inherited, and often other family members have allergic conditions as well, although not necessarily allergic rhinitis (see Chapter 4). Most afflicted persons are sensitive to *inhalants,* such as pollen, dust, mold, or smoke, but *foods* (chocolate, eggs, wheat) and drinks (milk, wine, beer) occasionally trigger allergic rhinitis attacks.

The condition exists in two forms: *seasonal* allergic rhinitis, which is bothersome only during the hay fever season; and *perennial* allergic rhinitis, which produces year-round symptoms. Thus, seasonal allergic rhinitis occurs during the spring and fall, when the pollen count is the highest. Perennial allergic rhinitis is often somewhat less severe in the winter, although symptoms continue throughout the year.

The pathogenesis of allergic rhinitis involves a typical IgE-mediated immune reaction, with mast cell rupture and release of histamine (see Chapter 4).

Symptoms and Signs

The classical features of acute inflammation are seen. There is edema and erythema of the nasal mucosa, along with a profuse, watery nasal discharge (Fig. 18–4). Pain is absent, but there is a

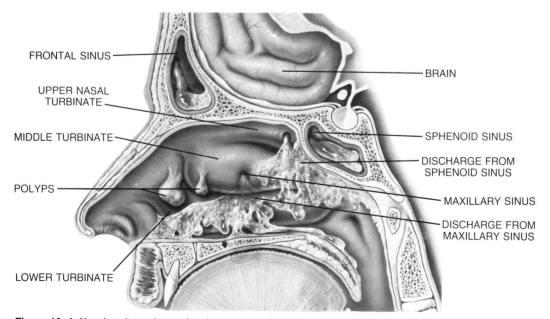

FRONTAL SINUS

UPPER NASAL TURBINATE

MIDDLE TURBINATE

POLYPS

LOWER TURBINATE

BRAIN

SPHENOID SINUS

DISCHARGE FROM SPHENOID SINUS

MAXILLARY SINUS

DISCHARGE FROM MAXILLARY SINUS

Figure 18–4. Nasal cavity and associated structures. (Reproduced with permission from Merck Sharp & Dohme, Division of Merck & Co., Inc.)

feeling of discomfort from pressure and congestion in the nasal tissues. Loss of function of the nose occurs in that the sense of smell is impaired and the warming effect of the nasal passages to incoming air is lost because of congestion.

Symptoms of allergic rhinitis include sneezing, nasal congestion, itching of the nose (and often the roof of the mouth), discharge (rhinorrhea), and headache, from sinus congestion. Allergic conjunctivitis often coexists with allergic rhinitis, adding the symptoms of eye itching, redness, and lacrimation to the existing misery.

Diagnosis   Allergic rhinitis is usually diagnosed easily, often by patients themselves. In addition to a history of allergy, particularly seasonal allergy, there are increased numbers of eosinophils in the nasal discharge, suggesting allergy. Skin tests reveal sensitivity to inhalants or other allergens. Examination of the nose using rhinoscopy shows a boggy, red, or pale-blue nasal mucosa. Sinusitis often coexists with allergic rhinitis, as mentioned, since it can be caused by allergy as well. The major confusing condition is *acute rhinitis* (common cold), which is caused by infection with one of the 30 or more upper respiratory tract viruses. The common cold is a short-term condition (it goes away in 7 days with treatment or in a week without!) and is more prevalent in winter than in spring or fall. Many children are thought to have repeated "colds" when they actually have allergic rhinitis. They respond well to antiallergy therapy.

Treatment   Allergic rhinitis is treated in three major ways: avoidance of allergen, symptomatic treatment, and hyposensitization.

Allergen Avoidance. If the individual is allergic to dust or pollen, relief can be obtained by using air conditioning, static precipitators to remove dust particles from the air, foam rubber pillows and mattresses, and a dust mask for outside activities, such as mowing the grass. Sometimes pets or overstuffed furniture are sources of allergy within the house. If foods or drinks are a major problem, the diet can be modified to eliminate these.

Treatment of Symptoms. Many individuals with allergic rhinitis experience excellent symptomatic relief with antihistamines, such as chlorpheniramine (Chlortrimeton), and decongestants, such as pseudoephedrine (Sudafed). These medicines do not alter the immune process causing the allergic state but do reduce the symptoms of allergic rhinitis. Antihistamines block histamine receptors and prevent its action on the nasal mucosa. This treatment may be completely adequate, especially if the person has seasonal allergic rhinitis. For more severe cases, corticosteroids, such as dexamethasone (Decadron), can be tried for short-term use. These drugs block the inflammatory response resulting from the effect of histamine on the nasal mucosa. Both oral and topical (spray or drop) forms are used. Some ENT specialists use injections of corticosteroids into the nasal turbinates (Fig. 18–4) to cause shrinkage of tissue and relieve congestion. Often, several months of benefit are obtained in this way with minimal systemic absorption and practically no side effects.

Hyposensitization. For those who have perennial allergic rhinitis or who do not benefit from other forms of seasonal treatment, this therapy is often used (see Chapter 4). Injections should be begun 3 to 6 months before the beginning of the hay fever season to attain the serum antibody titers necessary for protection.

Complications　　Allergic rhinitis is usually a self-limited condition, with few long-term complications. However, *sinus infection* can result from prolonged blockage of sinus openings as a result of allergic rhinitis. This requires antibiotic therapy and attention to the underlying allergic condition. *Hypertrophic rhinitis,* a thickening of the nasal mucosa often associated with polyp formation (Fig. 18–4), results from long-standing inflammation and is a complication of allergic rhinitis. The nasal mucosa is unresponsive to decongestants or antihistamines and permanent nasal obstruction is present. Treatment is difficult, but removal of causes of allergy and local treatment with corticosteroids often causes some shrinkage of nasal tissues. For resistant cases, surgical treatments are available. Surgical removal of part of the nasal turbinate, called a partial turbinectomy, has been used in the past and is still done, but many specialists prefer application of a supercooled probe to the nasal mucosa, producing a tissue shrinkage that may be permanent.

SINUSITIS　　Inflammation of the paranasal sinuses is usually caused by allergic reaction or infection. It frequently coexists with *allergic rhinitis,* since the etiologic basis for both can be allergy. In addition, pathogenic organisms in the upper respiratory tract, especially beta-hemolytic streptococci and pneumococci, often move into the sinuses and are trapped there because of impaired sinus drainage. Thus, sinusitis is also commonly associated with *acute rhinitis.* A third etiologic factor in sinusitis is exposure to irritating fumes (smoke, chemicals), and chlorinated water, especially when diving. In all cases, it is more common to find involvement of all eight sinuses (pansinusitis) than only one. Occasionally, however, one sinus is predisposed to infection because of an anatomic drainage defect. In general, infection is a less common cause of sinusitis than is allergy or exposure to irritating fumes.

Symptoms and Signs　　Common symptoms of sinusitis include headache, which results from pressure generated by edema within the rigid sinus cavities, and pain and tenderness on either side of the nose (maxillary sinuses) or in the eye orbits (frontal sinuses). Symptoms of allergic rhinitis are also common. If infection is present, purulent nasal discharge, fever, and aching joints are often seen. Many patients complain that the upper teeth hurt or feel "long"; this is due to the close proximity of the upper teeth to the maxillary sinuses.

Diagnosis　　Sinusitis is diagnosed by x-ray studies of the sinuses or by use of transillumination (see Chapter 15). Infected or congested sinuses appear cloudy. Dental abscess, erupting third molars, and tumors or polyps in the sinuses can all mimic the symptoms of sinusitis. Dental films will differentiate problems relating to the teeth from sinusitis. Tumors or polyps within the sinuses are uncommon and can usually be seen on sinus films. In infectious sinusitis, there is usually leukocytosis and a positive culture of the nasal discharge; in allergic sinusitis, the eosinophil count in the nasal discharge is high.

Treatment　　Helpful measures in the treatment of sinusitis include the use of decongestants (e.g., pseudoephedrine) and analgesics (aspirin, acetaminophen) to relieve symptoms. Antihistamines are especially useful if allergy is the major underlying cause. Several excellent combination antihistamine-decongestant products are available, including Dimetapp and Actifed. Many products also contain an analgesic as well (e.g., Sinubid). Elimination of allergens or the use of hyposensitization injections is sometimes necessary, in addition. If infection is present, cure can usually be attained with penicillin, ampicillin, erythromycin, or tetracycline. The drugs are administered orally for 5 to 7 days. Corticosteroids, such as dexamethasone, can be used to block inflammatory reactions, resulting in faster shrinkage of tissue and reduction of symptoms.

Complications   Acute infectious sinusitis can become a chronic problem, especially if factors such as nasal obstruction or organism resistance are present. In cases not responding to short-term antibiotic therapy, culture of secretions should be done and the most effective antibiotic chosen. Attention to allergy and nasal polyps will help to prevent chronic sinusitis. Sinus irrigation and, occasionally, surgery to improve sinus drainage may be required. Severe chronic infectious sinusitis sometimes results in infection of bone or other tissue in the vicinity of the sinuses. Surgery to remove necrotic tissue, along with specific antibiotic therapy, is usually curative.

THE THROAT

PHARYNGITIS   The pharynx (throat) becomes inflamed for a variety of reasons, and pharyngitis is one of the most common clinical findings. Most cases of pharyngitis are caused by viral infection—by the same organisms that cause acute rhinitis. Bacterial pharyngitis, especially that caused by beta-hemolytic streptococci, is an important clinical finding, since it can lead to rheumatic fever or glomerulonephritis. Many childhood diseases, such as scarlet fever or measles, often start with pharyngitis. A day or two later, the characteristic skin eruption occurs. Allergy is another important cause of pharyngitis. Constant drainage into the pharynx resulting from allergic rhinitis (postnasal drip) leads to irritation. Purulent drainage from infected sinuses has a similar effect. Inhalation of fumes or ingestion of spicy liquids can also cause pharyngitis.

Symptoms and Signs   The individual with pharyngitis complains about throat pain; dryness of the throat; and a thick, tenacious mucus (resulting from inflammation) covering the throat. Infectious pharyngitis also results in fever and malaise, along with other "cold" symptoms, such as swollen lymph nodes. Rhinitis, sinusitis, and laryngitis often coexist with pharyngitis, since infection, allergy, and irritation can be causes of all three conditions. Examination of the pharynx demonstrates the mucous exudate and erythema of the pharyngeal mucosa.

Diagnosis   Diagnosis is not difficult, but it is important to rule out streptococcal pharyngitis ("strep" throat) because of its possible serious complications. Streptococcal pharyngitis can be diagnosed by the finding of a positive throat culture for streptococci and the usually associated high fever.

Treatment   The treatment of pharyngitis depends upon its cause. Contributing causes should be eliminated, if possible. These include smoking, exposure to irritating fumes or air pollution, and ingestion of spicy liquids. Inhalation of steam from a vaporizer soothes and moistens irritated pharyngeal tissues. Throat lozenges or cough drops have a similar effect, as do gargles. Mild analgesics relieve the pain associated with pharyngitis. Control of rhinitis or sinusitis will help to reduce drainage and throat irritation. For bacterial pharyngitis, treatment for 4 to 5 days with penicillin, ampicillin, or erythromycin is usually effective.

Complications   Aside from the complications associated with streptococcal pharyngitis, most cases of pharyngitis are self-limited. However, chronic pharyngitis can develop if factors causing the acute condition are not controlled. Important among these are control of allergy and reduction of pharyngeal irritation caused by smoke or air pollution.

LARYNGITIS   In general, factors that cause or promote pharyngitis also lead to laryngitis. Thus infection, allergy, and inhalation of irritating fumes are important causes. Irritation resulting from smoking and/or alcohol ingestion is extremely common. In addition, since the larynx is the organ of voice, vocal abuse is a frequently seen etiologic factor in laryngitis. Shouting, screaming, or excessive use of the voice causes vocal cord inflammation, leading to symptoms of laryngitis. Laryngitis is an occupational hazard among singers, ministers, teachers, lecturers, and others who use the voice extensively in their daily work. Laryngitis often exists along with pharyngitis, rhinitis, or sinusitis, since these conditions have a common etiologic basis.

Symptoms and Signs   The chief symptom of laryngitis is hoarseness, caused by vocal cord edema. The swollen cords vibrate poorly, causing a husky quality to the voice. In more severe cases, swelling prevents any vocal cord motion and complete loss of voice (aphonia) results. This swelling may partially block the airway, resulting in dyspnea and breathing noises (respiratory stridor). Pain is usually absent in laryngitis, but cough and a sensation of something in the throat are commonly seen. Examination of the larynx with a curved mirror (indirect laryngoscopy) shows erythema and edema of the vocal cords and adjacent laryngeal mucosa, sometimes with slight bleeding resulting from rupture of small surface vessels. Other laboratory tests are not helpful, except that leukocytosis occurs with bacterial laryngitis.

Diagnosis   The major concerns in the diagnosis of laryngitis are the possibilities of ulcer, polyp, or malignant tumor of the vocal cord, which can produce similar symptoms.

Ulcers. Ulcers are caused by vocal abuse and occur on the contact surfaces of the vocal cords. Shouting, screaming, or incorrect singing technique are the usual causes.

Polyps. Polyps occur for similar reasons and are times referred to as "singers' nodes." Chronic irritation from tobacco smoke is another important cause of polyp formation. Polyps are benign and can be removed surgically. They also often regress spontaneously when the cause for the irritation is removed. Some children develop multiple laryngeal polyps, causing hoarseness and dyspnea and requiring repeated surgery for removal. This condition, called *juvenile papillomatosis,* is thought to be caused by a virus, as are certain other papillomas, e.g., warts.

Malignancy. The greatest concern in the differential diagnosis of laryngitis is the possibility of malignant laryngeal tumors. These usually occur in men over 40 who are heavy smokers. Early diagnosis and treatment are essential, since most malignant laryngeal tumors can be cured in the early stage. Irradiation of the affected area or surgery is frequently curative. In advanced cases, laryngectomy and removal of surrounding lymph nodes is necessary to halt the spread of the cancer.

Treatment   Voice rest, control of infection, and avoidance of irritating fumes or smoke are essential for recovery of inflamed laryngeal mucosa. Steam inhalation and control of aggravating allergic factors will hasten recovery. Topical medication is not effective in laryngitis, as it is in pharyngitis, since the epiglottis and cough reflex prevent materials from entering the larynx.

Complications   Acute laryngitis, normally short-term, becomes chronic if predisposing factors are not controlled. Careful attention to factors such as allergy, smoking, and overuse or misuse of the voice can result in prompt resolution of acute laryngitis.

SUMMARY

The eyes, ears, nose, and throat are affected by the same disease processes as those that affect other body areas, namely inflammation and infection. In addition, allergy, environmental factors, and anatomic abnormalities often predispose toward disease of these organs. Ear, nose, and throat disorders are usually primary and self-limited, whereas eye disorders such as cataract and glaucoma are often secondary to other factors. A number of systemic diseases are detected by retinal changes, giving the eye specialist the opportunity to diagnose some disorders that might be otherwise elusive at first.

Ear, nose, and throat disorders often occur together. This is because of similar etiologic factors in the conditions and also because of the anatomic proximity of the involved structures. Thus, nasal obstruction leads to ear infection and sinus infection because of reduced drainage from these areas. Allergic rhinitis or sinus infection can cause pharyngitis and laryngitis as a result of the irritation caused by drainage into the pharynx and larynx. The organisms that commonly cause sinus infection also cause otitis media, pharyngitis, and laryngitis. Treatment of these conditions, therefore, often involves correction of underlying contributing conditions to prevent recurrence of symptoms.

Questions
1. Speculate on possible reasons why a diabetic individual is more prone to cataract than a nondiabetic.
2. Comment on the possible consequences in a person with narrow-angle glaucoma who takes an antiulcer product containing atropine.
3. How would you distinguish among external otitis, otitis media, and myringitis bullosa?
4. How are allergic rhinitis and sinusitis alike? Different?
5. Discuss the similarities and differences between pharyngitis and laryngitis. How do differences in the anatomy of the two structures relate to causative factors and treatments?

Additional Reading

Bergman, H. D.: Otitis media—The disease, major complications and appropriate therapy. Southern Pharmacy Journal, 72:39, 1980. (*Good overview of the disorder.*)

Ferguson, G. G.: Common ear, nose and throat disorders and their treatment. Southern Pharmacy Journal, 70:15, 1978. (*Overview of common ENT disorders.*)

Mullarkey, M. F.: Allergic and non-allergic rhinitis. Postgrad. Med., 65:97, 1979.

Soll, D. B.: Glaucoma. American Family Physician, 9:125, 1974. (*Good article on types and diagnosis of glaucoma.*)

Speer, F.: Food allergy: The 10 common offenders. American Family Physician, 13:106, 1976. (*Easy-to-read article about causes of food allergy.*)

CHAPTER 19

DISEASES
OF THE
ORAL CAVITY

Diseases affecting the teeth, gingivae (gums), tongue, and associated structures within the oral cavity are generally considered together. Their diagnosis, prevention, and treatment are in the realm of the dentist, dental hygienist, and oral surgeon. The entire spectrum of disease processes, including inflammation, infection, immune response, and neoplasia, is represented by various oral diseases. In a sense, the oral cavity is a microcosm of the total body and serves as a model for the study of disease processes. The obvious advantage here is that oral structures are more visible and accessible than are most other body tissues. Thus, diagnosis can usually be made by direct observation, in contrast to the diagnosis of many "internal" diseases. In addition to visual diagnosis, a number of other diagnostic techniques are also available to the dental practitioner. X-ray studies are extremely useful for the identification of abnormalities of the teeth or bony structures of the oral cavity. Staining techniques, using fluorescein or other dyes, help to identify areas of accumulated deposit on the teeth and aid in its removal.

In dealing with oral diseases, one should not subscribe to an isolationist policy. That is, it should be continually remembered that oral conditions can reflect systemic diseases. While it is true that most oral disorders are confined to structures within the oral cavity, there are a number of systemic diseases that have an oral component. *Measles,* for example, frequently produces characteristic lesions (Koplik's spots) on the buccal (cheek) mucosa, usually before the identifiable skin rash appears.

Since the skin and oral mucosa have a common embryonic origin, a number of dermatologic conditions have oral manifestations. *Lupus erythematosus* often causes oral lesions similar to those seen on the skin (see Chapter 17). *Lichen planus,* which usually affects the skin as well as the oral cavity, is characterized by a grayish-white, netlike lesion that may erode and become red upon irritation. Other skin disorders, such as *herpes zoster* (shingles), also frequently cause oral lesions.

It is commonly observed that the oral cavity responds to measures that benefit other body areas and suffers when the general health is poor. The results of good nutrition are seen in the oral tissues as well as in other body tissues. *Herpes labialis* (cold sore) often occurs in an individual with a specific infectious disease already present or with general debility. Likewise, diabetics suffer from poor tissue healing, greater chance of oral infection, and deterioration of tissues supporting the teeth. Thus, the oral cavity should always be considered in the context of the whole body and with careful consideration of any other disease processes present.

STOMATITIS

The term stomatitis (stoma = mouth) is a general one and refers to inflammation of all or part of the oral cavity. Some authorities separate gingivitis from the general category of stomatitis if no other oral tissues are involved. In this discussion, we will consider gingivitis under the topic of periodontal disease.

Pathogenesis

Stomatitis can result from *traumatic injury* to the oral tissues. Common causes are biting of the tongue, lips, or buccal mucosa or irritation from projecting teeth or dental restorations. Pressure or friction from full or partial dentures affects the palate or gingival tissues. Injury from toothbrushing is often seen, especially if the brush is too stiff or too vigorously used on the gingivae. Hot foods or drinks cause thermal injury to the oral cavity, especially to the tongue and palate mucosa. A variety of chemical agents are irritating to the oral mucosa. Reactions to flavorings (e.g., cinnamon) or antibacterial agents (e.g., hydrogen peroxide) used in mouthwashes are common. Irritating substances used as toothache drops (e.g., oil of cloves) can inflame soft tissues adjacent to the affected tooth. A popular home remedy for toothache is to hold an aspirin tablet against the sore tooth. This causes injury to the buccal membrane and tongue because of the strong acidity of aspirin. Caustic agents that are used to "cauterize" oral tissues, such as silver nitrate, can produce inflammation. Likewise, chewing tobacco or "dipping" snuff often leads to chronic oral cavity inflammation (nicotine stomatitis).

Many forms of stomatitis are caused by *infection*. Viral infection is especially common, and the usual causative organism is *herpes*. Herpes infection exists in two forms:

1. *Primary herpetic gingivostomatitis* is an acute illness characterized by widespread lesions on the oral mucosa and skin, associated with involvement of the pharyngeal and regional lymph nodes.

2. *Recurrent herpetic stomatitis* (Fig. 19–1) is a milder condition that often develops in those who have recovered from the first illness. A substantial antibody titer develops following the primary condition, and some immunity persists for a long time, making subsequent infections less severe. The condition consists of lesions

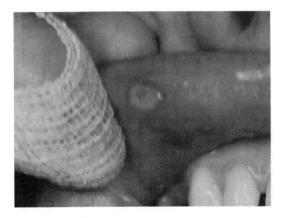

Figure 19–1. Recurrent herpetic stomatitis. (From Shafer, W. G., Hine, M. K., and Levy, B. M.: *A Textbook of Oral Pathology*, 4th, ed. Philadelphia, W. B. Saunders Company, 1983.)

on the lips ("cold sores") or in the mouth ("canker sores"). Exacerbation of the condition often follows infection, fever, gastrointestinal upset, or onset of menstruation. It appears that the herpes virus resides permanently in the affected tissues but becomes active only when conditions are favorable.

Less common forms of infectious stomatitis include *candidiasis* (thrush) and *actinomycosis*. Candidiasis (Fig. 19–2) results from infection with *Candida* (Monilia) *albicans,* a yeastlike fungus, and consists of whitish patches on the palate and other structures. A common cause of candidiasis is overtreatment with broad-spectrum antibiotics (see Chapter 2). Actinomycosis affects the jaws and produces abscesses that drain into the oral cavity. A similar condition (lumpy jaw) occurs in cattle.

Rare causes of stomatitis include tuberculosis and syphilis, in which the oral involvement is part of a systemic condition. Syphilitic stomatitis is usually seen in the secondary stage of syphilis (see Chapter 9).

Treatment   The treatment of stomatitis depends upon its cause. Since many forms are caused by traumatic injury, removal of damaging factors results in cure. This includes elimination of chemicals, foods, and drinks that may be irritating to the oral tissues. Careful brushing with a soft toothbrush, smoothing of projections from the teeth, and careful fitting of dentures help to reduce chronic irritation of the oral tissues.

Viral stomatitis is not directly treatable, but the pain can be relieved by application of local anesthetics (e.g., Xylocaine Viscous) to the affected areas. Drying of the areas by application of an alcohol-ether mixture for cold sores or an anti-inflammatory ointment (e.g., Kenalog in Orabase) for canker sores may speed healing.

Oral candidiasis usually responds to mycostatin (Nystatin) oral suspension. The drug is rinsed in the mouth and then swallowed.

Actinomycosis responds to high doses of penicillin, usually given intramuscularly and then followed by oral administration. Treatment of the oral manifestations of tuberculosis and syphilis requires control of the underlying systemic condition.

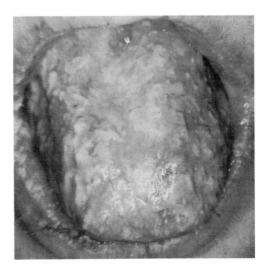

Figure 19–2. Candidiasis involving nearly the entire oral cavity. Thick plaques cover the tongue. (From Shafer, W. G., Hine, M. K., and Levy, B. M.: *A Textbook of Oral Pathology,* 4th ed. Philadelphia, W. B. Saunders Company, 1983.)

DENTAL PLAQUE AND CALCULUS

The normal mouth has considerable self-cleaning action, which reduces the tendency for stains or deposits to form on the teeth. The natural smoothness of tooth surfaces discourages deposition of materials. There is a constant washing action of saliva that removes food particles from teeth and associated areas. In addition, saliva contains *ptyalin,* which digests starches remaining on the teeth after eating. Saliva also inhibits growth of organisms that may contribute to the formation of deposits on the teeth. Mastication, especially of rough, coarse foods, exerts a cleaning effect on teeth and surrounding structures.

Counteracting the natural cleansing action of the mouth are numerous factors that promote stains or deposits on the teeth: a soft diet, improper oral hygiene, the use of tobacco, coffee or tea, insufficient saliva production, and alterations in the shape or position of the teeth. Thus, missing or malpositioned teeth undermine the self-cleaning ability of the oral cavity. Likewise, chipped teeth or those with uneven restorations accumulate debris more readily than do smooth tooth surfaces.

Tooth debris is of two types: stains and accretions.

Stains

Stains result from the action of colored materials on oral structures. Tobacco, coffee, tea, and certain foods are common offenders. Other stains result from contact with iron in drinking water (brown stain) and various bacteria (orange stain). These are called *exogenous stains,* since they result from contact with the external surface of the teeth. *Endogenous stains* result from internal changes in the tooth. A common example is grayish-brown discoloration associated with the use of tetracyclines during tooth development (before age 12). Damage to the tooth pulp and breakdown of materials in blood within the tooth causes black discoloration of the affected tooth. If a great deal of the tooth material has been lost, the pulp may show through the thin remaining tooth wall causing pink discoloration.

Accretions

Accretions are divided into two types: soft, such as *dental plaque,* and hard, such as *calculus (tartar).*

Soft Accretions. These are easily removed by brushing, whereas hard accretions must be removed by scaling, that is, scraping away the material with a sharp instrument. If oral hygiene is poor, the initial soft accretion formed is called *materia alba,* consisting of food debris, dead cells, bacteria, and other materials. Dental plaque (Fig. 19–3) forms in areas of poor hygiene a few days later. Whereas materia alba is white and soft, dental plaque is transparent and somewhat harder, although still removable by brushing. Plaque consists of materials from glycoproteins in the saliva combined with bacteria and bacterial products. The initial plaque structure is termed a *pellicle.* Cocci grow on the surface of the pellicle and form polysaccharides. With time (weeks to months), many bacteria die, leaving a large number of cell wall remnants and other structures that are incorporated into the plaque material. Probably, the initial event in plaque formation is the adsorption of glycoproteins (mucin) onto the tooth surfaces, leading to attachment of cocci to the glycoprotein surface.

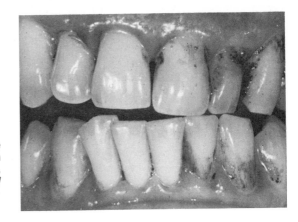

Figure 19–3. Dental plaque. The appearance of the teeth in all quadrants is similar, although the teeth on one side were not brushed for 3 days. (From Shafer, W. G., Hine, M. K., and Levy, B. M.: *A Textbook of Oral Pathology,* 4th ed. Philadelphia, W. B. Saunders Company, 1983.)

Hard Accretions. Dental calculus (Fig. 19–4) represents plaque that has become infiltrated with mineral deposits. It is extremely hard and not removable by brushing alone. Structurally, calculus resembles bone tissue and consists of calcium phosphate along with other materials, such as magnesium salts, proteins, bacteria, cellular debris, and water. The tendency to form calculus increases with age.

Calculus may be *supragingival* (above the gum line) or *subgingival* (below the gum line). Supragingival calculus is visible and can usually be easily removed by scaling. Subgingival calculus can be felt with a probe or detected by x-ray films and tends to be more difficult to remove.

There is a difference of opinion as to the exact mechanism of calculus formation. However, it appears that calcification of existing plaque is enhanced by alkalinization of the saliva, which reduces the solubility of calcium salts in the saliva and promotes their deposition on plaque structures. There is considerable difference among individuals in the tendency to form calculus and this difference is partly related to the inherent pH of the oral cavity.

Treatment   The formation of plaque and calculus can be discouraged by good oral hygiene, both with good home care and with regular professional prophylaxis. In addition, the inclusion of rough foods in the diet (carrots, celery, apples, whole grains) will help to constantly clear tooth surfaces of retained soft foods. The maintenance of smooth surfaces of teeth and restorations will avoid foci for plaque and calculus accumulation.

Figure 19–4. Dental calculus. (From Shafer, W. G., Hine, M. K., and Levy, B. M.: *A Textbook of Oral Pathology,* 4th ed. Philadelphia, W. B. Saunders Company, 1983.)

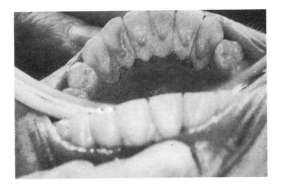

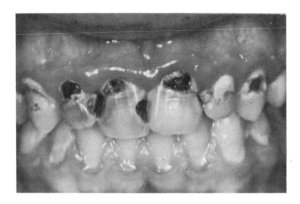

Figure 19–5. Dental caries. (From Shafer, W. G., Hine, M. K., and Levy, B. M.: *A Textbook of Oral Pathology,* 4th ed. Philadelphia, W. B. Saunders Company, 1983.)

A number of chemical agents have been tried to control plaque formation. These act by inhibiting bacterial growth or by interfering with attachment of bacteria or glycoprotein to tooth surfaces. The most promising of these drugs is *chlorhexidine.* When used in a mouthwash, chlorhexidine retards plaque formation. It is used extensively in Europe but has not been approved for use in the United States because it stains the teeth and may drastically alter the normal flora of the mouth.

Various antibiotics, including penicillin and erythromycin, have been tried for plaque control; however, they cause eventual development of resistant organisms in the oral cavity.

DENTAL CARIES

Tooth decay is the most common oral disease—and the most common chronic disease of the whole body—affecting more than 95 per cent of the United States population (Fig. 19–5). It has been observed in all races for as long as there has been recorded history. The fact that primitive societies generally have a lower incidence of dental caries ("cavities") is attributed to a diet containing more unrefined foods and less sugar than is seen in the more "civilized" cultures. In studies conducted among the Eskimos, the incidence of caries was approximately 1 per cent among those living on a native diet (high fat and low sugar) but increased to 18 per cent in those who began following a typical American or European diet.

The incidence of dental caries is highest among children between the ages of 5 and 15. It slowly declines between the ages 15 and 25, then decreases more rapidly so that those in the 35-year-and-older age group are much less vulnerable. Occasionally, the incidence increases drastically in the elderly, possibly because of alterations in diet (containing more soft foods) and reduced home care (with less attention to brushing) in the very old.

Pathogenesis

Many theories have been proposed as to the etiology of dental caries. The most widely accepted is that of W. D. Miller, whose extensive studies began in 1882, and is referred to as the *acidogenic* or *chemicoparasitic* theory. This theory holds that acids are formed by bacterial action on carbohydrates, leading to destruction of tooth enamel. This process is aided by direct bacterial action on vulnerable areas of the tooth surface and subsurface. Both lactobacilli and streptococci have been implicated in the etiology of dental caries.

In addition, plaque promotes tooth decay by providing a surface for bacterial attachment and by trapping acids formed as a result of bacterial action. Acids trapped under plaque, therefore, operate virtually undisturbed on the tooth surface. Dental caries is encouraged by a high sugar intake, particularly by eating sugar between meals so that it is not removed by other foods.

Other important factors include the texture and hardness of the tooth surfaces, making them more or less resistant to the effects of acid, the position and shape of the teeth, and the nature of the saliva. Malpositioned teeth retain food materials and are difficult to clean, thus promoting caries. Thin, voluminous saliva washes away food debris and discourages decay, whereas thick saliva sticks to teeth and holds food materials and bacteria, thus encouraging dental caries. Brushing immediately after meals or snacks greatly reduces the rate of caries formation, as does regular professional plaque removal. Individuals living in an area in which the water contains fluoride compounds or who use fluoride supplements have additional protection against dental caries, presumably because of the increased hardness of tooth enamel resulting from absorption of fluoride into the tooth.

In addition to these factors, there are inherent differences among people in their tendency toward dental caries. The cause of these differences is unknown, despite many speculations and studies regarding increased bacterial resistance or alterations in composition of the saliva in those more resistant to caries.

Sites for Caries   The most common sites for dental caries are the top surfaces of the bicuspids and molars (back teeth), the areas just above the contact points between teeth (interproximal areas), and the cervical (neck) areas of the teeth near the gum line. All of these areas are difficult to clean and thus retain plaque, which encourages decay. While visual inspection is often adequate for the diagnosis of caries, dental films of the involved areas are also quite useful. The carious area is decalcified and thus more transparent, resulting in a darker x-ray image when compared with the surrounding normal tooth.

Treatment   Since recalcification of damaged teeth occurs only to a slight degree, dental caries does not "heal," as do most other damaged areas in the body. Repair of the carious area must be accomplished by removing all of the decayed tooth material, sealing the restored area to prevent further decay, and filling the cavity with durable material.

A number of caries-preventive measures have been explored in past years. Chlorhexidine, which retards plaque formation, and antibiotic-containing mouthwashes are promising. Fluoride compounds, administered orally or applied to the teeth in solutions, gels, or toothpastes are effective in reducing the incidence and severity of dental caries. The greatest benefit obtains from the use of fluoridated drinking water (in the ratio of 1 part per million) or oral fluoride supplements from the prenatal period until age 14 or 15, along with application of fluoride compounds to the teeth several times during tooth development and the use of fluoridated toothpaste. Some fluoride is absorbed into the tooth enamel by topical contact with solutions, gels or toothpastes and systemically administered fluoride is incorporated into the enamel of the developing teeth.

Thus, while dental caries is not totally preventable, its course can be modified and its severity lessened by the use of preventive measures in conjunction with a low-sugar diet and excellent oral hygiene.

PULP DISEASE

The soft inner portion of the tooth containing the nerve and vascular supply is called the *pulp*. Normally protected by the outer surfaces of the tooth, it is nevertheless vulnerable to injury. Extremes of temperature, traumatic injury (such as a blow to the tooth), and extension of caries into the inner tooth can result in pulp damage. Initially, toothache results; later, however, with extensive pulp destruction, pain is absent. The pulp chamber becomes calcified with age, so that the pulp is often less sensitive to pain in the elderly.

Pulpitis

The most common pathologic condition involving the pulp is inflammation, resulting in *pulpitis*. The usual features of inflammation, including hyperemia, pain, and exudate formation are seen. Generally, pain is worsened by application of cold and partially relieved by application of heat. In more severe pulpitis, pain is continuous and requires narcotic drugs for relief.

Types of Pulpitis

A number of variations of pulpitis exist:

1. *Suppurative* pulpitis is associated with abscess formation, as is the case in other body areas with suppurative lesions. This often occurs when a carious lesion extends into the pulp, permitting entry of bacteria.

2. *Gangrenous* pulpitis usually results from ischemia of the pulp caused by stasis of blood or by vascular damage that disturbs the blood supply. Necrosis of the pulp results from the impaired circulation in either case.

3. *Ulcerative* pulpitis occurs when the pulp is exposed by caries or when a large portion of the tooth is broken away. Pain is usually minimal, since there is no pressure developed as a result of exudate formation as there is if the pulp chamber is closed. That is, the chamber is open and pressure is dissipated. If the opening is blocked by food so that pressure can develop, pain results.

4. *Chronic productive* pulpitis develops when the pulp is severely exposed, as with extensive caries. Granulation tissue forms in the exposed pulp, often extending through the carious area into the oral cavity. Shed epithelial cells from the tongue or buccal mucosa grow on the granulation surface and eventually cover it. This lesion is termed a *pulp polyp* and usually must be treated by extraction of the tooth.

Complications of Pulpitis

A number of complications to pulpitis can develop. Pulp injury can stimulate resorption of materials from the hard outer tooth with an increase in the size of the pulp chamber until only a shell remains. (Occasionally, this occurs in the absence of obvious pulp injury.) The tooth has a pink spot where the pulp is visible through the transparent remaining tissue. Often, the pulp is eventually exposed

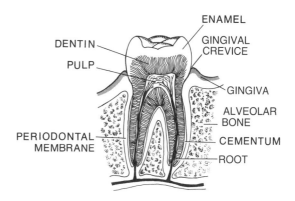

ENAMEL

DENTIN

GINGIVAL CREVICE

PULP

GINGIVA

ALVEOLAR BONE

PERIODONTAL MEMBRANE

CEMENTUM

ROOT

Figure 19–6. Structure of tooth and periodontium. (Adapted from Leonard, P.: *Building a Medical Vocabulary*. Philadelphia, W. B. Saunders Company, 1983.)

as more and more of the tooth wall is resorbed. This requires tooth extraction for treatment.

The increased pressure within the pulp cavity in suppurative or gangrenous pulpitis may force material from the inner tooth to areas surrounding the root of the tooth *(periapical areas)*. This results in inflammation of the surrounding tissue, often with abscess formation (periapical abscess). The tooth is pushed upward (or downward) slightly as a result and is painful when the person bites down on it. Likewise, slow pulp degeneration may result in formation of a *periapical granuloma,* representing attempted repair of damaged tissue. Periapical granulomas can become infiltrated with epithelial cells, producing *radicular cysts,* whereas periapical abscesses can extend further into soft tissues, causing *cellulitis.* If the bone marrow of the jaw or facial area is invaded, it is termed *osteomyelitis.* A periapical abscess that breaks through the gingival mucosa and drains into the oral cavity is called *parulis* or *gum-boil.* Occasionally, such an abscess forms a *fistula* through the external tissue and drains from the skin around the oral cavity.

Treatment

Dental pulp disease can be prevented by avoiding traumatic or thermal injury to the teeth and by using care in the restoration of carious teeth, thus avoiding trauma to the pulp. Mild pulpitis usually resolves when the cause is removed. If the pulp is extensively damaged and beyond recovery, complete pulp extraction (root canal surgery) is necessary.

PERIODONTAL DISEASE

The areas of the oral cavity comprising the periodontium include the gingivae, alveolar bone, periodontal membrane, and cementum (Fig. 19–6). The major function of the periodontium is to support the teeth. Without this support, even healthy teeth become loose and prone to disease. Periodontal disease is uncommon in children, but the prevalence increases with age. By age 30, approximately 70 per cent of the population have it to some degree and by age 45, virtually 100 per cent of the population are affected. It is the most common cause of loss of teeth after age 35.

In general, periodontal disease is initiated by the accumulation of irritating materials on tooth surfaces, especially below the gum line. Rough tooth surfaces, either spontaneously occurring or created by improper dentistry, also cause local irritation of periodontal

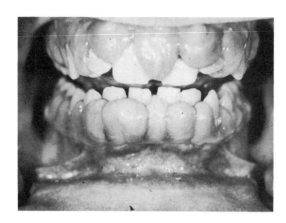

Figure 19–7. Phenytoin-induced hyperplastic gingivitis. (From Shafer, W. G., Hine, M. K., and Levy, B. M.: *A Textbook of Oral Pathology,* 4th ed. Philadelphia, W. B. Saunders Company, 1983.)

tissues. Thus cracked or chipped teeth or those with uneven restorations irritate tissues below the gum line. Breathing through the mouth encourages drying of the gingivae, which predisposes to irritation. Inflammation results from all these situations. Infection is not generally a direct cause of periodontal disease, but bacterial products may contribute to periodontal inflammation. The habit of vigorously brushing back and forth across the gingivae with a stiff brush irritates the tissues and may lead to gingival recession and the development of periodontal disease. In addition, irritating materials taken into the oral cavity (tobacco, alcohol, aspirin) may cause periodontal inflammation.

Many other factors contribute to the development of periodontal disease. Malocclusion of the teeth, missing teeth, and grinding of the teeth (bruxism) result in damage to or inflammation of periodontal supporting structures. Systemic conditions, such as diabetes mellitus; deficiency of vitamin C; or the hormone imbalance associated with puberty, pregnancy, or menopause may encourage the development of periodontal disease. However, these conditions do not *cause* periodontal disease; rather, they accentuate the effect of factors, such as those previously described, that have a primary effect in its development.

Phenytoin (Dilantin) can stimulate inflammation and overgrowth of gingival tissue with long-term use (Fig. 19–7). Again, though, it appears that the drug merely sensitizes the tissues to primary sources of inflammation, such as deposits, poor hygiene, or faulty dental work.

The two major types of periodontal disease are gingivitis and periodontitis.

Gingivitis

Gingivitis may be further classified as simple, hyperplastic, hormonal, or atrophic.

1. *Simple gingivitis* is characterized by swelling and bleeding of gingival tissues. Bleeding is often detected as a pink coloration of the toothbrush.

2. *Hyperplastic gingivitis* results from the gingival response to chronic irritation, resulting in proliferation of gingival tissue. A form of this occurs upon chronic exposure to phenytoin, as stated previously.

3. *Hormonal gingivitis* occurs during pregnancy, at puberty, or after menopause and is related to changes in hormone levels, resulting in increased gingival sensitivity to local irritants. Stabilization of hormone levels often lessens the degree of inflammation.

4. *Atrophic gingivitis* consists of gingival inflammation associated with recession (shrinkage) of gingival tissue, exposing the necks of the teeth and encouraging further periodontal disease. It is usually caused by incorrect brushing technique or by conditions that promote tooth movement (bruxism, malposition of teeth).

A severe form of acute gingivitis is called *acute necrotizing ulcerative gingivitis,* also known as Vincent's infection or trenchmouth (Fig. 19–8). It is caused by infection with a spirochete but requires contributing factors for infection to occur. That is, the organism is usually present in the oral cavity but becomes pathogenic when the tissue resistance is lowered. Debility, poor oral hygiene, tobacco, and local irritation are frequently seen predisposing factors. In addition to the usual symptoms of gingivitis, the gingivae are extremely painful and sloughing of gingival tissue occurs, often associated with a foul breath odor. Fever, malaise, and enlargement of regional lymph nodes are also common. The term "trenchmouth" derives from the common occurrence of the disease among combat troops, in which many of the contributing factors are operating.

Periodontitis

Periodontitis is commonly a result of uncontrolled gingivitis and represents spread of the inflammatory process into underlying periodontal structures. There is resorption of alveolar bone, along with separation of the gingivae from the roots of the teeth, leading to formation of *periodontal pockets.* The presence of periodontal pockets can be detected by probing the gingival crevice with a thin, dull instrument. Loss of support to the teeth results, and the teeth become loose. Under pressure of chewing, they drift, especially side-to-side, and this further damages the periodontium and weakens their support. If severe alveolar resorption occurs, the alveolar ridge may be too small to support dentures adequately. The patient then loses the teeth and usually cannot be fitted with dentures. If it is possible to wear dentures, it is usually impossible to obtain a good fit.

Figure 19–8. Acute necrotizing ulcerative gingivitis (trenchmouth). (From Shafer, W. G., Hine, M. K., and Levy, B. M.: *A Textbook of Oral Pathology,* 4th ed. Philadelphia, W. B. Saunders Company, 1983.)

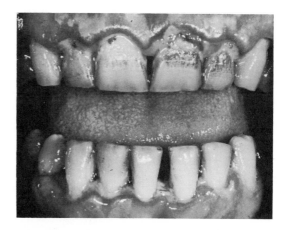

Treatment of
Periodontal Disease

The etiologic factors that favor development of gingivitis also predispose to periodontitis. Therefore, gingivitis generally develops before periodontitis, as mentioned. Control of factors that promote gingivitis (poor oral hygiene, faulty dentistry, direct irritation of the gingivae) usually prevent or lessen the severity of periodontitis. As stated previously, periodontal disease is less common in young people than in older individuals. However, a severe form, called *juvenile periodontitis,* is occasionally seen in teenagers. It may be that immune reaction, rather than the factors just discussed, is the major cause of this condition.

In addition to causing loss of tooth support, periodontal pockets are also prone to impaction with food material or other items. The infection that often results from this is called a *periodontal abscess.* Such abscesses may require incision and drainage and antibiotic therapy for cure.

PROLIFERATIVE ORAL DISEASE

There are a wide variety of conditions in which proliferation of oral tissues is the major feature. They can be roughly divided into three categories: granulomas, benign tumors, and malignant tumors.

Granulomas

Granulomas are not technically tumors, even though the name ends in *-oma,* but represent inflammatory lesions (see Chapter 6). Their nomenclature arose at a time when the nature of the inflammatory process was not well understood. A common oral granuloma is *pyogenic granuloma,* which commonly forms on the gingivae, tongue, or lips. Pyogenic granuloma represents an overgrowth of granulation tissue, usually in response to local injury. The lesion is soft, red, or bluish in color and highly vascular, bleeding easily if disturbed. A variation of pyogenic granuloma is *pregnancy "tumor"* (granuloma gravidarum), which forms on gingival tissue during pregnancy. The lesion is stimulated by the high levels of hormones circulating during pregnancy and regresses when pregnancy ends.

Benign Tumors

Common benign oral tumors include papillomas, fibromas, epulis lesions, torus lesions, and exostosis.

Papillomas. Papillomas are raised, firm lesions occurring virtually anywhere in the oral cavity (Fig. 19–9). Their surface has a rough, cauliflowerlike appearance. The cause of papilloma formation is not known, but a viral etiology has been suggested because they closely resemble *warts,* which are external papillomas thought to be caused by viruses.

Fibromas. These occur in most intraoral areas and are composed primarily of fibrous tissue, as their name indicates. They are pale, firm lesions that grow slowly. A variety of fibroma, *traumatic fibroma,* occurs primarily in the buccal mucosa in response to injury and consists mainly of scar tissue.

Epulis Lesions. These usually result from chronic irritation below the gum line (calculus or foreign material) and arise in the gingivae. If the bulk of the lesion is fibrous material, it is called a *fibroid epulis;* if the lesion also contains bone tissue, it is referred to as an *ossifying fibroid epulis.* A lesion containing large, multinucleated cells (giant cells) that are involved in bone destruction and repair is called a *giant cell epulis.* Giant cell epulis is more deeply attached and more difficult to remove than the other forms of epulis. It also grows faster and reaches a larger size.

Torus Lesions. These are outgrowths of normal oral bone tissue that are covered with mucosa.

Two common forms exist: *torus palatinus,* which arises from the palate, and *torus mandibularis,* whose origin is the inner surface of the mandible (jawbone) below the gum line. The major difficulties caused by torus lesions are damage to the covering mucosa caused by mechanical trauma (hard foods) and problems in fitting dentures. In most cases, the lesions are not removed but have to be dealt with nevertheless.

Exostosis. These are similar to torus lesions, except that bony growth occurs on the outer (buccal) areas of the mandible and maxilla (upper facial bone). The condition often develops in those who put excessive stress on the teeth (heavy chewing, grinding of the teeth, cracking nuts, or the circus trick of bending bars with the teeth). Injury to overlying tissue often results from mechanical trauma, as it does with torus lesions.

Malignant Tumors

Malignant lesions of the oral cavity arise in any area, but common sites are the tongue and floor of the mouth. There is often a history of heavy alcohol and/or tobacco use or of chronic irritation from broken teeth or jagged dental work. The habit of chewing tobacco or "dipping" snuff increases the risk of oral cancer. In some Asian countries, the practice of chewing *betel nuts* is common. Betel nuts contain a mild stimulant similar to caffeine; however, they also are carcinogenic, especially to the buccal area of the mouth where they are held for long periods.

Many malignant oral tumors are preceded by the development of *leukoplakia* (Fig. 19–10) (see Chapter 3). The finding of leukoplakia in the oral cavity should stimulate a search for its cause and cure, since this may prevent the development of oral cancer.

Squamous cell carcinoma (Fig. 19–11) is the most common malignant oral tumor. Its incidence is approximately 20 per 100,000 in men and 5 per 100,000 in women in the United States. Squamous cell carcinoma occurs in most intraoral areas, as well as on the lower lip in smokers or those exposed to excessive sunlight. The lesions are ragged, ulcerated, and usually whitish in appearance.

Figure 19–9. Papilloma of the tongue. (From Shafer, W. G., Hine, M. K., and Levy, B. M.: *A Textbook of Oral Pathology,* 4th ed. Philadelphia, W. B. Saunders, Company, 1983.)

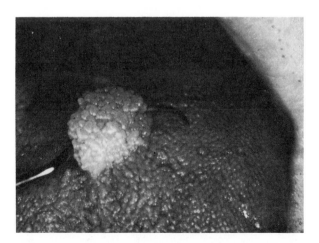

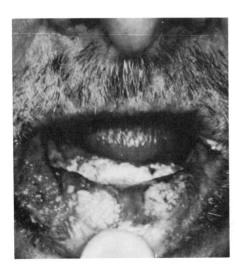

Figure 19–10. Oral leukoplakia. (From Shafer, W. G., Hine, M. K., and Levy, B. M.: *A Textbook of Oral Pathology,* 4th ed. Philadelphia, W. B. Saunders Company, 1983.)

A variety of oral carcinoma is *verrucous carcinoma* (Fig. 19–12), characterized by warty growths in areas of chronic irritation. The lesions are especially common in heavy users of chewing tobacco or snuff.

Adenocarcinoma of the salivary gland is a less commonly seen oral malignancy. It produces swelling of the affected area. If the parotid salivary gland is affected, swelling occurs in the midfacial area. Many salivary gland tumors contain both benign and malignant cells and are thus called *mixed tumors*.

Treatment of Oral Tumors

The treatment of most oral tumors involves surgical removal of the lesion. Some carcinomas that cannot be completely removed can be treated by x-ray therapy or by implantation of radioactive materials into tumor areas, such as implantation of radium "seeds" for carcinoma of the floor of the mouth.

X-ray therapy is also useful as a preoperative or postoperative treatment measure. The area can be irradiated before surgery to destroy small numbers of cells outside the surgical area or after surgery to destroy any cells that escaped removal. Such adjunctive use of x-ray therapy with surgery often improves the rate of successful treatment.

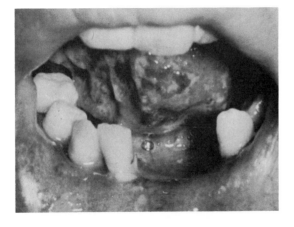

Figure 19–11. Squamous carcinoma of the tongue. (From Shafer, W. G., Hine, M. K., and Levy, B. M.: *A Textbook of Oral Pathology,* 4th ed. Philadelphia, W. B. Saunders Company, 1983.)

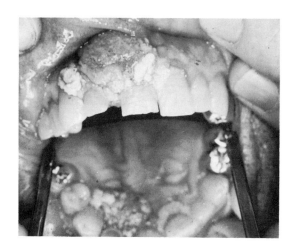

Figure 19–12. Verrucous carcinoma of the oral cavity. (From Shafer, W. G., Hine, M. K., and Levy, B. M.: *A Textbook of Oral Pathology,* 4th ed. Philadelphia, W. B. Saunders Company, 1983.)

SUMMARY

Oral disorders represent a complete assortment of disease processes and in this manner are similar to disorders of most other body areas. The common oral diseases demonstrate infection, inflammation, immune response, and neoplasia as the major pathologic changes. In addition, there are oral manifestations to many systemic diseases, including infectious childhood diseases, herpes zoster, and lupus erythematosus.

Many oral conditions are caused by common etiologic factors, including poor oral hygiene, chronic irritation of oral tissues, and improper diet. In almost all cases, early prevention and treatment measures forestall the development of more serious conditions. For example, early treatment of gingivitis prevents development of periodontitis and loss of teeth. Nowhere is the saying "an ounce of prevention is worth a pound of cure" more appropriate than in the oral cavity.

Questions

1. How might allergic stomatitis develop? What are some common materials that would likely cause allergy in the susceptible individual?
2. Describe the processes by which dental plaque and calculus are thought to form. Would an acidic saliva enhance or retard calculus formation?
3. Explain why extensive internal tooth damage is often painless, while less severe damage is usually extremely painful. How does a pulp polyp develop?
4. Using the principles of autoimmunity discussed in Chapter 4, describe how periodontal disease could develop as an autoimmune disorder.
5. Compare and contrast epulis and torus lesions, papillomas and fibromas, leukoplakia and verrucous carcinoma.

Additional Reading

Brown, W. E.: Physicochemical mechanisms of dental caries. J. Dental Res., 53:204, 1974.

Gibbons, R. J., and Van Houte, J.: On the formation of dental plaque. J. Periodontol., 44:347, 1973.

Page, R. C., and Shroeder, H. A.: Pathogenesis of inflammatory periodontal disease. Lab. Invest., 33:235, 1976.

Shafer, W. G., Hine, M. K., and Levy, B. M.: *A Textbook of Oral Pathology.* Philadelphia, W. B. Saunders Company, 1974. *(Excellently detailed, well-illustrated text.)*

Smith, C. J.: Global epidemiology and aetiology of oral cancer. Int. Dental J., 23:82, 1973.

CHAPTER 20

ANEMIAS

GENERAL CONSIDERATIONS

Red Blood Cell Formation

Development of the red blood cell (erythrocyte) begins in the bone marrow and continues through six stages:

1. Initial cell formation occurs as a result of the stimulating action of *erythropoietin,* produced by the kidney, on bone marrow tissue. The cell is called a *proerythroblast.* Proerythroblasts correspond to myeloblasts, lymphoblasts, and monoblasts in the leukocytic series and to megakaryoblasts in the thrombocytic series.

2.–4. In the next three stages, the red cells are called *normoblasts* (early, intermediate, late) and remain within the bone marrow areas.

5. In this stage, the cells are transformed into *reticulocytes,* also called *immature erythrocytes.*

6. The final step is the formation of *mature erythrocytes.* Both reticulocytes and mature erythrocytes are found primarily in the circulating blood.

All red cells except the proerythroblast contain *hemoglobin.* In the mature erythrocyte, hemoglobin functions as a carrier of oxygen and carbon dioxide, binding with oxygen in the capillary network of the lung and carrying it to the tissues. Carbon dioxide from body tissues attaches to hemoglobin and is carried back to the lung for removal by means of exhalation.

Hemoglobin consists of four subunits, each containing two parts: the *heme* portion, which contains iron as Fe^{+2}, and the *globin* portion, a complex polypeptide. The normal hemoglobin in adult humans is *hemoglobin A* (HbA). In the fetus, hemoglobin is in the form of *fetal hemoglobin* (HbF). This is replaced shortly after birth with HbA, except in a few individuals who retain HbF throughout life. This condition, which is common among those of Mediterranean descent (Italians, Greeks) is called *thalassemia major.* Other forms of thalassemia also exist in which other types of hemoglobin are present. *Sickle cell anemia* is also characterized by the presence of an abnormal hemoglobin, *HbS.* Generally, abnormal hemoglobins do not represent 100 per cent of the affected individual's total hemoglobin content but are mixed with some HbA. The severity of symptoms depends largely on the percentage of abnormal hemoglobin present.

A complex interaction of many influences is needed for normal erythrocyte formation. The bone marrow machinery for red cell production must be functional. Erythropoietin must be produced in adequate amounts. Minerals such as iron, cobalt, and copper must be available in sufficient quantities. In addition, certain vitamins, such as cyanocobalamin (vitamin B-12) and folic acid, are required for normal cell maturation. Inadequacy in any area leads to impaired red cell synthesis.

Red cell synthesis can be both overactive and underactive.

Polycythemia. Overproduction of erythrocytes (*polycythemia*) occurs to a slight degree under conditions of chronic hypoxia as a result of increased release of erythropoietin. Thus, the individual living at a high altitude or suffering from chronic lung disease, such as emphysema, develops a degree of polycythemia (*secondary polycythemia*) in these cases. *Primary polycythemia* (polycythemia vera) is caused by spontaneous overproduction of erythrocytes. In both types, the blood viscosity increases as a result of the high red cell count and complications can result from obstruction of small capillaries. The heart often hypertrophies, especially in polycythemia vera, as a result of the extra work needed to circulate the viscous blood. Interestingly, some polycythemia patients eventually develop *leukemia,* indicating an abnormality of leukocyte formation as well. Secondary polycythemia improves when its cause is corrected. The treatment of polycythemia vera involves periodic removal of blood to reduce the red cell count and the use of myelosuppressive drugs, such as radioactive phosphorus (^{32}P), to suppress the abnormally high rate of red cell formation.

Anemia. If the formation of erythrocytes or hemoglobin is at an abnormally low rate, or if the erythrocyte count or hemoglobin value is low despite adequate bone marrow function, the condition is termed *anemia*. Anemia develops for a variety of reasons (Table 20–1). Anything that interferes with a step necessary for red cell formation can cause anemia. Thus, impaired bone marrow activity, reduced production of erythropoietin, inadequate supplies of minerals (such as iron), or insufficient stimulation of erythrocyte maturation results in anemia. In addition, conditions that increase red cell loss or destruction also cause anemia. Although some anemias are relatively easy to diagnose, others require the expertise of the hematologist.

Common Tests for Anemias

Among the routine tests (Table 20–2) performed when anemia is suspected are the *erythrocyte count, hemoglobin determination,* and *hematocrit value.* The normal erythrocyte count is 4 to 6 million/mm³ and is slightly lower for females than for males. The normal hemoglobin content of blood is 12 to 18 gm/dl in adults, again somewhat lower for females than for males. The hematocrit value represents the percentage of packed erythrocytes in a known volume of blood. This is determined by filling a capillary tube with blood and then centrifuging it to force the heavier cell fraction to the bottom of the tube, leaving the clear plasma layer on top. Since the tube is the same diameter along its length, the height of the column of cells is proportional to its volume. In practice, other cells are also included in the column when the sample is centrifuged but their

Table 20–1. MECHANISMS OF ANEMIA DEVELOPMENT

Blood loss
Red cell hemolysis
Deficiency of necessary factor
Impaired bone marrow function
Decreased formation of erythropoietin

Table 20–2. COMMON BLOOD TESTS FOR ANEMIA

Test	Normal Value
Erythrocyte count	4 to 6 million/mm^3
Hemoglobin content	12 to 18 gm/dl
Hematocrit value	35 to 55 per cent
Mean corpuscular hemoglobin concentration	32 to 36 per cent
Serum iron level	75 to 170 μg/dl
Unsaturated iron binding capacity	60 to 70 per cent
Reticulocyte count	1 per cent of erythrocytes

relative volume is negligible. Normal hematocrit value is 35 to 55 per cent, slightly lower for females than males.

These three values often parallel each other, since all are dependent upon the number of erythrocytes and the content of hemoglobin of each. A rule of thumb is that the hemoglobin value is usually three times the erythrocyte count (e.g., 15 gm/dl versus 5 million cells/mm^3) and the hematocrit value is three times the hemoglobin value (e.g., 45 per cent versus 15 gm/dl).

Another useful test is the *mean corpuscular hemoglobin concentration* (MCHC), calculated from the hemoglobin and hematocrit values. MCHC tells whether the erythrocytes contain a normal amount of hemoglobin (normochromic) or have reduced amounts of hemoglobin (hypochromic). The normal value for MCHC is 32 to 36 per cent.

Several other tests are used in the diagnosis of anemias:

1. The *serum iron level* is helpful in determining whether the anemia is due to iron deficiency or to other cause, such as increased red cell destruction. The normal serum iron level is 75 to 170 μg/dl.

2. The *unsaturated iron binding capacity* (UIBC) represents the percentage of available binding sites on the iron-carrying compound transferrin. Since transferrin is normally saturated 30 to 40 per cent, the unsaturated capacity is 60 to 70 per cent, or approximately 200 μg/dl of iron. This value indicates whether iron is being circulated in normal amounts and gives a clue as to the type of anemia present. For example, in iron deficiency anemia, UIBC is abnormally high because there are many available unbound sites on transferrin.

3. The *reticulocyte count* represents the percentage of reticulocytes in the circulating blood. The normal value is approximately 1 per cent. Since reticulocytes are the final step in erythrocyte production before the mature red cell, the reticulocyte count is a measure of the rate of red cell production. A high reticulocyte count indicates rapid cell formation, probably because mature erythrocytes have been destroyed or lost. A low reticulocyte count indicates impaired bone marrow activity, usually because the marrow has been damaged.

4. *Bone marrow hemosiderin*, the common storage form of iron in the body, is examined in difficult anemia cases. It is absent in iron deficiency anemia but is normal or increased in all other anemias. The application of the tests for anemia will be covered with each type of anemia discussed.

IRON DEFICIENCY ANEMIA

Anemia due to iron deficiency is the most common type, in spite of the fact that the daily iron requirement is relatively low. Most of the iron from hemoglobin is "recycled" from red cells that have lived out their lifespan (120 days) to newly formed red cells. Adult men and postmenopausal women require only about 1 mg of iron per day to keep iron stores constant. Premenopausal females, adolescents, and children require 15 to 20 mg/day. This increased requirement is due to menstrual blood loss in adult premenopausal women and to rapid growth with constant increases in the total number of erythrocytes in children and adolescents. Accordingly, adult males and postmenopausal females develop iron deficiency much less often than premenopausal females, adolescents, or children; thus, such a deficiency in the former group is of greater concern, since it is more likely due to a serious condition.

Pathogenesis

Iron deficiency anemia develops for a variety of reasons. Chronic blood loss (bleeding ulcer, hemorrhoids, excessive menstruation, gastrointestinal cancer) can deplete body iron stores faster than they can be replaced by the average diet. In all of these conditions, careful investigation of the cause of the bleeding should be made and appropriate treatment instituted. *Acute* blood loss (hemorrhage) can also cause iron deficiency anemia as the body uses up iron stores for replacement of lost red cells.

Diets deficient in iron can eventually result in iron deficiency anemia because the small daily iron loss finally depletes iron stores. Diets that eliminate all common sources of iron, such as meat and spinach, will eventually lead to anemia. Many people follow unusual diets for weight control or other reasons. They should make sure that they have adequate iron intake. Occasionally, compulsive eating of starch or other iron-poor substances is the cause of anemia. This condition is called *pica*.

A common problem in infants and toddlers is *milk anemia,* caused by living primarily on cow's milk (which has very little iron content) in place of solid foods. Breast-fed infants fare somewhat better, since human milk contains more iron than cow's milk; however, both groups need iron supplementation, as do those on milk formulas.

Symptoms and Signs

Symptoms of iron deficiency anemia are more common in adults than in children. In fact, the pediatrician often suspects the condition by noting pallor of the nail beds, palms, or mucous membranes in a child who seems normally active and alert. In adults, symptoms are more common and include easy fatigue, listlessness, and loss of appetite. Signs often include brittle hair and fingernails, along with pallor of the skin. *Chlorosis* refers to the greenish color of the skin. An older term for iron deficiency anemia, chlorosis literally means "green around the gills," a good description of the appearance. In more severe cases, the extreme drop in hemoglobin and red cell count impairs tissue oxygenation, and tachycardia, dyspnea, or angina develops.

Laboratory Findings

Common laboratory findings include reduced erythrocyte count, reduced hemoglobin and hematocrit values, reduced serum iron

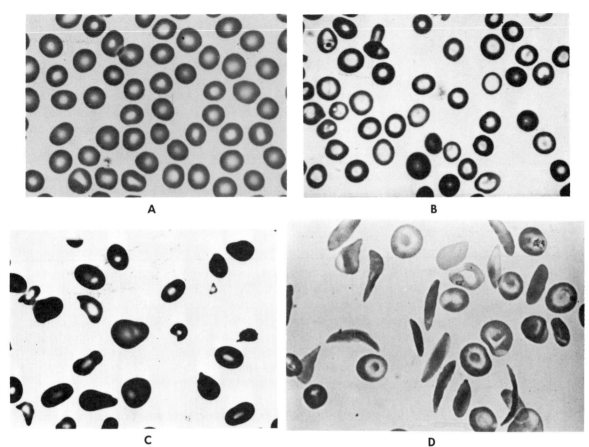

Figure 20–1. Types of red blood cells. *(A)* Normal. *(B)* Microcytic. *(C)* Macrocytic. *(D)* Sickle-shaped. *(A, B,* and *C* from Henry, J.: *Clinical Diagnosis and Management by Laboratory Methods,* 16th ed. Philadelphia, W. B. Saunders Company, 1979; *D* from Raphael, S. S.: *Lynch's Medical Laboratory Technology,* 4th ed. Philadelphia, W. B. Saunders Company, 1983.)

level, and increased UIBC. The red cells are small (microcytic) (Fig. 20–1) and pale in color (hypochromic). Examination of the bone marrow, if done, shows no hemosiderin. In iron deficiency anemia associated with ·gastrointestinal bleeding, the stool is positive for occult blood.

Diagnosis   The finding of hypochromic, microcytic anemia with absence of bone marrow hemosiderin is specific for iron deficiency anemia. Anemia associated with chronic infection appears similar, but hemosiderin is present in the marrow. A history of unusual diet or chronic blood loss is extremely helpful in diagnosis.

Treatment   The treatment of iron deficiency anemia has a long and colorful history. The Greeks used to drink water in which swords had been allowed to rust and thought that they derived strength from the sword, rather than from its iron content. Thus, their treatment was correct but for the wrong reason. In the old West, water used to quench metal in a blacksmith's shop was drunk for its iron content. The French added an elegant touch by steeping iron filings in wine and then drinking the wine. (This way, they did not have to wait for the iron to correct the anemia—they felt better right away!) Some of our more modern products (e.g., Hadacol, Geritol) have also employed iron and vitamins, liberally laced with alcohol. Pierre Blaud, another Frenchman, is credited with the development of the first iron pill, a combination of ferrous sulfate and potassium carbonate (Blaud's pills), in 1830. This proved more efficacious, although less tasty, than the iron-wine extracts.

Current therapy for iron deficiency anemia utilizes ferrous sulfate (Feosol), ferrous gluconate (Fergon), and other iron salts alone or in combination with other minerals, vitamins, or both. The recommended doses are more than adequate to promote maximal gastrointestinal absorption of iron in deficiency states. For those who experience severe gastric irritation and cramping with oral iron products (a common side effect), an intramuscular iron preparation containing iron dextran (Imferon) is available. It is important to remember that iron therapy should be continued for at least 3 months *after* erythrocyte count, hemoglobin, and hematocrit values return to normal. This is needed to replenish hemosiderin stores and thus to prevent relapse of anemia when therapy is discontinued.

Complications and Prognosis

Patients with angina pectoris, congestive heart failure, or severe respiratory disease are adversely affected by anemia, since the oxygen-carrying ability of blood is impaired. Sometimes anemia is the underlying cause in "refractory" heart or respiratory disease. Occasionally, iron deficiency anemia results from gastric cancer and associated chronic blood loss. The presence of anemia may lead to diagnosis of the underlying condition.

For most individuals with iron deficiency anemia, the prognosis is excellent once the cause is identified and treated. With additional attention to cause, relapse can usually be prevented.

PERNICIOUS ANEMIA

Pernicious, or Addisonian, anemia is of a type called *megaloblastic* or *macrocytic*. In place of a small red cell, as seen in iron deficiency anemia, there is a large oval-shaped red cell (macrocyte) in the blood and a large red cell precursor (megaloblast) in the bone marrow. The condition develops because there is insufficient influence of vitamin B-12 on the developing red cell. The cell continues to grow instead of completing maturation at a normal size. Such red cells are easily destroyed and are functionally poor in spite of their large size, and anemia results. The term *pernicious* is somewhat outmoded, since it originally was used to indicate the relentless nature of the disease. Today, the condition is easily treated and its complications can be prevented.

Pernicious anemia is more common in people of Anglo-Saxon and Scandinavian descent than in other ethnic groups and is slightly more common in males than females. It is not clear whether there is a genetic tendency toward it, but its clustering in certain families and its prevalence in ethnic groups that have historically intermingled suggests such a possibility. The disease usually surfaces after age 35, often between 50 and 80 years of age.

Pathogenesis

Vitamin B-12 is absorbed from the diet through the action of *intrinsic factor of Castle,* secreted by gastric parietal cells. Absorption of vitamin B-12 occurs primarily in the ileum. Current theory regarding the development of pernicious anemia proposes that the afflicted individual develops antibodies against the gastric parietal cells, antibodies affecting binding of vitamin B-12 to intrinsic factor, or antibodies affecting the absorption process itself.

Three different antibodies have been identified. The basis of antibody formation is presumably an autoimmune reaction. Regardless of which antibody or combination of antibodies is formed, the result is impairment of absorption of vitamin B-12, leading to depletion, even though the dietary supply is adequate ("starvation in the midst of plenty"). The gastric mucosa atrophies, leading to reduced or absent secretion of hydrochloric acid (achlorhydria) and various digestive enzymes. Systemic depletion of vitamin B-12 results, and there is eventual demyelinization of nerve fibers, beginning with nerves of the extremities. Finally, the central nervous system is affected.

Gastrectomy or ilectomy can also result in pernicious anemia, since the parietal cells, which secrete intrinsic factor, or the absorption areas of the ileum are lost. Another form of pernicious anemia occurs in an individual who harbors a particular type of tapeworm (*Diphyllobothrium latum*), usually obtained by eating raw fish. The worm resides in the gastrointestinal tract and ingests vitamin B-12 entering by way of the diet, thus creating a deficiency in the host. In these three situations, pernicious anemia is said to be secondary, whereas the "classical" type, characterized by immune reaction, is primary.

Symptoms and Signs

Three types of symptoms occur with pernicious anemia. There are typical *anemia symptoms,* including easy fatigue and lethargy, dyspnea, and tachycardia. In this way pernicious anemia resembles other anemias. However, *digestive symptoms* also occur, as a result of the lack of hydrochloric acid and digestive enzymes. Indigestion, belching, and diarrhea are common, and the tongue is red and sore (glossitis). In addition, *peripheral neuropathy* is seen. Loss of the myelin sheath in peripheral nerve fibers causes tingling, numbness, and loss of vibratory sense in the extremities. If the central nervous system (CNS) is involved, mental disturbances and even paralysis can result. However, most cases are diagnosed and treated long before CNS demyelinization occurs.

Laboratory Findings

The characteristic blood finding in pernicious anemia is macrocytosis, often associated with considerable variation in size of the red cells (poikilocytosis). There is often mild leukopenia and decreased platelet count (thrombocytopenia) (normal = 200,000 to 500,000/mm³). Bone marrow examination shows large numbers of megaloblasts and increased bone marrow hemosiderin. The serum vitamin B-12 content is decreased (normal = 300 to 400 pg/ml) (a picogram is one millionth of a microgram). Two specialized tests are used in the diagnosis of primary pernicious anemia.

Histalog Test. This test measures the ability of gastric cells to secrete hydrochloric acid after stimulation with betazole (Histalog). Like histamine, Histalog stimulates acid secretion by normal gastric cells. In pernicious anemia, however, the atrophic gastric mucosa is incapable of responding. Thus, the test gives indirect evidence of the presence of pernicious anemia.

Schilling Test. This test measures the gastrointestinal absorption of radiolabeled vitamin B-12. A known quantity is given orally and followed later by a larger amount of unlabeled vitamin B-12 to force the labeled material from the body. Labeled vitamin B-12 absorbed orally appears in the urine and can be measured by collecting all urine for 24 hours after administration. In pernicious anemia, very little radiolabeled vitamin B-12 appears in the urine, since there is virtually no absorption of it after oral administration. To confirm the test results, intrinsic factor is given and the test is repeated, thereby resulting in much improved absorption of vitamin B-12.

Diagnosis

The major condition that must be differentiated from pernicious anemia is folic acid deficiency anemia. The blood picture is virtually identical with both. However, the Histalog and Schilling tests are normal in folic acid deficiency anemia, as is the serum vitamin B-12 content.

Treatment

Pernicious anemia resulting from fish tapeworm infestation can be cured by eliminating the worm. Other types must be treated by the administration of vitamin B-12 by intramuscular injection to bypass the faulty oral absorption route. Typical products include cyanocobalamin (Rubramin PC) and hydroxocobalamin (Neobetalin 12). Treatment must be continued for life. Digestive disturbances can be partially overcome by the oral administration of dilute hydrochloric acid. The preparation should be taken using a glass straw to avoid contact of the acid with tooth enamel. Dietary adjustments and the use of antacids are often necessary, as well, to control digestive symptoms.

Complications and Prognosis

Cases diagnosed early can be treated promptly with avoidance of complications. Severe, untreated cases result in CNS damage. If symptoms have persisted for more than 6 months, they may be irreversible, as remyelinization of nerve fibers does not occur.

FOLIC ACID DEFICIENCY ANEMIA

Pathogenesis

Most cases of folic acid deficiency anemia occur as a result of dietary deficiency. Diets poor in green vegetables, liver, and other sources of folic acid induce deficiency. Alcoholics are especially prone to the condition, probably as a result of a combination of poor diet, increased utilization of folic acid, and impaired absorption resulting from gastrointestinal damage. Pregnant women have an increased demand for folic acid from the developing fetus and can easily become deficient unless they supplement folic acid. In addition, they often diet to control their weight during pregnancy, which may restrict folic acid intake.

Less commonly, folic acid deficiency develops as a result of drug administration. Phenobarbital (Luminal) and phenytoin (Dilantin), used in the treatment of epilepsy, can impair absorption of dietary folic acid. Other drugs, which include methotrexate, an anticancer agent, and triamterene (Dyrenium), a diuretic, prevent the conversion of folic acid to folinic acid. Folinic acid is the active form of folic acid in the body.

Rarely, folic acid deficiency anemia is caused by malabsorption in an individual with a faulty or diseased digestive tract. In this case, multiple vitamin deficiencies usually exist.

Symptoms and Signs

The symptoms and signs relating to anemia are quite similar to those of pernicious anemia. However, because there is no demyelinization of nerve fibers, neurologic symptoms are absent. The gastric mucosa is normal, except in the rare cases caused by gastrointestinal malabsorption, and digestion is normal. Most complaints relate to easy fatigability, lethargy, and other symptoms of anemia.

Laboratory Findings

The blood picture in folic acid deficiency anemia closely resembles that of pernicious anemia. The bone marrow shows megaloblastosis and increased hemosiderin content, as with pernicious anemia. Serum vitamin B-12 content is normal, but folate activity is reduced (normal = 5 to 20 ng/ml) (a nanogram is one thousandth of a microgram). Histalog and Schilling tests are normal, reflecting normal gastric acid secretion and vitamin B-12 absorption.

Diagnosis

As previously mentioned, the major diagnostic choice is between folic acid deficiency anemia and pernicious anemia. The former is diagnosed primarily by the normal Histalog and Schilling tests and the reduced serum folate activity.

Treatment

Treatment of folic acid deficiency anemia depends upon its cause. A well-balanced diet that contains sources of folic acid will correct dietary deficiency. Control of alcoholism and the use of folic acid supplements will reverse the condition in the alcoholic. Drugs that block absorption of dietary folic acid or prevent its conversion to folinic acid can often be withdrawn, and other agents can be substituted.

Supplemental administration of folic acid is desirable in almost all cases of deficiency, since it will speed recovery from anemia and rebuild stores in the body. Multivitamins contain small amounts of folic acid. Larger amounts are available on prescription (e.g., Folvite). Prenatal vitamins, obtainable on prescription, contain large amounts of folic acid along with other factors needed during neonatal development. If malabsorption of folic acid exists, supplementation beyond the quantity obtainable in the normal diet is mandatory.

For those who must continue to take drugs that block conversion of folic to folinic acid, folinic acid is available as Leukovorin. This is given by intramuscular injection and bypasses the effects of such drugs. The duration of treatment of folic acid deficiency anemia varies, depending upon the cause, and may be lifelong in some cases, such as in those with gastrointestinal malabsorption.

Complications and Prognosis

There are few complications to folic acid deficiency anemia, since neuropathy does not occur. Severe anemia of any type can be incompatible with life, but prompt recovery in most cases of this type occurs after therapy is instituted.

A word of caution is in order regarding the treatment of folic acid deficiency anemia, however. Since folic acid and vitamin B-12 perform similar functions in red cell formation and maturation, a deficiency of one can be overcome by administration of large amounts of the other. Thus, folic acid can "spare" vitamin B-12 and *vice versa,* resulting in a normal blood picture. If vitamin B-12 is taken by a person suffering from folic acid deficiency anemia, the blood picture is corrected and no harm results. However, if folic acid is taken by an individual who has pernicious anemia, the blood picture is corrected but neuropathy continues unabated. Serious neurologic damage can result. Furthermore, the condition is then difficult to diagnose, since the blood picture is normal and time is wasted before proper treatment with vitamin B-12 is instituted. This points up the need for correct diagnosis before any treatment is begun.

SICKLE CELL ANEMIA

In the United States black population, approximately 8 per cent carry a single trait for type S hemoglobin (HbS), rather than HbA. These individuals are heterozygous for sickle cell disease; i.e., they have received the trait from only one parent. They are said to have *sickle cell trait.* Approximately 0.2 per cent have received the trait from both parents. These homozygous individuals have *sickle cell anemia.* In some parts of Africa, the incidence of sickle cell trait is much higher, with as many as 30 per cent of the population affected. Occasionally, those of Mediterranean heritage are also affected. Other ethnic groups are rarely affected and there is no sex preference for either sickle cell trait or sickle cell disease.

Pathogenesis

Sickle cell disease is classified as a *hereditary hemoglobinopathy.* That is, there is a defect in the formation of HbA. In this case, the amino acid *valine* is substituted for *glutamine* in HbA, forming HbS. This relatively minor alteration has serious consequences: The HbS molecules tend to stack together because of increased bonding between molecules, and long chains of stacked HbS molecules are formed. The red cell is forced out of shape by the molecular chains and assumes a sickle or crescent configuration. Sickling occurs under conditions of hypoxia, when bonding between HbS molecules is greatest. The sickled red cells tend to stack together like coins (rouleaux formation) and form clumps that obstruct small blood vessels. The HbS that leaks from damaged red cells tends to precipitate in blood because of reduced solubility, and blood viscosity increases. The overall effect is a sludging of blood, associated with reduced circulation and the development of ischemia in areas of small blood vessel circulation. Eventually, tissue necrosis develops from repeated ischemic episodes. Anemia develops primarily because the spleen detects the presence of the abnormally shaped red cells and destroys them.

Individuals with sickle cell anemia (homozygous) have almost all HbS and very little HbA. Those with sickle cell trait (heterozygous) have only about 40 per cent HbS and the rest HbA. Consequently, they are less affected and usually show no symptoms unless subjected to extreme hypoxia. Unless a blood test detects the trait, these persons are generally unaware of their condition. Those with sickle cell disease can experience an attack of sickling (sickling crisis) as a result of minor changes in blood oxygen tension, such as mild hypoxia during sleep. Exposure to high altitude, respiratory depression, exercise, infection, pregnancy, dehydration, and systemic acidosis can also trigger off sickling crisis.

It is ironic that the sickle cell trait was probably initially a helpful abnormality. In areas of Africa where malaria is endemic, carrying the sickle cell trait would offer some protection against the disease. The malaria parasite resides for part of its life cycle in the red cell. As the malaria organism uses up oxygen from the erythrocyte, intracellular hypoxia develops. This does not alter the normal cell, but it causes sickling in cells in an individual with sickle cell trait. The sickled cells are detected by the spleen and destroyed, and the malaria parasite is eliminated. Unfortunately, in those with sickle cell *anemia,* the condition itself is worse than the malaria against which it protects.

As more people with sickle cell trait marry and have children, the incidence of sickle cell disease increases. The incidence is about 25 per cent in children born of parents who are each heterozygous for the trait. This points up the great need to identify those with sickle cell trait.

Symptoms and Signs

Symptoms of anemia are present in sickle cell anemia, as expected. Jaundice develops as a result of the high level of bilirubin formed from hemoglobin released during cell destruction. In blacks, the yellow skin color of jaundice is not easily noticed. However, the sclera of the eye becomes yellow (scleral jaundice) and is quite noticeable. Pain in the abdomen and extremities is common, resulting from hypoxia owing to ischemia. Fever is common during an attack, presumably because of cell destruction and release of pyrogens. Sickle cell anemia patients are often tall and slender, but the connection between this finding and their underlying condition is not clear.

Laboratory Findings

In addition to the presence of sickle-shaped red cells in sickle cell anemia, there is also a decrease in erythrocyte count and hemoglobin value. Electrophoresis of blood shows HbS to be the predominant hemoglobin, with only small amounts of HbA. Marked increase in reticulocyte count is seen (reticulocytosis), often approaching 20 per cent of the erythrocyte count. This reflects the body's effort to replace cells destroyed by the spleen. Serum bilirubin is elevated, resulting from massive erthyrocyte destruction, as previously mentioned. Those with sickle cell trait usually have normal laboratory findings, unless the cells are subjected to severe hypoxia.

The screening tests for sickle cell trait are based upon the use of a strong reducing agent, such as sodium metabisulfite, to create the necessary cellular hypoxia. When cells from an individual with sickle cell trait are mixed with such a compound, sickling and clumping occur and this can be verified with microscopic observation. Newer tests, such as Sickle-Quik, do not require a microscope. The blood sample is mixed with a reducing agent, and the resulting turbidity of the solution can be observed by placing the sample in front of a lined card and observing blurring of the lines. This type of test is excellent for screening large numbers of people for sickle cell trait without sophisticated equipment.

Diagnosis The finding of anemia in a black person does not guarantee the presence of sickle cell anemia. The person could have iron deficiency anemia, iron deficiency anemia with sickle cell trait, thalassemia, or one of the rarer anemias caused by formation of HbC or HbD. Occasionally, a mixture of HbS and HbD is seen, representing two simultaneous anemias. Differential diagnosis of sickle cell anemia is based upon electrophoresis of the blood to detect the presence of HbS, positive results in the sickle cell detection test, and the invariable finding of reduced erythrocyte count. The widespread nature of symptoms, involving many organ systems, seen in sickle cell anemia is often a source of confusion because attention may be directed to the affected organ as the primary, rather than secondary, source of difficulty.

Treatment and Prevention Treatment of sickle cell disease is, unfortunately, symptomatic. No successful means of converting HbS to HbA or of reducing the tendency for HbS molecules to bind has been developed. Blood transfusions are given when anemia becomes severe, as after a major sickling crisis. Adequate hydration to increase the solubilization of red cells and hemoglobin in blood is helpful. Anti-infectives are needed for the infections commonly associated with reduced circulation. Analgesics are often required for the severe pain of hypoxia.

The greatest hope lies in prevention. If all individuals with sickle cell trait could be identified and refrained from marrying others with the trait, sickle cell disease would eventually become extremely rare. Widespread screening programs being conducted at the present time are designed with these goals in mind.

Complications Most people with sickle cell disease die before age 40. Cerebral hemorrhage or thrombosis, kidney damage, bone destruction, and leg ulcers are common complications to the condition. The heart usually hypertrophies, as a compensation for hypoxia and as a result of the extra effort expended in circulating the viscous blood. Severe infections are often seen, brought about by tissue hypoxia and necrosis. Multiple complications are the rule, owing to the widespread organ involvement seen with the disease. Those with sickle cell trait have a normal life span and rarely develop any complications to their condition.

APLASTIC ANEMIA Anemia caused by failure of bone marrow cells is termed *aplastic anemia*. In almost all cases, there is failure to form leukocytes and platelets as well as erythrocytes. The combination of erythrocytopenia, leukocytopenia, and thrombocytopenia is called *pancytopenia*. This term describes the blood picture; aplastic anemia refers to the underlying bone marrow defect (*aplasia* is the opposite of *hyperplasia*.) The incidence of aplastic anemia is only about 4 per million, but it is a frequently fatal form of anemia. There is no particular sexual or racial preference.

Pathogenesis Approximately half the cases of aplastic anemia are idiopathic. The rest result from an odd assortment of etiologic factors. Exposure to radiation, especially whole-body x-ray treatment or accidental contact with high-powered radiation sources, is a cause. Infection with hepatitis virus is occasionally a cause, as is exposure to dichlorodiphenyltrichloroethane (DDT) or benzene.

Some cases of aplastic anemia are associated with the use of specific drugs, such as chloramphenicol (Chloromycetin), phenyl-butazone (Butazolidin), or certain anticancer drugs. Most anticancer drugs are directly toxic to bone marrow cells, since they suppress the ability to form rapidly growing cells in general. The harmful effect they exert on the tumor cells also extends to the host, and the bone marrow depressant effect is largely *dose-related*. With most other drugs that cause aplastic anemia, the effect is not dose-related but occurs as an unusual response in the affected individual (idio-syncrasy). Chloramphenicol, however, seems to have both effects.

The mechanism of pathogenesis in aplastic anemia is not known, but it is assumed that the toxic agents directly damage the bone marrow cells. Perhaps individuals who develop the disease are unusually susceptible to the effects of toxic agents; i.e., the "climate" is right for disease development. In any event, the bone marrow becomes infiltrated with nonfunctional fatty tissue, which replaces the normal functioning marrow.

Symptoms and Signs

The victim of aplastic anemia develops the usual symptoms of anemia but also suffers from the effects of leukopenia and throm-bocytopenia. The tendency toward infection increases, as does its severity. Bleeding tendency develops, and the blood fails to clot normally. Any of these three major problems can occur first and cause the individual to seek medical attention.

Laboratory Findings

The blood count of erythrocytes, leukocytes, and thrombocytes is abnormally low. Leukocyte counts often fall below 2000/mm^3 and thrombocyte counts below 30,000/mm^3. The reticulocyte count is usually low, reflecting impaired ability to form erythrocytes. Bone marrow examination shows a paucity of cells, with fatty infiltration of marrow tissue. There is increased hemosiderin content of the marrow, resulting from impaired utilization of iron in the formation of erythrocytes, and this is also reflected in a drop in UIBC.

Diagnosis

Several conditions present some of the clinical findings of aplastic anemia. In myelofibrosis, the marrow is replaced by fibrous, rather than fatty, tissue. In addition, leukocytosis and hepatosple-nomegaly are present. Early forms of leukemia ("aleukemic" leu-kemia) may give a blood picture similar to aplastic anemia. However, marked leukocytosis usually follows. Lymphomas, such as Hodgkin's disease, can cause a clinical condition similar to aplastic anemia when there is invasion of bone marrow. In all cases, bone marrow biopsy provides the information needed for diagnosis.

Treatment

There are four primary types of treatment in aplastic anemia:

1. *Elimination of any possible toxic agent* should be the first step.

2. *Blood transfusions* temporarily correct the anemia and supply platelets and leukocytes as well. Specific blood products, such as

packed red cell concentrates or platelet concentrates, can also be used.

3. *Anabolic steroids,* such as methandrostenolone (Dianabol), are sometimes successful in stimulating bone marrow activity. These should be tried for at least 2 months before being abandoned.

4. *Bone marrow transplants* between compatible individuals are now being performed in some medical centers. The marrow must be typed, as are blood and other tissues, for a correct match. As with kidney transplants, an identical twin is the most ideal donor. The technique is complicated, expensive, and somewhat painful, but successful enough to warrant its use where possible.

Complications and Prognosis More than half of those with aplastic anemia die, usually from severe hemorrhage or overwhelming infection. Some patients are maintained for years, using repeated transfusions and careful antibiotic therapy for infections. A few spontaneously recover some or all of their bone marrow function.

SUMMARY

Red cell development requires a functioning bone marrow, adequate stimulation of marrow cells with erythropoietin, and the presence of normal amounts of specific vitamins and minerals. If any of these elements is missing, anemia results.

Common causes of anemia include iron deficiency, folic acid deficiency, and impaired absorption of vitamin B-12. Less common causes include hereditary abnormalities of hemoglobin formation, red cell hemolysis, and impaired bone marrow function. The anemia associated with renal failure is caused by reduced formation of erythropoietin.

Many anemias can be treated by supplying the deficient element. This is the case with anemias associated with iron deficiency, folic acid deficiency, or impaired absorption of vitamin B-12. Hemoglobin abnormalities are not correctable at present, but damaged bone marrow can sometimes be stimulated to function with the use of drugs, or replaced with suitable donor tissue. The complications of anemias are more effectively treated today than in the past, giving an improved prognosis in most cases.

Questions
1. Hereditary spherocytosis is a condition characterized by spherically shaped erythrocytes and hemolysis of red cells. Using information obtained from the discussion of sickle cell anemia, explain why red cell hemolysis occurs.
2. What would be the effect of removing blood as a treatment for polycythemia in an individual with severe emphysema? Severe angina pectoris?
3. Compare and contrast pernicious anemia and folic acid deficiency anemia as to laboratory findings, symptoms, and complications.
4. In earlier times, pernicious anemia was treated by having the anemic person eat several pounds of raw or lightly cooked liver per day. Why couldn't the liver be cooked more thoroughly?
5. Complete exchange of blood (exchange transfusion) is used in infants with erythroblastosis fetalis, a hemolytic condition caused by incompatibility between the blood of the mother and fetus. Explain why exchange transfusion is not effective as a treatment for sickle cell anemia.

Additional Reading   Ferguson, G. G.: Anemias and their treatments. Southern Pharmacy Journal, 70:10, 1978. (*Overview of the well-known anemias.*)

Good, R. A.: Aplastic anemia-suppressor lymphocytes and hematopoiesis. N. Engl. J. Med., 296:10, 1977.

Kass, L.: *Pernicious Anemia.* Philadelphia, W. B. Saunders Company, 1976.

MacLean, W. C., and Graham, G. G.: Vegetarianism in children. American Journal of Diseases of Children, 134:513, 1980. (*Discussion of iron-poor diets.*)

Sheehy, T. W., and Plumb, V. J.: Treatment of sickle cell disease. Arch. Intern. Med., 137:779, 1977.

CHAPTER 21

MALIGNANT DISORDERS

GENERAL CONSIDERATIONS   Probably no word strikes more fear in our hearts than the word "cancer." We immediately think of the spread of a malignant tumor throughout the body, progressing inexorably to death. Yet, such a gloomy prognosis is not always warranted. Cancer occurs in more than 100 different forms, some of which are easily diagnosed at an early stage and completely curable. Basal cell carcinoma of the skin, for example, an extremely common type of cancer, is 100 per cent curable if treated at an early stage. Even neglected lesions do not metastasize, although they invade locally, and thus rarely cause death. There are now apparent cures of acute lymphoblastic leukemia, Hodgkin's disease, choriocarcinoma (a tumor composed of placental tissue), and Wilms' tumor (a childhood kidney tumor). Many other types of cancer, if detected early, can be cured with surgery, drugs, radiation, or a combination of treatments. To automatically sound the death knell with the word cancer makes no more sense than to do the same with "heart disease." Heart disease can consist of only a mild arrhythmia, easily controllable with drugs, or it can represent intractable congestive heart failure.

Incidence of Cancer   Approximately 20 per cent of deaths in the United States are due to cancer and its complications, second only to heart disease. More than a million new cases of cancer are diagnosed each year, of which about a third are skin cancers and generally easily treated. An exception is malignant melanoma, a highly dangerous form of skin cancer that strikes 10,000 people per year and kills about 5000. However, malignant melanoma represents only 3 per cent of skin cancers and 1 per cent of cancer cases in general. If all types of cancer are considered together, the overall survival rate is approximately 50 per cent. Thus, the excellent survival rate in basal cell carcinoma of the skin is counterbalanced by the poor survival rate in carcinoma of the lung, pancreatic carcinoma, malignant melanoma, and anaplastic carcinoma of the thyroid gland.

   The incidence of the common types of cancer varies considerably from country to country and between males and females in the same country. Native Japanese, for example, have a much lower rate of cancer of the lung, breast, prostate, colon, and bladder than the United States population does, but they have a greater frequency of cancer of the stomach and esophagus. These differences can be partly explained by differences in diet or environment, but genetic factors may also be important in some cases. Japanese persons living in the United States have rates of common types of cancer between

327

the incidence among native Japanese and the incidence among native Americans. This suggests that the lifestyle is important in determining susceptibility to certain forms of cancer. White American women have eight times the incidence of breast cancer of Israeli women. Such factors as the number of children borne, the age at birth of the first child, and whether or not the children are breast-fed may be important influences on the tendency toward breast cancer, in addition to the obvious dietary and cultural differences. Within the United States, the incidence of lung cancer is higher for men than women, as is the case for Hodgkin's disease and most leukemias. The difference in incidence of lung cancer is explained by the fact that women have smoked cigarettes for a shorter period of time than men and have probably been exposed to fewer occupational carcinogens than men. Conversely, breast cancer in males is only 1 per cent as common as in females. Differences in hormonal effects in the two sexes may be important here.

Etiology   A mind-boggling array of etiologic factors for cancer has been accumulated. Many of these are discussed in Chapter 1. It is usually very difficult to prove that a particular factor causes cancer, however, since it is generally not possible in human populations to eliminate all variables except the one in question. A butcher exposed to vinyl chloride fumes in the packaging of meat may also drink more alcohol and eat different foods than another butcher similarly exposed to vinyl chloride. In addition, there may be variations in the type of water ingested, in the amount of pollution in the air, and in the exposure to chemicals related to hobby activities. This does not even consider genetic differences that might alter the susceptibility to vinyl chloride carcinogenesis in the liver.

Some factors seem to be obvious causes of cancer. The amount of sunlight exposure is directly proportional to the susceptibility to skin cancer. Chewing betel nuts (Chapter 19) increases the risk of buccal cancer, apparently because of direct contact between the nut and the buccal tissue. Cancer of the lower lip appears in the area where a cigarette, cigar or pipe is held. Even in these cases, though, other influences may be operating in concert with the obvious factor.

In spite of the fact that there seems to be a direct cause-and-effect relationship between the cancer-causing factors (*carcinogens*) and cancer development, the process may be somewhat more complex. With many carcinogens, another agent is needed to act along with the primary stimulus in order to produce a malignant lesion. The carcinogen is called the *initiator,* and the helper agent is termed the *promoter.* Thus 3,4-benzpyrene, a carcinogen, may have little effect if painted on a mouse's skin in small doses. If the skin is then painted with croton oil (promoter), skin cancer readily develops. Croton oil by itself is irritating but not carcinogenic.

If this line of thought is carried a step further, we can see that a carcinogen might "prime" the tissue for malignancy later on. If there then were exposure to a promoter at a later time, cancer would develop. This might explain why some carcinogens have an extremely long latency period between exposure and the development of cancer. For example, exposure to asbestos often causes pleural cancer years later, even though there may be no exposure during the intervening period. Perhaps the asbestos-primed pleural tissue is then affected by promoters causing the eventual development of cancer.

Theories of Cancer Development

There are two major schools of thought regarding the development of cancer: the *somatic mutation theory* and the *aberrant differentiation theory*. Both are well supported by experimental evidence.

Somatic mutation refers to the change in cellular chromosomes that occurs following exposure to radiation, certain drugs, and specific viruses. Alterations or breaks in chromosomes can change the characteristics of cell growth. The cell could then mutate into a malignant or premalignant cell. If premalignant, it might be more vulnerable to the influence of other carcinogens and/or promoters in the environment. Individuals with certain hereditary disorders that increase the rate of chromosome breakage, such as *Bloom's syndrome,* are much more susceptible to certain forms of cancer, possibly because of chromosome damage. There is evidence that the body detects many chromosome breaks and attempts to repair them. Perhaps in these cases, however, the rate of breakage exceeds that of repair. Most types of cancer are more common in older people. It is possible that there is an accumulation of chromosome defects that cannot be corrected, along with reduced repair ability, in the older person.

Aberrant differentiation refers to abnormal specialization of developing cells. A cell destined to become a gastric mucosal cell differentiates into a gastric carcinoma cell. A bone cell becomes an osteosarcoma cell. A lymphocyte differentiates into a leukemic cell. This theory of cancer development recognizes the fact that all cells develop from an embryonic stage through steps to the mature, specialized cell. A defect anywhere in the differentiation process could lead to malignancy. A carcinogenic factor might thus induce such a defect as the cell develops. In support of this theory are the observations that malignant tumors occasionally differentiate into benign tumors or, in rare instances, back into normal tissue. Perhaps the body recognizes certain cells as being abnormal and makes alterations in them or eliminates them entirely. What a weapon we would have if we could convert malignant cells to normal cells!

Regardless of which mechanism is operating for a given type of cancer, the process must continue through many generations of cells in order for a tumor to develop. It is thought that tumor cells go through several stages, becoming more and more malignant with each generation. There may also be a selection process operating, whereby strong cells are allowed to continue growing and weaker cells are eliminated. In this manner the tumor would gain strength as it grew and would finally overcome any existing body defenses. It is apparent that time is required for cancer to develop. Time is needed for the initiator/promoter actions to take place, for abnormal cells to develop, and for the tumor to gain size and momentum. Interference with the developmental process might prevent or arrest cancer in the early stages.

Body Defenses Against Cancer

We live in a virtual sea of carcinogens, but most of us do not develop cancer. It is obvious that there must be a resistance factor in operation, as is the case with infectious organisms. Those with immunologic deficiencies have a 1000-fold increase in the frequency of cancer, especially forms of lymphoma. Immunosuppressed individuals, for example those with kidney transplants, have an 80-fold increase in cancer incidence. This points up the importance of the immune system in cancer prevention.

Recently, *tumor antigens* have been isolated from malignant cells. These antigens evoke an immune response in the normal individual, leading to formation of sensitized T lymphocytes ("killer" cells) that attack the cancer cells. The process is a type of cell-mediated immunity (see Chapter 4). Additional support for this idea comes from the clinical observations that spontaneous regression of tumors occasionally occurs and that tumors heavily infiltrated with lymphocytes do not spread as rapidly as those devoid of lymphocytic cells. Recent attempts to improve the immune response against cancer cells using bacille Calmette-Guérin (BCG) vaccine have been interesting, although not particularly successful. Perhaps the procedure requires modification and refinement to become more effective.

The other apparent body defense against cancer, previously mentioned, is the ability to repair damaged or broken chromosomes and to avoid malignant changes in the cells. Thus caffeine, a known mutagen in cell culture preparations, is consumed in large quantities by most people without harmful effect. The exact nature of this repair process is unknown.

Diagnostic Tests for Cancer

Malignant lesions occurring in visible body areas, such as the skin or oral cavity, can be directly seen and felt and are often diagnosed early for that reason. Other tumors, e.g., in the digestive and respiratory tracts, can be visualized with the help of specialized instruments, usually lighted tubes inserted into the affected area.

Some lesions can be detected with the use of *radioactive isotopes*, by noting the difference in uptake between the malignant and nonmalignant areas. Thus, thyroid tumors are detected with a radioactive iodine scan, pancreatic tumors can be diagnosed with the use of radioactive selenium, and bone tumors can be pinpointed by using radioactive phosphorus. The isotope chosen is one that readily incorporates into the affected tissue.

X-ray studies are useful for detecting many solid tumors in the brain, gastrointestinal tract, and other areas, but are made more sensitive if a contrast medium or dye is used to outline the involved area. Obtaining barium contrast x-rays of the lower intestinal tract is a more definitive technique than using conventional x-rays. Computer-assisted tomography (CAT or CT scan) is a form of x-ray in which a computer-directed composite of multiple x-rays taken from different angles is made. It can also be augmented with dyes or contrast media (Fig. 21–1).

Ultrasound techniques can now detect solid tumors or perform other functions. The advantage of ultrasound is that it is apparently harmless to the body, unlike x-ray or isotope administration.

Cells shed, scraped, or washed from a lesion can be examined for malignancy. This is the basis of the Papanicolaou (Pap) smear

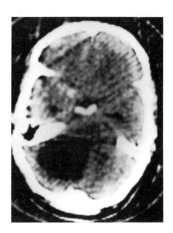

Figure 21–1. Computed tomographic scan of brain showing cerebellar tumor. (From Ramsey, R. G.: *Neuroradiology with Computed Tomography.* Philadelphia, W. B. Saunders Company, 1981.)

for cervical cancer. The technique is called *exfoliative cytology.* For lesions that are not directly accessible, as in the gastrointestinal or respiratory tract, an instrument can be used to remove a few cells for examination. Often, this instrument is combined with the instrument for visualization of the tumor.

Biopsy of tissue involves removal of a sample for microscopic study. For some tumors close to the surface of the body (e.g., peripheral lung and breast tumors), a *needle biopsy* can be used. A sample of tissue or fluid from the tumor area is removed, using a special large-bore needle. *Surgical biopsy* is the surgical removal of tissue for study. It is often used for tumors of the breast, lung, intestine, or other areas. The biopsy specimen can be mounted in paraffin and sliced into very thin sections using an instrument called a *microtome.* If time is of the essence, a frozen section can be obtained and the pathologic report rendered immediately while the patient is still anesthetized. This avoids the need for additional anesthesia and trauma to the patient. For those malignancies affecting the bone marrow, a *bone marrow biopsy* is often used to facilitate diagnosis. A small quantity is removed from a hollow bone using a special needle.

Some tumors synthesize compounds that serve to identify them. *Alpha-fetoprotein* (AFP), a type produced by fetal liver cells, is also secreted by malignant liver tumors (hepatocarcinomas). Thus, the appearance of AFP in the blood stream of an adult aids in the diagnosis of liver cancer. Colon carcinomas and other malignant tumors produce *carcinoembryonic antigen* (CEA). The serum level of CEA roughly parallels the size of the tumor. The CEA disappears from the serum if the tumor has been completely excised but persists if some tumor tissue remains. Both AFP and CEA are useful in following patients with certain types of cancer, but the tests are not completely diagnostic. Perhaps in the future a sensitive test can be developed to detect the presence of any type of cancer and therefore serve as a screening test in apparently healthy people.

Classification of Cancer   The nomenclature of benign, intermediate, and malignant tumors is discussed in Chapter 6. In general, the ending *-oma* is used for benign tumors and *-carcinoma* or *-sarcoma* for malignant tumors.

Table 21–1. TYPICAL STAGES IN TUMOR SPREAD

Stage	Description
I	Tumor cells found only in original site
II	Tumor cells found in original site plus in regional lymph nodes
III	Tumor cells found in original site and regional lymph nodes plus in distant lymph nodes
IV	Metastatic tumor cells found in many body areas

Besides determining whether the tumor is benign or malignant, it is important to know its characteristics and stage at the time of diagnosis. The characteristics of benign tumors are contrasted with those of malignant tumors in Chapter 6. In clinical practice, a tumor is *staged* (assigned to a particular stage) after diagnosis (Table 21–1). This helps in the selection of appropriate treatment and in determining the prognosis. In general, stage I lesions have a more favorable prognosis than stage II, III, and IV lesions, since they have spread less. Staging is not completely accurate, since metastatic tumors seeds may have spread but not yet become detectable at the time of diagnosis. Thus, the tumor is staged at a lower number, but with time greater spread is apparent. Nevertheless, staging is a useful technique in cancer treatment.

A more precise system of grading malignancies currently in use is the *TNM system*. With this system, *T* refers to the size of the primary tumor (T1 through T4); *N* represents the regional lymph node involvement (N0 through N2); and *M* denotes distant metastases (M0 through M2). This system gives more standardization in reporting results of treatment than just indicating the stage and permits better comparison of different forms of treatment for the same type of cancer.

Types of Cancer

Of the hundred or so types of cancer, some are quite rare. Of course, having a rare form of cancer is little comfort to the afflicted person, who feels singled out from 10,000 or 100,000 people, often with no rhyme or reason for it. Specific types of tumors often have fairly uniform properties and may follow a similar course in several different body tissues. Thus, an adenocarcinoma of the stomach may be similar to an adenocarcinoma of the colon and require a similar form of treatment.

A general distinction made in cancer terminology is between solid tumors and cancer involving the bone marrow or lymphatic system. Solid tumors, such as adenocarcinomas, begin from a single cell or group of cells and spread from that point. Malignant diseases of the bone marrow or lymphatic system often do not present as solid lesions but as infiltrations of abnormal cells in normal tissue. For example, in Hodgkin's disease a cervical lymph node is often infiltrated with atypical cells. These disorders often begin with more widespread proliferation of abnormal cells than is the case with solid tumors. There may be no primary source of cells that can be removed surgically in some cases. X-ray and drug therapy are the mainstays of treatment if surgery is not possible. Proliferative malignant diseases of the bone marrow are called *leukemias,* whereas those of the lymphatic system are called *lymphomas*. Bear in mind that in advanced disease many different body areas may be infiltrated with abnormal cells; i.e., leukemic cells may be found in the lymphatic system and lymphoma cells may be found in the bone marrow. In these cases, diagnosis is difficult.

This chapter considers cancer of the breast, lung, and colorectal area, representing the three most common solid tumors in the United States population. (Skin cancers, although more common in total incidence, are often excluded from cancer statistics, since hospitalization is rarely required.) The four common types of leukemia are also discussed, as is Hodgkin's disease, the most common lymphoma.

Treatment of Cancer

Surgery, radiation treatment (radiotherapy), and drug treatment (chemotherapy) are the main forms of treatment for malignant disease.

Surgery

Surgery is generally preferable, if it can be used, since it offers the greatest chance of removal of all tumor cells. Even with wide surgical excision, however, some cells may remain, since malignant tumors contain fingerlike projections extending into surrounding tissues. In addition, metastasis may have occurred prior to surgery, making removal of all malignant cells impossible.

Radiotherapy

Radiotherapy, using x-ray, cobalt isotopes, or other forms of damaging radiation, destroys tumor tissue (as well as normal tissue) and is useful in areas not accessible to surgery. Irradiation of tissues around the area of tumor infiltration, in conjunction with surgical excision of the tumor, may kill residual cells and prevent metastasis. Irradiation of enlarged lymph nodes in lymphomas may destroy trapped cells and result in shrinkage of lymphoid tissues. In acute leukemias, the central nervous system (CNS) is often irradiated in conjunction with chemotherapy. Most anticancer drugs do not enter the CNS to any great extent and are ineffective against leukemic cells retained within the CNS. Irradiation of the CNS, therefore, destroys a pool of cells not accessible to chemotherapy.

Chemotherapy

Chemotherapy is useful as an adjunct to surgery to destroy residual cells and is the major form of treatment for leukemias, late-stage lymphomas, and widespread metastatic cancer. In addition, chemotherapy is useful for certain solid tumors having such a rapid rate of growth that they are inoperable at the time of diagnosis (e.g., oat cell carcinoma of the lung).

There are several important considerations regarding the use of drugs for cancer treatment. Unlike bacterial infections, cancer often evokes little immune response. That is, drugs receive little help from the body in the eradication of abnormal cells. In a bacterial infection, if the bacterial count is greatly reduced by drug therapy, body defenses can eliminate the remaining organisms and cure the infection. With cancer, it is necessary to kill virtually every cell with the chemotherapy, a goal that may be impossible to reach without also killing the host as a result of drug toxicity. Resistance develops with chemotherapy of cancer, as it does with the chemotherapy of infection, and the new wave of cells proliferates in spite of repeated administration of formerly effective drugs. Additional drugs must then be tried, and eventually all are ineffective.

Combination chemotherapy helps to prevent resistance, since it employs several drugs acting by different mechanisms on various phases of the cycle of the malignant cells. It is much more difficult for resistance to develop in this case and more cells are killed. Combination chemotherapy has led to vastly improved survival times for Hodgkin's disease and acute leukemia within the last 20 years.

Another principle of cancer chemotherapy is that drugs are generally more effective against rapidly growing than slowly growing tumors. Thus leukemias and lymphomas, characterized by rapid cell proliferation, are better controlled with drugs than are slowly growing tumors of the lung or prostate. The difference in growth rate between normal and malignant cells usually allows for greater "leverage" to be applied to the malignant cells. That is, the malignant cells incorporate the drug more quickly and are damaged more than the slowly growing normal cells. Normal body cells that have an inherently rapid growth rate or have a high replacement ("turnover") rate are damaged more by chemotherapy than are slowly growing normal cells. Therefore, chemotherapy often causes bone marrow depression (pancytopenia), loss of hair (alopecia), and sloughing of gastrointestinal mucosal tissue. These fast-turnover tissues are affected more than slow-turnover tissues, such as bone or cartilage.

BREAST CANCER

Cancer of the breast is the leading cause (20 per cent) of cancer deaths in women in the United States and is the most common cause of death from all causes in women 40 to 44 years of age. The incidence of breast cancer is approximately 1 in 11, and the mortality rate of those afflicted is about 1 in 3. Thus, one in 30 to 35 women will die from breast cancer. The average age of those with the disease is 60 years. If cancer develops in one breast, there is a tenfold increase in the risk of a new tumor (not metastasis) in the other breast. The factors promoting cancer in one breast act similarly on the other breast. Males also develop breast cancer, but the incidence is only 1 per cent of that in females. Interestingly, males who have had sex change operations and received estrogens as a part of the conversion treatment become much more vulnerable than before.

Pathogenesis

A large number of factors influence the occurrence of breast cancer, but their exact roles are generally unclear (Table 21–2). The chance of developing the disease increases two to three times if the mother or a sister of the individual has had breast cancer. If two or

Table 21–2. KNOWN RISK FACTORS IN BREAST CANCER

Breast cancer in mother or sister
Never married
No children
Early onset of menstruation
Late menopause
Endometrial cancer
Cystic breast disease
Obesity

more close relatives have had breast cancer, the risk is even greater. Unmarried women and those who have never had children have a slightly greater risk of developing the disease. Early onset of menstruation (before age 12) and late menopause (after age 50) also increase the risk of breast cancer. It appears from these findings that there is some hereditary tendency toward the disease and that the action of female hormones may exert some influence on its development.

Women who have had uterine (endometrial, not cervical) cancer have an increased risk of breast cancer. Those with cystic breast disease (mammary dysplasia) or obesity also develop the disease more often than normal individuals without these conditions. Estrogen administration, in the form of replacement during or after the menopause or in oral contraceptives, does not clearly increase the risk of breast cancer. However, the long-term effects of such drugs are not known, and it is possible that they might be harmful after 10 or more years of continuous use, particularly if used in the postmenopausal patient.

Symptoms and Signs In the vast majority of cases, the breast cancer victim detects the disease herself, usually by noting a painless lump. Other common symptoms include retraction of the skin over the lesion, change in the nipple area (puckering, retraction), erosion or itching of surface tissue, redness, and edema. Often the surface contour of the breast changes and the change is apparent when looking in a mirror. Self-examination should be done after menstruation ceases for the month, at a time when estrogen and progesterone levels are at a low point. This avoids confusion of cystic breast nodules, induced by increased hormone activity during the premenstrual period, with *bona fide* tumors.

In more advanced cases, enlarged axillary lymph nodes are seen, indicating that tumor cells have infiltrated the regional nodes. Unfortunately, this is commonly seen, since the breast area is richly supplied with lymphatics. In late-stage breast cancer, symptoms of bone involvement (pain), liver metastases (jaundice), or lung infiltration (pulmonary effusion) are often seen.

Laboratory Findings Routine laboratory tests are normal in early-stage breast cancer. In metastatic disease, the erythrocyte sedimentation rate (ESR) may be increased and the serum alkaline phosphatase level is often elevated (normal = 30 to 85 IU/ml), reflecting liver and/or bone involvement. Likewise, hypercalcemia occurs if there is excessive bone destruction. Bone metastases may be detected with scans using radioactive technetium, strontium, or fluorine, all of which are preferentially absorbed into bone tissue. Liver scans, using isotopes or ultrasound, can detect metastatic lesions as well.

Mammography and *thermography* are both used to detect breast cancer. Mammography, which is considered the more sensitive of the two tests, is a specialized x-ray of the breast (Fig. 21–2). Tumor tissue has a different density than the surrounding normal tissue, and this is detectable on x-ray examination. Thermography is based upon the difference in heat production between normal and malignant tissue. Malignant tissue is metabolically more active and gen-

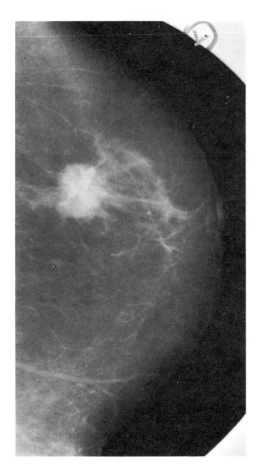

Figure 21–2. Mammogram showing breast cancer. (From Griffiths, H. T., and Sarno, R. C.: *Contemporary Radiology: An Introduction to Imaging.* Philadelphia, W. B. Saunders Company, 1979.)

erates more heat than normal tissue. Thermography does not expose the patient to radiation (which itself can cause breast cancer) and is a good screening technique if backed up by mammography.

Biopsy, via needle or surgical excision, gives definitive proof of the existence of breast cancer. Needle biopsy can be performed in the doctor's office, but it is less accurate than surgical biopsy.

Diagnosis

Not all breast lumps are malignant, and the finding of a benign breast lesion is sometimes the happy ending to an otherwise tragic story. Cystic breast disease is often confused with breast cancer but waxes and wanes in response to hormonal stimulation (see *Symptoms and Signs*). Fibroadenoma of the breast is a common benign tumor, as is intraductal papilloma. These lesions can be excised with no long-term risk to the patient. Biopsy gives the final answer in the differentiation of breast lumps.

Treatment

After staging the tumor, the choice of treatments can be made.

Surgery. Surgery is the treatment of choice, where possible. Several levels of surgery can be performed, depending upon the classification of the tumor.

1. *Local excision* (lumpectomy) is restricted to a highly selected group of patients with a localized tumor of very limited invasive

potential. Unfortunately, most breast cancers do not fall into this category.

2. *Simple mastectomy* (removal of only the breast) is useful if the lesion is confined to the breast with no spread to regional tissues. This is often difficult to determine.

3. *Modified radical mastectomy* is currently the most widely used procedure for unselected cases of breast cancer. This includes removal of the breast, regional lymph nodes, and nearby muscle and connective tissue, with preservation of the pectoralis major muscle.

4. *Standard radical mastectomy* is similar to the modified procedure but also includes removal of the pectoralis major muscle. This produces a sunken area beneath the clavicle (collar bone) and is much more disfiguring than the modified procedure. While this operation has been performed most frequently in the past, there is evidence that the modified operation is equally curative for most types of breast cancer.

Radiotherapy. Radiation therapy is used in several ways in the treatment of breast cancer. It is occasionally the only treatment modality in some early-stage breast lesions but is more commonly used an adjunct to surgery. Preoperative radiation treatment destroys tumor cells that have spread into regional tissues. Postoperative radiotherapy destroys cells that have spread from the primary site or been disseminated as a result of surgical manipulation of the tissue. In late-stage breast cancer, radiotherapy is used to treat bone lesions and enlarged lymph nodes caused by metastatic tumor deposits.

Chemotherapy. Chemotherapy of breast cancer has many facets. In addition to standard anticancer agents, a wide variety of hormones and hormone antagonists are also employed.

Estrogen. Breast tumors containing estrogen receptors are usually responsive to hormonal manipulation. It is important that breast tumor tissue be assayed for estrogen receptors to determine the suitability of hormone treatment. Estrogens, such as estradiol (Aquadiol), are used in postmenopausal women with advanced breast cancer and cause tumor regression in about 65 per cent of those with a positive estrogen receptor assay. Estrogens should not be given to premenopausal women or to those in or recently through the menopause, as this generally increases tumor growth in these cases.

Antiestrogens. Antiestrogens, such as tamoxiphen (Novaldex), are useful in premenopausal women, since they reduce the stimulating effect of endogenous estrogens on the tumor.

Androgens. Androgens, such as calusterone (Methosarb) or testolactone (Teslac), are useful in both premenopausal and postmenopausal breast cancer patients to induce regression of metastatic bone lesions. In addition, androgens may cause tumor regression in premenopausal women.

Corticosteroids. Corticosteroids, such as prednisone, are used occasionally in breast cancer treatment. These reduce inflammation associated with tumor invasion and increase appetite and the sense of well-being. Reduced inflammation often decreases bone pain associated with advanced cancer, but these drugs cause little tumor regression.

Combinations. A variety of specific anticancer drugs have been employed for breast cancer treatment, usually in advanced cases. The combination of doxorubicin (Adriamycin) and cyclophosphamide (Cytoxan) is currently the most effective. Limited studies, using cyclophosphamide, methotrexate, and fluorouracil (CMF) as a postsurgical treatment in premenopausal women with no obvious distant metastases, have shown beneficial results. This treatment apparently destroys metastatic cells undetected at the time of surgery.

Complications

Metastasis from the primary breast lesion is the most important complication to breast cancer. The bones and liver are common metastatic sites. Often, metastatic seeds are spread by the time the disease is diagnosed, even though no obvious lesions are present. As mentioned, scans of the bones and liver help to detect metastatic deposits in these areas. Metastasis or direct spread of the breast lesion into the pleural cavity is also common, leading to pleural effusion. Pleural fluid can be drained by means of thoracentesis and anticancer drugs can be applied directly to the involved area.

Hypercalcemia, caused by bone destruction with leakage of calcium into the blood stream, is often seen in late-stage breast cancer. Nausea, vomiting, and the possibility of renal stones result. This complication can be partly corrected with the use of a low-calcium diet (avoidance of dairy products and spinach) and a large fluid intake, which maintains solution of calcium in the urine.

Lymphedema (swelling of the arm on the affected side) often results following surgery or radiotherapy for breast cancer because these treatments destroy regional axillary lymph channels and interfere with drainage from the arm. Some lymphedema may be unavoidable, but it can be minimized by using care in surgery and by irradiating only necessary areas. The swollen arm often normalizes with time and can be improved with the use of an elastic bandage and diuretic drugs.

Prognosis

The 5-year survival rate in breast cancer with no apparent spread beyond the breast is approximately 80 per cent. If there are infiltrated axillary lymph nodes at the time of diagnosis, the 5-year survival rate is about 50 per cent. The chance of cure depends largely upon the exact location of the tumor, degree of malignancy, and presence or absence of obvious lymph node involvement.

Even with no apparent spread beyond the primary tumor, metastasis often develops (in 25 per cent of the patients), making cure difficult if not impossible. Early diagnosis and appropriate treatment offer the greatest hope of cure.

LUNG CANCER

Cancer of the lung and accessory structures is the leading cause (30 to 35 per cent) of cancer death in men in the United States and the second leading cause in women. The same is true in most other industrialized nations. Lung cancer has grown from a rare disease to one that affects more than 100,000 previously healthy individuals each year. The late Dr. Alton Ochsner, a pioneer in the study of lung cancer, wrote of seeing a case of lung cancer as a young medical resident in the late 1920s. He was told to observe it carefully, since he would likely never see another!

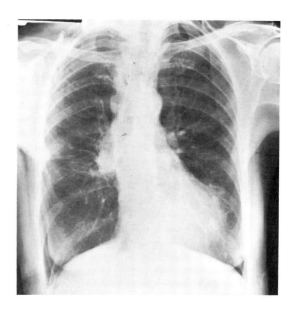

Figure 21–3. Bronchogenic carcinoma. (From Griffiths, H. T., and Sarno, R. C.: *Contemporary Radiology: An Introduction to Imaging.* Philadelphia, W. B. Saunders Company, 1979.)

Types of Lung Cancer

The common type of lung cancer (90 per cent of cases) is called *bronchogenic carcinoma* (Fig. 21–3), since it originates in the bronchial mucosa. It usually affects males over age 40 who are heavy smokers and is most often a squamous cell carcinoma.

A much less common type of lung cancer (5 per cent of cases) occurs equally in males and females over 40 and and consists of multiple lesions, often bilateral, in the alveoli and bronchioles. This type, called *bronchiolar carcinoma* (Fig. 21–4), tends to grow more slowly and metastasizes later than the bronchogenic type.

Bronchial carcinoid (formerly called bronchial adenoma) is an intermediate tumor that represents about 5 per cent of the cases. It is generally benign but metastasizes in about 10 per cent of the cases, thus warranting the term "carcinoid" rather than "adenoma."

Figure 21–4. Bronchiolar carcinoma. (From Griffiths, H. T., and Sarno, R. C.: *Contemporary Radiology: An Introduction to Imaging.* Philadelphia, W. B. Saunders Company, 1979.)

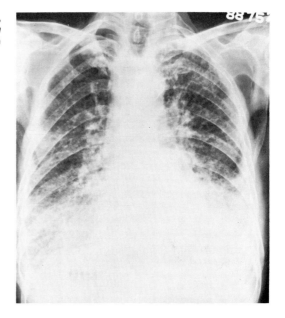

It also has equal incidence in men and women and is most commonly seen in those over 40.

Among the bronchogenic carcinomas, *oat cell carcinoma*, a small cell anaplastic tumor, is an extremely rapidly growing lesion. It is often inoperable at the time of diagnosis but can be treated with chemotherapy and/or radiotherapy.

Pathogenesis

There is no question that inhaling tobacco smoke is the major cause of lung cancer. Countless studies have proven this beyond any doubt. The Report of the Surgeon General in 1964 and again in 1978 extensively documented tobacco smoke as the leading cause of lung cancer, as well as a major cause of cancer of the oral cavity, pharynx, larynx, esophagus, and bladder. Pack-a-day smokers have a tenfold increased risk of lung cancer and heavy smokers (two or more packs a day) have a 20-fold increased risk, compared with nonsmokers. Those who have stopped smoking for 10 years or more revert to nonsmoker statistics. Thus, it is nearly always advantageous to stop smoking, even after a long time, if cancer has not yet developed.

Although more than 1200 promoters or inducers of cancer have been found in tobacco smoke, it is not clear which of these cause human lung cancer. Therefore, removal of substances from tobacco, if possible, is not currently practical. The use of filtered cigarettes probably reduces the risk of lung cancer by 25 per cent over that of nonfiltered cigarettes, presumably because the filter traps some tobacco carcinogens.

While smoking is the major cause of lung cancer, other etiologic factors are important as single influences or in conjunction with smoking. Air pollution or industrial exposure to asbestos, uranium, nickel, arsenic, and even coal significantly increases the risk of the disease. If lung tissue is scarred, as is the case with healed wounds, tuberculous lesions, or retained shrapnel, cancer is more likely to develop in those areas (scar cancer) than in normal tissues. The risk of lung cancer increases drastically if two or more factors are operating. Thus, nonsmoking uranium miners have a lung cancer rate four times that of the general population (smokers and non-smokers) and the incidence increases to ten times in uranium miners who smoke.

Extensive studies by Dr. Oscar Auerbach and others in the 1950s and 1960s have shown that there is a series of histologic steps in the development of lung cancer. First, there is loss of bronchial cilia (squamous metaplasia), then hyperplasia of the basal epithelial tissue of the bronchial lining, then abnormalities in the nuclei of affected cells. Finally, local cancer (carcinoma *in situ*) develops and spread follows. If the stimulus for cancer development is stopped before cancer develops, the changes are usually reversible and the tissue may revert completely to normal in several years. This supports the clinical findings that the 10-year *ex-smoker* approaches the *nonsmoker's* risk for lung cancer.

Symptoms and Signs

Cough, wheezing, and hemoptysis (expectoration of blood) are the chief symptoms of lung cancer. Often, symptoms are absent until the disease is well established or are attributed to the effects of smoking ("cigarette cough"). Persistent or repeated chest infections are sometimes a clue to the presence of a lung tumor and the resulting loss of respiratory tract resistance and self-cleaning ability. Chest pain is not common, but it can result from metastatic lesions in the chest wall, ribs, or spine. Local effects of tumor growth include bronchial obstruction and lung collapse (atelectasis). Some tumors, especially oat cell carcinomas, often secrete antidiuretic hormone (ADH), or occasionally adenocorticotropic hormone (ACTH), leading to edema formation. Clubbing of the fingers is often seen with lung tumors but is poorly understood as to cause.

Because lung cancer often metastasizes prior to diagnosis, symptoms of secondary involvement of other body organs may be seen. A common finding is neurologic symptoms (headache, seizure, paralysis), caused by a brain tumor secondary to the lung tumor. Symptomatology referable to the liver or kidney is also occasionally seen.

Laboratory Findings   Routine laboratory tests are not generally helpful in lung cancer diagnosis. Chest x-ray studies detect larger tumors and may discover small, asymptomatic ("coin") lesions. The annual chest x-ray examination, long recommended by the American Cancer Society, is no longer recommended, except in high-risk individuals. The relative benefit of annual chest roentgenograms in nonsmokers, compared with the risk from the x-ray exposure, is small. Heavy smokers or those in occupational contact with respiratory carcinogens benefit considerably more, especially because lesions are often detected at an earlier stage than without routine x-ray examination.

Since most malignant lung tumors are bronchogenic (i.e., occur in the bronchial mucosa), it is possible to detect malignant cells in the sputum or by means of bronchoscopy. Peripherally located tumors can be examined using needle biopsy. *Mediastinoscopy* (observation and biopsy of the mediastinal area) is useful for centrally located tumors or those having mediastinal node involvement. Direct biopsy using a chest incision (thoracotomy) is the most definitive method in doubtful cases.

Diagnosis   Emphysema (see Chapter 14), lung infections, and benign lung tumors are the conditions most often confused with lung cancer. The symptoms of cough, wheezing, repeated chest infection, and atelectasis are frequently seen in emphysema. In addition, the victim is usually a heavy smoker and/or has been exposed to industrial or environmental pollution. Tuberculosis or fungal lung infections, such as histoplasmosis (see Chapter 9), often produce x-ray findings identical to those of lung cancer. However, the lesions are usually calcified and this can be detected using special tomographic techniques. Benign lung tumors (e.g., bronchial "adenoma") are not always entirely benign. They may yield x-ray findings similar to those of carcinomas and can produce local invasion, and even metastasis, in some cases. The differential diagnosis of all these conditions is based upon x-ray findings—often with the use of a CAT scan—and biopsy or sputum examination. With lung infections, culture of the pathogen is often possible and skin tests (e.g., the Mantoux test) frequently aid in diagnosis.

Treatment

Surgery. Several modes of treatment are beneficial. Surgery is the primary treatment for lung cancer, when possible, and offers the greatest hope for cure. For isolated carcinoid lesions, local excision is often satisfactory, since most do not metastasize. Bronchiolar carcinomas and bronchogenic carcinomas metastasize more readily and require more extensive surgical treatment, including wide excision and removal of regional lymph nodes. Many malignant lung tumors are inoperable at the time of diagnosis. The remaining lung tissue may not support life because of extensive emphysema. There may be bilateral tumor involvement or there may be evidence of metastasis.

Radiotherapy and Chemotherapy. Palliative chemotherapy or radiotherapy is somewhat helpful in inoperable cases. The most useful drug combination currently employed is cyclophosphamide (Cytoxan), doxorubicin (Adriamycin), methotrexate, and lomustine (CCNU). Fast-growing tumors, such as oat cell carcinomas, are most successfully treated by combining chemotherapy and radiotherapy.

Prevention. Most cases of lung cancer can be prevented. If smoking were stopped completely today, the disease would again become rare in 25 to 30 years. Our efforts to clean up the environmental atmosphere and to reduce occupational exposure to airborne carcinogens have been an additional help in the prevention of lung cancer.

Complications and Prognosis

The overall 5-year survival rate for those with bronchogenic carcinoma is 8 per cent. In those who have had surgical removal of the tumor with no evidence of metastasis or regional spread, the 5-year survival rate increases to 25 to 35 per cent. The most common complications are metastatic brain tumor, respiratory obstruction, and liver and kidney metastases. It is unlikely that detection or treatment methods will improve dramatically in the near future. The greatest hope lies in prevention, i.e., encouraging smokers to quit, discouraging nonsmokers from starting, and working to further reduce atmospheric and industrial pollution.

COLORECTAL CANCER

Cancer of the colon and rectum is the second leading cause of cancer death in males in the United States and the third in females, causing approximately 50,000 deaths per year. Tumors are found with equal frequency in men and women in all areas of the lower intestinal tract, with the exception of lesions confined to the rectal area, which affect males twice as often as females. The onset of colorectal cancer is generally after age 50, and the disease is slightly more common among blacks than whites and among urban rather than rural dwellers. In general, the disease is more prevalent in highly developed areas (North America, Europe) and lowest in incidence in Third World areas of Asia and Africa. The exception is Japan, with both a highly developed society and a low incidence of the condition. The majority of colorectal cancers occur in the sigmoid colon and rectum; 60 per cent of them are visible by sigmoidoscopy, and 10 per cent can be felt directly by rectal examination.

Pathogenesis   Two theories exist as to the method of development of colorectal cancer. One is that malignant tumors arise in previously existing polyps and that further change in the polyp gives rise to a tumor. Evidence for this is that malignant changes can often be seen in those with certain types of polyps who are followed for 5 to 10 years. The other line of thought is that polyps are already at an early stage of malignancy and therefore do not change into malignant tumors later on. In either case, with enough time, some polyps will become clearly malignant.

Those with multiple colonic polyps (familial polyposis coli) are much more prone to colon cancer than normal individuals. Long-standing ulcerative colitis (more than 10 years) and chronic granulomatous infection of the lower digestive tract are also risk factors for disease development.

Diet has also been strongly implicated in the development of colorectal cancer and other digestive conditions, such as diverticulitis (see Chapter 12). In theory, a diet containing a large amount of bulk would promote increased water absorption and a faster stool transit time, thus reducing contact of the bowel wall with carcinogens from the diet. Specifically, the fat content of food may be related to the development of colorectal cancer. A high-fat diet promotes secretion of a large amount of bile acid for fat digestion. Bile acid is acted upon by organisms within the intestinal tract to form several compounds known to be carcinogenic in animals. Thus, a high-fat diet would promote increased exposure to carcinogens. If meat is eaten to the exclusion of bulky foods, this would also provide greater contact of these compounds with the intestinal mucosa.

Symptoms and Signs   Most people with colorectal cancer have a change in bowel habits, yielding constipation, diarrhea, or more subtle alterations in frequency of bowel movements or stool consistency. These symptoms are attributed to obstruction or irritation caused by the lesion. Bleeding is common, since most lesions are on or near the surface of the bowel, and this results in occult fecal blood, obvious blood in the feces, or frank rectal bleeding. Anemia is a common result of the loss of blood. Weight loss is frequently seen in colorectal cancer, as is the case with most other malignancies. This can be attributed to decreased appetite, the nutritional requirements of the tumor, and other poorly understood mechanisms. Many lesions are palpable, either as abdominal masses or by rectal examination.

Laboratory Findings   In addition to iron deficiency caused by bleeding, most patients with colorectal cancer show a positive test for occult fecal blood (using Occultest, for example). The lesion is detectable with barium x-ray studies of the lower intestinal tract and with sigmoidoscopy or colonoscopy. Some authorities recommend annual sigmoidoscopy for all persons over 40 and especially for those with conditions predisposing them to colorectal cancer. Biopsy is possible prior to surgery with most lesions. Carcinoembryonic antigen is found in the serum of most individuals with colorectal cancer as well as in those with other malignancies. However, the usefulness of CEA assay is primarily in determining the effectiveness of treatment, rather than in initial diagnosis of the condition. It disappears from the serum when all tumor cells are destroyed.

Diagnosis   Obstruction of the colorectal area, diverticulitis, ulcerative colitis, and functional disorders of the colon may produce symptoms easily confused with those of rectal cancer. Generally, these conditions can be differentiated from colorectal cancer with the use of sigmoidoscopy or colonoscopy and barium x-ray films of the lower digestive tract.

Treatment   **Surgery.** This is the only curative treatment for colorectal cancer. Resection of the tumor with anastomosis of the bowel ends or with externalization of the colon (colostomy) is used, the choice between the two depending upon the location of the tumor and the amount of intestine involved. Regional lymph nodes are also removed during surgery and examined for tumor cells. Even in advanced cases, surgery is often necessary to relieve bleeding or obstruction, although it may offer only palliative treatment for the primary malignancy.

Radiotherapy and Chemotherapy. These are adjunctive treatments and may kill cells remaining after surgery or those already spread from the primary site. In addition, radiotherapy is employed prior to surgery as it is in breast cancer to destroy cells in the vicinity of the tumor. The current chemotherapy of choice is a combination of fluorouracil and semustine (Methyl CCNU).

Complications and Prognosis   Metastatic colorectal cancer frequently invades the liver, lungs, and bones. These areas can be examined with x-ray or scan techniques to determine the presence of tumor deposits. If there is widespread metastasis, chemotherapy is the treatment of choice. Local bowel obstruction or symptoms related to local spread of the tumor are frequently seen. These cases can often receive benefit from surgery.

Follow-up examination is extremely important after treatment for colorectal cancer. Routine barium x-ray studies and sigmoidoscopy should be performed at least annually to ensure that there is no recurrence of the disease.

The 5-year survival rate in surgically treated cases of colorectal cancer is about 50 per cent. If there is no lymphatic or regional vascular involvement, the 5-year survival rate is 60 to 70 per cent. The greatly increased 5-year survival rate in colorectal cancer, compared with that of lung cancer, lies primarily in earlier onset of symptoms and the greater accessibility of the lesion for biopsy with the former condition. Perhaps we can further reduce our chance of developing colorectal cancer by following a diet that emphasizes reduced fat intake and increased intake of bulky vegetables, grains, and fruit.

LEUKEMIA   Leukemia is the seventh leading cause of cancer death in the United States and the most common cause of cancer death in children under 15. The overall incidence is about 1 per 10,000 population.

The disease favors males over females in all forms, but with some types the difference in incidence is relatively slight. All ethnic groups are affected equally, with the exception that Orientals almost never develop one form, chronic lymphocytic leukemia.

The term "leukemia" means "white blood" and was used by Virchow to describe the extremely high leukocyte count seen in most cases. It is now known that there are cases of leukemia in which the white blood cell count is normal or abnormally low, as well. This is called *aleukemic leukemia* or *subleukemia.* The key features of the leukocytes in leukemia is that they are abnormal and immature, lacking the functional ability of the mature white cells. The abnormal leukocytes replace normal bone marrow cells and infiltrate the liver, spleen, and lymph nodes throughout the body. Replacement of normal bone marrow with leukemic cells leads to impaired formation of erythrocytes and thrombocytes, as well as normal leukocytes. The major characteristics of leukemias as a group are, therefore (1) infiltration of immature cells into the circulating blood, (2) anemia, and (3) thrombocytopenia. Leukemias generally cause death as a result of *infection,* because of impaired leukocyte formation, or *hemorrhage,* because of reduced platelet function.

Pathogenesis   Although the exact cause of leukemia is unknown, there are known predisposing factors in its development. Chronic, low-level exposure to radiation is associated with an increased risk of leukemia. Radiologists, x-ray technicians, and others who receive small, daily doses of radiation have approximately twice the risk of developing the disease. Massive exposure to radiation, as seen in survivors of atomic blasts, also increases the risk of leukemia but is more likely to completely destroy bone marrow activity (aplastic anemia). Exposure to benzene increases the chance of developing leukemia as well as aplastic anemia. Certain genetic disorders also increase the risk of leukemia. Down's syndrome is associated with a 20-fold increased chance of developing leukemia. Bloom's syndrome, associated with excessive chromosome breakage, increases the risk of leukemia. Identical twins show concordance for leukemia; that is, if one develops it, the other has a greatly increased risk. Within certain families, the incidence of leukemia is unusually high, suggesting a genetic factor that increases susceptibility. A viral etiology for leukemia is suspected in some cases, since a number of primates as well as other animals develop leukemia after viral infection. However, this association has not been proven in humans.

These factors appear to share the commonality of causing a loss of control over normal leukocyte development, resulting in failure of the cells to mature. Studies have shown an abnormally long life of leukocytes in most types of leukemia, indicating that immature cells are accumulating, rather than continuing their maturation and dying after a normal life span. Whereas the life span of a normal lymphocyte is about 100 days, the figure is extended to 200 to 500 days in chronic lymphocytic leukemia. It appears that a genetic defect occurs in some leukemic cells, leading to loss of cell control. In chronic myelocytic leukemia, a characteristic chromosome alteration (Philadelphia chromosome) is usually seen.

Table 21–3. COMMON TYPES OF LEUKEMIA

Type	Age Group
Acute lymphoblastic leukemia (ALL)	Under 15
Acute myeloblastic leukemia (AML)	Over 15
Chronic myelocytic leukemia (CML)	Over 30
Chronic lymphocytic leukemia (CLL)	Over 50

Common Types of Leukemia

There are four common types of leukemia (Table 21–3). Two are classified as *acute* and two are *chronic* diseases. "Acute" refers to the sudden, dramatic onset of the disease and the rapid downhill course without treatment. Chronic leukemias have an insidious onset and a much slower course without treatment.

The conditions are further classified according to the type of abnormal cell produced: lymphocyte, monocyte, or other cell form. In acute leukemias, the abnormal cell is in a primitive (blast) form; in chronic leukemias, the cell represents a later stage of development (although still abnormal). Acute lymphoblastic leukemia (ALL) is primarily a childhood disease; acute myeloblastic leukemia (AML) usually affects adults. Chronic lymphocytic leukemia (CLL) and chronic myelocytic leukemia (CML) are both adult diseases, with CLL occurring especially in the elderly and CML primarily in young adults. These generalizations are not absolute, and it is possible for any person to develop any type of leukemia.

Current Treatment of the Common Leukemias

Since leukemias represent a proliferation of abnormal cells into many body areas rather than a condition involving localized tumors, surgery is not feasible. Chemotherapy and radiotherapy are the treatments of choice.

Chemotherapy. Chemotherapy differs somewhat between acute and chronic leukemias. With *acute* leukemias, the aim is to destroy as many leukemic cells as possible, ideally to produce complete remission of the disease. Combination chemotherapy is widely used, since this gives the best chance of destroying all leukemic cells. In *chronic* leukemias, the aim is to control the disease but not necessarily to destroy all leukemic cells. Since cell proliferation is occurring at a lower rate in chronic leukemias than in acute leukemias, it is not usually possible to destroy all leukemic cells without reaching a level of toxicity with chemotherapy that is dangerous or even lethal to the host. Accordingly, single-drug therapy is commonly employed. The drugs currently used in the chemotherapy of the common types of leukemia are outlined in Table 21–4. Bear in mind that techniques of chemotherapy change frequently, as better drugs are discovered or improved methods of administration are developed as a result of clinical experience.

Radiotherapy. Radiotherapy is used in several ways in the treatment of leukemia. Irradiaton of enlarged lymph nodes containing leukemic cells results in cell destruction and shrinkage of the involved tissue. Irradiation of the spleen bombards large numbers of trapped cells and results in massive cell death and reduction in size of the spleen. X-ray treatment of the brain and spinal cord area destroys cells that are retained there and are protected from the

Table 21–4. CURRENT CHEMOTHERAPY OF THE COMMON LEUKEMIAS

Type	Drugs Used
Acute lymphoblastic leukemia (ALL)	Vincristine (Oncovin) plus prednisone *for induction of remission,* mercaptopurine (Purinethol), methotrexate, or cyclophosphamide (Cytoxan) *for maintenance*
Acute myeloblastic leukemia (AML)	Doxorubicin (Adriamycin) plus cytarabine (Cytosar) *for induction of remission,* doxorubicin, cytarabine, thioguanine, or daunorubicin (Cerubidine) *for maintenance*
Chronic myelocytic leukemia (CML)	Busulfan (Myleran) or melphalan (Alkeran) *for control*
Chronic lymphocytic leukemia (CLL)	Chlorambucil (Leukeran), cyclophosphamide (Cytoxan), or prednisone *for control*

effects of chemotherapy. This greatly increases the effectiveness of chemotherapy. Whole body x-ray or isotope treatment (with ^{32}P) is used in CML and CLL to depress bone marrow activity and to reduce leukocyte count.

Adjunctive Drugs. A variety of adjunctive drugs are used in leukemia treatment. Corticosteroids, such as prednisone, are used to depress lymphocyte production in both ALL and CLL. Allopurinol (Zyloprim) blocks the formation of uric acid (see Chapter 17) and is useful in the adjunctive treatment of acute leukemias. With the massive cell destruction that accompanies chemotherapy and/or radiotherapy, purine compounds are released from the damaged cells and enter the uric acid pathway, leading to hyperuricemia. Allopurinol prevents hyperuricemia and its complications in the leukemia patient. A wide assortment of anti-infective drugs are employed for leukemia patients, since infection is a very common complication to the disease. Infection results from both the condition itself and its treatment, which compromise the normal immune response. Antibacterial, antifungal, antiviral, and antiparasitic drugs are used frequently in these immunosuppressed patients.

Other Forms of Treatment. Blood transfusions are given to correct the anemia associated with leukemia, and platelet transfusions are used to reverse the thrombocytopenia characteristic of the disease. Bone marrow transplants are now successfully performed for acute leukemias, as they are for aplastic anemia. The leukemic bone marrow must be completely destroyed and the donor marrow grafted in its place for effective results. Some patients are completely cured of leukemia by this treatment, although it is technically difficult.

Acute Lymphoblastic Leukemia

The peak incidence of ALL is in the first 5 years of life, and the disease is relatively common below age 15. The major symptoms are weakness, malaise, fever, and loss of appetite. Often, gingival bleeding, petechial hemorrhages, pallor, and bone pain are seen. The sternum is especially tender to the touch. Bone pain results from leukemic infiltration into solid bone tissue, whereas bleeding tendencies result from thrombocytopenia. Physical examination reveals hepatosplenomegaly and lymphadenopathy.

Laboratory Findings   The laboratory findings in ALL include anemia, thrombocytopenia and the presence of lymphoblasts in the circulating blood. Leukocytosis, leukopenia, or a normal leukocyte count may be seen, depending upon the case. Bone marrow examination reveals large numbers of lymphoblasts, with a corresponding decrease in the population of other cells. X-ray or bone scan often shows bone lesions and associated decalcification (osteoporosis).

Diagnosis   Acute lymphoblastic leukemia can be confused with aplastic anemia, especially if the leukocyte count is low. Mononucleosis or other infections causing a "leukemoid" reaction may also superficially resemble ALL. However, there is no thrombocytopenia or anemia with leukemoid reaction. Metastatic spread from a solid tumor into the bones, liver, and spleen can mimic leukemia closely in terms of symptoms and laboratory findings. Bone marrow biopsy, plus a search for the primary location of cancer, usually permits accurate diagnosis.

Treatment   The drugs most commonly used for ALL are outlined in Table 21–4. Generally, a combination of drugs is used to induce a remission, then single-drug therapy is used for maintenance of the remission state. In addition, irradiation of the CNS is used adjunctively to destroy trapped cells, as previously mentioned.

Complications and Prognosis   As with other leukemias, the major complications of ALL are hemorrhage, especially involving the gastrointestinal tract and brain, and infection resulting from impaired immune response. The outlook is generally positive, however, since in over 90 per cent of those under 20 years of age, remission can be induced with combination chemotherapy and CNS irradiation. Approximately a third of the patients on intensive therapy appear to be cured.

Acute Myeloblastic Leukemia   Acute myeloblastic leukemia is quite similar to ALL in symptoms and signs, laboratory findings, and complications. However, the treatment and prognosis are quite different and the condition is usually seen in adults rather than children. The aberrant cell in this case is a myeloblast, the precursor of the myelocyte, the cell that eventually matures to form a granulocyte. Differentiation between ALL and AML on the basis of blood smear is difficult, since myeloblasts and lymphoblasts are similar in appearance, but peroxidase-staining granules are found in AML and not ALL. This difference permits a distinction to be made between the two conditions.

Treatment   Drug therapy of AML emphasizes combination chemotherapy (Table 21–4) in conjunction with CNS irradiation to induce remission, but the specific anticancer agents employed are different than with ALL. There is currently a controversy as to whether repeated cycles of high-dose chemotherapy or low-dose maintenance therapy is best in the long run. High-dose cycling of chemotherapy causes more destruction of leukemic cells but also destroys a larger number of normal cells than does low-dose maintenance therapy.

Prognosis   The outlook in AML is not as optimistic as in ALL. About 50 per cent of the patients with AML are brought into remission with intensive therapy, but remission periods average 1 year or less. Cures are rare, and the duration of survival is usually only 1 to 2 years.

Chronic Myelocytic Leukemia   Chronic myelocytic leukemia is primarily a disease of young adults. The symptoms and signs are similar to those of the other leukemias, but develop slowly, often requiring months to years before the disease is clinically apparent. Many cases are discovered accidentally, during a routine physical examination, in an asymptomatic individual. The high leukocyte count (often over 500,000/mm^3), plus the usual hepatosplenomegaly, are a tipoff.

The characteristic cell found in CML is an abnormal myelocyte. Leukemic myelocytes carry the Philadelphia chromosome in about 90 per cent of the cases and are deficient in alkaline phosphatase. The bone marrow shows replacement of normal cells with leukemic myelocytes and granulocytes (the next step in myelocyte maturation). Anemia and thrombocytopenia are also seen, as with the other leukemias.

Diagnosis   Leukemoid reaction resulting from infection is occasionally confused with CML, but more accurately mimics acute leukemias. Myelofibrosis (replacement of bone marrow tissue with fibrous tissue) causes leukocytosis and splenomegaly, but Philadelphia chromosome is absent and alkaline phosphatase content of the leukocyte is normal.

Treatment   X-ray or ^{32}P therapy and chemotherapy are used (Table 21–4). Since the goal is long-term control rather than cure, single-drug therapy is usually employed. Treatment is not necessary until the white blood cell count reaches a certain point or symptoms become bothersome. Overtreatment encourages general bone marrow depression and rapid development of resistant cells.

Complications and Prognosis   In addition to the usual complications of hemorrhage and infection seen with other leukemias, about half of CML patients eventually experience a "blastic crisis," usually several years after onset of their disease. This is a reversion to a more acute form of leukemia, with rapid proliferation of blast forms rather than more mature leukemic cells. Blastic crisis is almost always fatal, but temporary response to chemotherapeutic agents is sometimes seen. In general, the life expectancy after diagnosis of CML is 3 to 4 years.

Chronic Lymphocytic Leukemia   Although it occasionally is seen in younger people, CLL is largely an old-age disease. It favors men over women approximately 2:1 and is extremely rare in Orientals. The culprit in this case is an abnormal, small lymphocyte with a very long life span. The leukemic cells fail to divide at the normal rate and thus accumulate, leading to an extremely high lymphocyte count. The white blood cell count may exceed 500,000/mm^3, of which more than 90 per cent are lymphocytes. Large numbers of abnormal lymphocytes are also found in the bone marrow, lymph nodes, and spleen. Anemia is common, but thrombocytopenia is not as pronounced as with the other types of leukemia. Lymphadenopathy is usually seen, but hepatosplenomegaly is less common than with CML.

Symptoms and Signs   The symptoms of CLL include weakness and easy fatigue, relating mainly to the concurrent anemia. Often, these symptoms are attributed to old age in the typical patient, rather than to a disease state. The onset is insidious and diagnosis is often made accidentally, as with CML.

Diagnosis   Leukemoid reactions and certain lymphomas are occasionally confused with CLL because of the proliferation of lymphocytes seen in each case. However, blood smear, bone marrow biopsy, and lymph node biopsy, where applicable, aid in the establishment of the correct diagnosis.

Treatment   Radiotherapy and chemotherapy are used (Table 21–4), as in CML, with the major goal being long-term disease control. However, the drugs used in the two conditions are different. Corticosteroids are often used in CLL to reduce the abnormally high lymphocyte count.

Complications   Besides the complications of hemorrhage and infection, about a third of patients with CLL develop hemolytic anemia, presumably due to an immune reaction against red blood cells. This "adds insult to injury," since the individual is already anemic as a result of leukemia. Blood transfusions are usually required for treatment.

Prognosis   The outcome of CLL varies widely, depending largely upon the degree of infiltration of body organs and the severity of anemia and/or thrombocytopenia. In severe cases, the life expectancy is 1 to 2 years, but survival for 12 to 15 years is often seen in milder forms of the disease.

HODGKIN'S DISEASE   Malignancies originating within the lymphatic system are called *lymphomas,* a questionable term because it suggests a benign condition. The terminology developed at a time when the disorders were thought to be inflammatory rather than malignant conditions. Today, although inflammation may be involved as an initiating event, the diseases are considered malignant since they metastasize and eventually kill the patient if untreated.

Lymphomas can be roughly divided into *Hodgkin's disease* and *non-Hodgkin's lymphomas.* Non-Hodgkin's lymphomas are classified according to several systems and vary greatly as to histologic presentation. The Shah of Iran died of a type of non-Hodgkin's lymphoma called *histiocytic lymphoma.* Another well-known non-Hodgkin's lymphoma is *Burkitt's lymphoma,* found mostly in African children. Burkitt's lymphoma particularly affects the jaw and nearby lymph nodes. It is of special interest because it is thought to be caused by infection with the Epstein-Barr virus. In most people, infection with this virus causes mononucleosis, associated with only temporary cervical lymphadenopathy, but no malignancy.

Hodgkin's disease, the most common lymphoma in the United States, has two periods of peak occurrence. A number of cases occur between the ages of 15 and 35, and an even larger number are seen in those over 50. Males are affected more often than females.

Pathogenesis

The cause of Hodgkin's disease is unknown, but it is speculated that an initial inflammatory reaction may give rise to later malignant change in the affected tissues. There is some evidence that an infectious agent may trigger the condition, as seems to be the case with Burkitt's lymphoma. Occasional clustering of the disease among close, but unrelated, contacts suggests an infectious etiology. Likewise, the presence of several cases in some families suggests either an infectious agent or a hereditary etiology. It is quite possible that more than one etiologic factor functions in the development of Hodgkin's disease or even that it represents several similar, but not identical, diseases.

Some authorities propose that Hodgkin's disease develops as a result of an immunologic defect involving T lymphocytes. According to the theory, patients with Hodgkin's disease form an immunosuppressive factor that inhibits T lymphocyte activity. Such a factor has been isolated from affected individuals. Furthermore, these patients show reduced skin reaction to a variety of antigens, such as tuberculin, and are more prone to infection, suggesting reduced immune function compared with normal individuals.

A key finding in Hodgkin's disease is a characteristic multinucleated large cell called a *Reed-Sternberg* cell. This is considered by most authorities to be the malignant cell of Hodgkin's disease. If T lymphocyte activity is suppressed, any Reed-Sternberg cells that spontaneously arise will fail to be eliminated through T lymphocyte activity. Thus, proliferation of Reed-Sternberg cells and spread of the disease would occur (Fig. 21–5).

Symptoms and Signs

Hodgkin's disease usually presents as a unilateral lymphadenopathy, especially involving the cervical nodes. Often, a single node is enlarged and the swelling is firm and painless. Symptoms of fatigue, weight loss, and pruritus (itching) are also frequently present. In more advanced cases, hepatosplenomegaly and multiple lymph node involvement are seen. Fever is often an early sign of Hodgkin's disease, as it is with other malignancies, and probably represents cell destruction and release of pyrogens. If the disease begins within the chest, pressure from expanding lymph nodes may cause shortness of breath as an early symptom.

Laboratory Findings

The diagnosis of Hodgkin's disease is often established by lymph node biopsy. In addition to finding Reed-Sternberg cells, the pathologist frequently sees lymphocytes, eosinophils, plasma cells, and other cell forms in the affected node. A large population of lymphocytes in the node (lymphocyte predominance) is considered favorable, since it probably represents body defense against the disease. Chest x-ray films may show enlarged thoracic lymph nodes. Bone

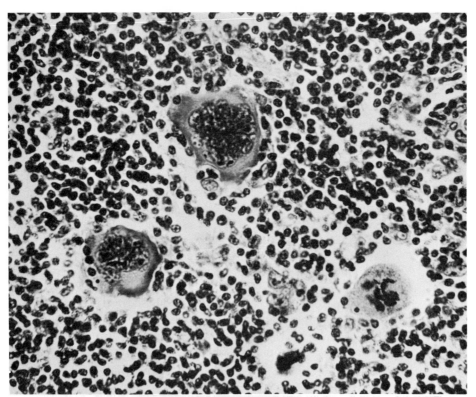

Figure 21–5. Reed-Sternberg cells surrounded by lymphocytes in Hodgkin's disease. (From Robbins, S. L., and Cotran, R. S.: *Pathologic Basis of Disease,* 2nd ed. Philadelphia, W. B. Saunders Company, 1979.)

marrow biopsy shows invasion of Reed-Sternberg cells in more advanced cases. Anemia often results from a combination of bone marrow damage and red cell hemolysis in later stages of disease.

Diagnosis   A number of conditions can produce unilateral lymphadenopathy. Mycobacterial infections (especially atypical forms) often cause swelling of lymph nodes on one side of the neck. A peculiar infection occurring after a cat scratch to the face (cat-scratch disease) causes unilateral lymphadenopathy. Phenytoin (Dilantin) causes lymphadenopathy as a side effect, but it is usually bilateral. Lymph node biopsy is the most reliable diagnostic technique and is absolutely necessary in the differentiation of the various forms of lymphoma.

Treatment   Before treatment is undertaken for Hodgkin's disease, it is important that the stage of disease be determined. Stage I disease is confined to only one lymph node; stage II disease affects two or more nodes on one side of the diaphragm; stage III disease occurs on both sides of the diaphragm but affects only the lymph nodes, spleen, or lymphoid tissue of the pharyngeal area (Waldeyer's ring); and stage IV disease implies widespread infiltration, affecting virtually any body area. Accurate staging requires all available information as to the extent of spread and may require exploratory laparotomy and biopsy of the liver and thoracic lymph nodes in addition to the usual laboratory workup.

Surgery. Surgery for Hodgkin's disease is limited to lymphadenectomy of isolated nodes and splenectomy in more advanced cases. Surgical removal of a solitary node in stage I disease offers the greatest hope of cure.

Radiotherapy. In stage I or II disease, radiotherapy destroys localized abnormal cells and is an excellent adjunct to surgery. Current therapy emphasizes the irradiation of apparently uninvolved nodes to destroy any metastatic cells. In stage III disease, radiotherapy can be used to shrink groups of nodes or to eradicate cells from other areas of infiltration.

Chemotherapy. Chemotherapy is most effective for stage III and IV disease, when the rate of cell proliferation is greatest. It is often combined with radiotherapy to enhance the destructive effect on malignant cells. The most widely used combination at the present time is the *MOPP treatment,* consisting of *m*echlorethamine (Mustargen), *v*incristine (*O*ncovin), *p*rocarbazine (Matulane), and *p*rednisone.

Complications

In addition to hemolytic anemia, which often develops in late-stage Hodgkin's disease, a common complication is the development of pressure from enlarged lymph nodes, causing pain, shortness of breath, or other symptoms. Hemolytic anemia is treated with blood transfusions, whereas enlarged lymph nodes can be reduced by localized irradiation of the affected area. With widespread chest involvement, pleural effusion is common, often requiring thoracentesis and drainage for relief of symptoms.

Prognosis

The current overall 5-year survival rate with Hodgkin's disease is about 80 per cent, dramatically better than it was even 3 years ago. The improvement comes as a result of earlier diagnosis, more accurate staging, and the use of combination chemotherapy in conjunction with surgery and radiotherapy. Many individuals live 15 to 20 years after diagnosis. Those with stage I disease have a good chance of being cured with appropriate therapy. In the last 20 years, the outlook for Hodgkin's disease has changed from one of hopelessness to one of optimism, especially if the disease is diagnosed in stage I.

SUMMARY

There are more than 100 types of cancer, ranging from highly curable skin lesions to extremely malignant carcinomas of the lung and thyroid gland. Although all types of cancer have certain features in common, we can only generalize about them to a certain point. To attach a hopeless prognosis to all forms of cancer is to use unwarranted pessimism. Great improvements have been made in the treatment of acute leukemias, Hodgkin's disease, choriocarcinoma, and other formerly fatal types of cancer, and many patients are now cured of these conditions. Cancer prevention is often more important than treatment. Efforts to clean up the atmosphere and water and to reduce industrial exposure to carcinogens and personal commitments to avoid smoking can dramatically change the cancer statistics in the near future.

The most common solid tumor malignancies in the United States are carcinomas of the lung, breast, and colorectal area. There are four types of leukemias frequently seen, two of which are acute forms and two chronic. Hodgkin's disease is the most common form of lymphoma in the United States. All of these conditions can be treated, using surgery, chemotherapy, and/or radiotherapy, with improved survival of the patient. Within the last 20 years, great strides have been made in the treatment of Hodgkin's disease and both types of acute leukemia, primarily as a result of combination chemotherapy in conjunction with radiotherapy. Early diagnosis of solid tumors offers the best hope of cure, since these tumors often metastasize early. Serum tests for cancer, now in their infancy, may be the wave of the future.

Questions

1. Argue for and against using the single term "cancer" to describe a heterogeneous group of more than a hundred diseases.
2. Compare and contrast the somatic mutation theory and the aberrant differentiation theory in carcinogenesis. Are the two mutually exclusive?
3. Explain the terms *leverage* and *turnover* as they apply to cancer chemotherapy. Why is it often not possible to destroy all cancer cells with chemotherapy?
4. What is the difference between an *initiator* and a *promoter* of cancer?
5. Compare and contrast acute and chronic leukemias as to symptoms and signs, laboratory findings, and outcome without treatment. Why is the chemotherapeutic approach to the two types of leukemias different?

Additional Reading

Cline, M. J.: Acute leukemia: Biology and treatment. Ann. Intern. Med., 91:758, 1979.

Desforges, J. F., Rutherford, C. R., and Piro, A.: Hodgkin's disease. N. Engl. J. Med., 301:1212, 1979.

Hardcastle, J. D. *et al.:* Screening for symptomless colorectal cancer by testing for occult blood in general practice. Lancet, 1:791, 1980.

Henderson, I. C., and Canellos, G. P.: Cancer of the breast: The past decade (two parts). N. Engl. J. Med., 302:17, 78, 1980.

Nystrom, J. S. *et al.:* Identifying the primary site in metastatic cancer of unknown origin. J.A.M.A., 241:381, 1979.

Rahwan, R. G.: Cancer mechanisms. U. S. Pharmacist 7:32, 1982. *(Very good refresher article on all aspects of cancer development.)*

CHAPTER 22

SPECIAL PROBLEMS IN PEDIATRICS AND GERIATRICS

PROBLEMS COMMON TO YOUNG CHILDREN AND OLDER ADULTS

The very young and very old have a great deal more in common than merely their existence at the extremes of the age spectrum. Both are vulnerable to overwhelming infection resulting from subnormal immune reactions. Both exhibit alterations in the action, metabolism, or excretion of many drugs, largely associated with immaturity or senility of organ functions. Both suffer from diseases peculiar to their age groups. In addition, both require more supportive care when ill than does a young adult. The old-saying that elderly people enter their "second childhood" has some basis in fact, both in terms of mental changes and in the increased vulnerability to disease.

Infections

Pneumonia and other serious infections are particularly devastating to infants and elderly people. The early observation that bacterial pneumonia was the "friend of the old and enemy of the young" (see Chapter 9) pointed up the tendency of those infections to overcome the weakened defenses of these two population groups.

Drug Effects

Drug metabolism is markedly different in both infants and geriatric patients, compared with young, healthy adults.

Older Adults

The elderly generally have reduced drug-handling ability, resulting from decreased organ function (Table 22–1). The processes of metabolism, largely in the domain of the liver, and excretion, primarily a kidney function, slow down with age, and drugs tend to remain in the body longer in their original form. Thus, it is often necessary to give less drug per dose and to give it less often to the elderly person. In addition, the elderly usually have less water and more fat per kilogram of body weight than young adults, increasing the concentration of water-soluble drugs and decreasing the concentration of fat-soluble drugs in the body.

Many older people have reduced amounts of plasma proteins, especially serum albumin. This results in less protein binding and more free drug in the blood stream for those drugs that are partly protein-bound (e.g., digitalis products, oral anticoagulants). Accordingly, the same dose of drug per kilogram may have a greater effect in the elderly individual than in a young adult. Interestingly, absorption of drugs via oral administration or injection does not greatly differ between the two.

Table 22–1. PHYSIOLOGIC AND ANATOMIC ALTERATIONS IN THE AGED*

Factor	Amount Remaining at Age 75† (%)
Water content of body	82
Maximum work rate	70
Vital capacity	56
Brain weight	56
Blood flow of brain	80
Resting cardiac output	70
Glomerular filtration rate of kidney	69

*Based on a comparison of a 75-year-old man with a 30-year-old man.
†Based on a total value of 100 per cent.

Older people often react differently to certain types of drugs than do young adults. Sedatives, such as phenobarbital, may cause excitation. Antidepressants, such as imipramine (Tofranil), may have exaggerated or prolonged effects. Analgesic drugs, such as morphine or codeine, often have more pronounced effects in the elderly than in young adults. Drugs used to lower blood pressure, including reserpine (Serpasil) and methyldopa (Aldomet), can cause an excessive reduction of blood pressure, leading to syncope (fainting). A general rule in drug administration to the elderly is to give 75 per cent of the normal adult dose and watch for unusual reactions. The dose and/or frequency of drug administration can then be adjusted for the particular individual.

Young Children   Children are not "small adults" when it comes to drug administration. There are distinct differences in drug absorption, distribution, binding, metabolism, and excretion between children and adults.

Absorption. The thinner skin and the altered gastric pH of infants change the absorption of drugs administered both by topical and oral routes. For example, hexachlorophene is toxic when applied topically to infants but is much less toxic in older children and adults. Oral absorption is better in children under 3 years of age for penicillin G (Pentids) but worse for phenobarbital and acetaminophen (Tylenol) because of the lower acid content (higher pH) of the stomach.

Distribution. The portion of body weight composed of body water changes from 85 per cent in premature infants, to 75 per cent in full-term newborns, to 55 per cent in those over 1 year of age. This means that water-soluble drugs have a larger volume of distribution in the extremely young, while fat-soluble drugs have a smaller volume of distribution and are, therefore, at higher concentration. This alters the normal effects and toxicity of drugs administered to children of different ages.

Binding. In general, infants have a lower concentration of albumin and other proteins in plasma. Therefore, protein-bound drugs exist more in the free (unbound) state in the very young. This increases their effects and toxicity.

Metabolism. Liver function is generally subnormal in young children (especially premature infants) and reaches adult values only after several years of life. Drugs requiring liver metabolism can thus accumulate and cause toxicity if given at "normal" doses. A tragic example of this was seen in the late 1950s and early 1960s, when chloramphenicol (Chloromycetin) was administered to newborns with resistant infections. The drug, although dosed correctly for the size and weight of the infants, caused toxicity and death because it was not metabolized at a normal rate and it accumulated, causing a very high blood level. This condition, called the "gray baby sickness," resulted in increased attention of the medical and scientific community to the metabolic differences between infants and adults.

Excretion. Excretion of most drugs is reduced in infants, compared with the excretory function in normal adults. The kidney is not yet fully developed and, in addition, receives a smaller fraction of blood from the heart for the first year of life. Antibiotics and other drugs that depend heavily upon renal excretion must be given less frequently and in lower doses in infants than in older children or adults. The odd exception to this rule is digoxin (Lanoxin), a digitalis product that is *more* rapidly excreted and must be given in proportionally higher doses in infants than in older children or adults.

Various formulas for dosage calculation in children have been developed, based upon age, weight, or body surface area. However, although these formulas work well for some drugs, they fail miserably for others. Through experience and, unfortunately, some trial and error, current doses for most drugs have been established. Many drugs can now be monitored on the basis of blood level (e.g., digoxin, phenytoin), and this is a great help in establishing the correct dosage regimen in a particular case.

DISORDERS ESPECIALLY PREVALENT IN INFANTS

Immediately after birth, most physiologic functions must change radically in the newborn for survival as an independent being. Respiration must become autonomous, the route of circulating blood changes drastically, and the neonate begins to control body temperature for the first time. It is not surprising that this is an extremely vulnerable period for disease development, even in those of normal birth weight (over 2500 gm). Premature infants, especially those weighing less than 1000 gm at birth, are even less well equipped to deal with the stresses of neonatal life. The infant mortality rate in this group is ten times higher than in the 1000- to 2000-gm group and 150 times higher than in those infants weighing over 2500 gm at birth.

Prematurity/ Immaturity

The term "immaturity" is often used to describe many of the specific problems existing in the low-weight infant. The respiratory system is immature. The alveolar tissue does not exchange gases normally, and contains more fluid than in the full-term infant. Additionally, respiratory controls are not fully developed, and periods of cessation of breathing (apnea) are more likely to occur. Two common respiratory system-related problems, *respiratory distress syndrome* and *sudden infant death syndrome,* are seen more frequently in low-birth weight infants.

The brain, kidneys, liver, and gastrointestinal tract are also incompletely developed in the premature infant. The brain substance is more fragile and there is less myelinization of nerve fibers. Control of vital functions is less precise, and motor activity is markedly reduced. Impaired digestion of fats and fat-soluble vitamins (A, D, E, K) is seen, but most other gastrointestinal functions are essentially normal. The greatly reduced function of the liver and kidney affects not only drug handing but also the ability to metabolize and excrete endogenous compounds, such as bilirubin (see Chapter 13). As a result, jaundice is extremely common in premature infants.

Infants with a low birth weight are now placed in a *neonatal intensive care unit* in most areas of the United States. This specialized treatment facility provides monitoring and maintenance of physiologic functions, accurate blood level determinations for drug administration, and carefully calculated administration of nutrients and fluids. Many units have specially equipped vans or helicopters to transport such infants from outlying areas to the facility. Special self-contained life support systems can also be used to transport the infants by standard airplane or ambulance. The widespread availability of neonatal intensive care units has resulted in a 10 to 15 per cent reduction in infant mortality within the last decade.

Respiratory Distress Syndrome/Hyaline Membrane Disease

Respiratory distress syndrome (RDS) affects 10 per cent of the premature infants and has a mortality rate of 20 to 50 per cent, highest in those with a birth weight of less than 1000 gm. The term RDS denotes a nonspecific condition that can be caused by a variety of factors, including oversedation of the mother during delivery, immature respiratory system development, and brain damage. However, the most common cause of RDS is hyaline membrane disease (HMD). In HMD, there is a deficiency in the formation of *pulmonary surfactant,* a lecithin material that reduces alveolar surface tension and permits full expansion of the alveoli and therefore the lungs, in the newborn. When the lungs fail to expand completely, excessive respiratory effort is required of the infant for ventilation. In addition, hyaline material is formed in the lungs as a result of cell necrosis and leakage of protein material into the alveolar spaces, caused by the reduced production of surfactant. Hyaline material interferes with gas exchange by covering alveolar surfaces and causes hypoxia and dyspnea (Fig. 22–1).

Respiratory distress syndrome/hyaline membrane disease is more common in premature infants, in those born to diabetic mothers, and in those delivered by cesarean section than in normal infants. Prematurity/immaturity may result in subnormal secretion of pulmonary surfactant. Diabetes mellitus and the resulting hyperglycemia in the mother can cause formation of high levels of insulin (hyperinsulism) in the fetus as a compensation. High levels of insulin have been shown to depress the formation of pulmonary surfactant. Cesarean section increases the risk of RDS/HMD, but the cause-and-effect relationship is unclear. While it was originally thought that the risk in infants delivered by cesarean section was higher because they were, as a group, less healthy, this idea has been discounted by later studies. When infants delivered by cesarean section were compared with another group of vaginally delivered infants with similar health problems, the risk was still greater in the cesarean-delivered group. Thus, cesarean delivery itself appears to increase the risk of RDS/HMD.

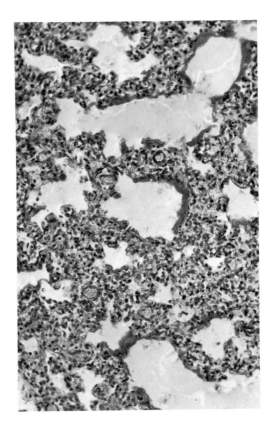

Figure 22–1. Infiltration of hyaline membrane material in respiratory distress syndrome/hyaline membrane disease. The hyaline membrane covers the alveolar surface and plugs air passages in the lung. (From Robbins, S. L., and Cotran, R. S.: *Pathologic Basis of Disease.* Philadelphia, W. B. Saunders Company, 1979.)

Infants with RDS/HMD can now be diagnosed *in utero* by analyzing the amniotic fluid and noting the deficiency in lecithin. They can be treated before and after delivery with corticosteroids, which stimulate the production of pulmonary surfactant. Respiratory assistance for 3 or 4 days after delivery increases the chance of survival. Caution must be used in the administration of oxygen, since arterial partial pressures of over 80 mm Hg often induce damage to the lens of the eye (retrolental fibroplasia) and to lung tissue. All efforts should be made to provide adequate control of diabetes mellitus in the mother to prevent hyperglycemia and its effects on the fetus. Premature delivery, especially via cesarean section, should be avoided if at all possible.

Sudden Infant Death Syndrome

Approximately 10,000 infants die each year in the United States of a mysterious ailment that has a worldwide incidence of about 2 per 1000 live births. The babies are usually less than 6 months old and are well or have only a mild respiratory infection. The typical victim comes from a large family of lower economic status, is often premature, and has a very young mother. Great variation exists in the pattern, however, and no one factor correlates perfectly with an increased risk of disorder. Autopsy of the victims discloses no cause of death, although the infants as a group are smaller, lighter, and slightly less well developed than normal infants. There is also a fivefold increased risk of recurrence of the condition in families having lost one child to it.

The term *sudden infant death syndrome* (SIDS) has been coined to denote these tragic cases. Most infants die while in a crib or bed, and the term "crib death" is also used. Not all infants die while asleep. In those cases that have been observed, the infant stops breathing, becomes cyanotic, and dies without a cry or struggle.

This ailment has been explored from every angle: viral infection, allergy, suffocation from bedding, malposition of oral and pharyngeal structures causing respiratory obstruction, and others. No one factor is responsible in the majority of cases, and such "causes," in fact, may be incidental findings. The most plausible etiologic theory for SIDS at the present time is that the affected babies have abnormalities in cardiac or respiratory control. Since they are often premature or developmentally slower than unaffected infants, it is conceivable that the conduction system in the heart or the respiratory control centers in the brain are still in the process of maturation within the first 6 months of life. During this time, temporary stoppages of the conduction of pacemaker impulses to the ventricles or medullary respiratory impulses could likely occur. The cardiac or respiratory activity would simply stop.

Those fortunate infants who have been saved from an episode of SIDS with artificial respiration and those judged to be at higher risk for the condition can now be monitored during sleep with a special instrument. A buzzer sounds if there is a sudden drop in respiratory or cardiac activity and an adult can administer artificial respiration and/or external cardiac massage. A number of lives have been saved in this way, frequently with the bare minimum of assistance. Often, merely jiggling the baby is enough to restart cardiac or respiratory activity. Research is now under way to better identify those infants at risk of developing SIDS and thus to avert the devastation of this family tragedy.

Erythroblastosis Fetalis
(Hemolytic Disease of Newborn)

Incompatibility of antigenic blood factors between parents can lead to an immune reaction in the fetus, characterized by red blood cell hemolysis. In the usual situation, the father is Rh positive and the mother is Rh negative. The fetus inherits the Rh factor from the father and thus has Rh incompatibility with the mother. Significant placental bleeding (greater than 1 ml) can cause absorption of fetal blood containing Rh antigen by the mother. This leads to sensitization of the mother to Rh antigen and the formation of Rh antibodies in her blood stream. Normally, because significant bleeding does not occur until delivery, the first pregnancy is not affected. In subsequent pregnancies, however, maternal Rh antibodies formed during the first delivery (or miscarriage) react with Rh antigen in Rh-positive fetuses, leading to red cell hemolysis *(erythroblastosis fetalis)*. In mild cases, no symptoms develop because the bone marrow rapidly replaces hemolyzed red cells. In more severe cases, anemia develops because hemolysis occurs faster than replacement. Additionally, hemoglobin accumulates from hemolyzed red cells and is converted to bilirubin, leading to hyperbilirubinemia and jaundice. If the serum level of bilirubin is extremely high, bilirubin enters the brain across the incompletely developed blood-brain barrier and central nervous system (CNS) damage (kernicterus) develops. This can result in mental retardation or motor disorders in the young infant.

Erythroblastosis fetalis can now be prevented by noting the original incompatibility in the parents through careful blood typing. After the first delivery (within 72 hours), the mother can be given an Rh immunoglobulin preparation (RhoGAM), which ties up Rh antigen and prevents the development of maternal Rh antibodies. After the short-term effect of RhoGAM wears off, as is the case with all passive immunoglobulin preparations (see Chapter 4), the mother is no longer sensitized to Rh antigen. RhoGAM is also used after miscarriages, since these can trigger sensitization, and before delivery, if maternal sensitization is occurring. This can be determined by testing the mother's blood for Rh antibody and by assaying the amniotic fluid for elevated bilirubin level, which signifies red cell hemolysis in the fetus.

If erythroblastosis fetalis occurs because of laboratory errors, inadequate prenatal care, or other reason, the infant can still be treated to prevent severe anemia and kernicterus. Exposure for several days to ultraviolet light (with the eyes protected) causes oxidation of bilirubin, rendering it much less harmful and readily excretable from the body. In more severe cases, the infant's blood can be completely exchanged to remove antigen-antibody complexes. This can be done even *in utero* before delivery if signs of erythroblastosis fetalis develop during pregnancy. The overall mortality of those who develop erythroblastosis fetalis is now only 5 per cent, largely because of improved methods of treatment.

Down's Syndrome   In about 1 in 800 births, the infant possesses an extra chromosome (47 instead of 46) and has *Down's syndrome*. This disorder is characterized by mental retardation and a flat facial profile superficially resembling the Mongol race (Fig. 22–2). (The older term "mongolism" has been largely abandoned.) In addition to these defects, children with Down's syndrome have a high frequency of congenital heart defects and acute leukemia, usually lymphoblastic (see Chapter 21). The parents are usually normal, and the condition

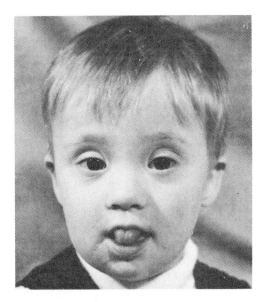

Figure 22–2. Down's syndrome. Note "mongoloid" appearance of tissue surrounding the eye. (From Behrman, R. E., and Vaughan, V. C. III: *Nelson Textbook of Pediatrics,* 12th ed. Philadelphia, W. B. Saunders Company, 1983.)

represents a mistake in formation of the ovum, rather than an inherited chromosomal defect. The risk of Down's syndrome rises with increasing maternal age. It is 1 in 2000 below age 30, but increases to 1 in 50 after age 45. The chances are great (1 in 60) of having a second child with the disorder. Studies have suggested that the father's age may be a factor in Down's syndrome, but the relationship is less clear than with the mother. In a few cases, it has been shown that the extra chromosome came from the father rather than from the mother.

Most children with Down's syndrome have intelligence quotients (IQs) ranging from 25 to 50 (normal = 100), although a few are very close to normal intelligence. All can be helped to become more productive and self-sufficient with special training and the support of loved ones.

Phenylketonuria   Phenylketonuria (PKU) is an inherited recessive disorder caused by a lack of phenylalanine hydroxylase, an enzyme that converts phenylalanine to tryosine (see Chapter 1). This condition is more prevalent in those of Scotch-Irish descent (1 in 5000) and rare in blacks (1 in 300,000). The disease is present at birth, but its complications develop largely after birth when the infant begins living on a normal diet containing phenylalanine. Since phenylalanine cannot be converted to tyrosine, it accumulates to high levels (above 50 mg/dl; normal = 1 mg/dl) in the blood stream. High levels of phenylalanine in the brain are associated with demyelinization of neurons and neurologic symptoms, including mental retardation and seizures. Often, the presence of large amounts of phenylalanine in body fluids causes a musty, mouselike odor that is easily noticed. Most children with PKU are blond, blue-eyed, and light-skinned, partly because of impaired synthesis of melanin pigment resulting from reduced formation of tyrosine.

Virtually all babies born in the United States and in many other developed countries are tested a few days after birth for PKU, using the *Guthrie test* on a serum sample. If PKU is detected, the infant is placed on a low phenylalanine diet for at least 6 years to avoid brain damage. Control of PKU is a major medical breakthrough, since it means prevention of a common form of mental retardation.

Cystic Fibrosis   Cystic fibrosis (CF) occurs once in about 1500 births in whites and once in 17,000 births in blacks. It is especially common in those of European heritage. The disorder is transmitted as a recessive trait, whereby homozygotes have the disease but heterozygotes have no symptoms, as is the case with sickle cell anemia. The disease affects exocrine glands, especially of the pancreas and respiratory tract, causing production of a thick, protein-rich secretion. In addition, the sweat glands are affected, resulting in production of sweat containing abnormally large amounts of sodium chloride and potassium. Since the condition is associated with cystic dilation of pancreatic ducts and fibrous atrophy of certain glands, the term "cystic fibrosis" was coined. It is now clear that the disease involves much more than just these abnormalities.

Most of the difficulty with CF comes from the obstruction caused by secretion of the thick mucus. Respiratory infections are common, since the self-cleaning ability of the lungs and upper respiratory tract structures, via the flow of mucus, is impaired. Obstruction of pancreatic ducts results in reduced secretion of pancreatic juice into the duodenum, leading to indigestion (especially of fats) and severe constipation. Intestinal obstruction is a frequent result and rectal prolapse, resulting from the straining associated with chronic constipation, is often seen. The absorption of fat-soluble vitamins is inadequate, and these must be supplemented in the diet. Eventually, chronic obstructive pulmonary disease (COPD) develops as a result of repeated infections and the resulting fibrosis.

Most children with CF are diagnosed within a year of birth on the basis of this symptomatology. In addition, analysis of the sodium chloride content of the sweat after stimulation of secretion with pilocarpine (sweat test) provides positive laboratory evidence of the disease. The condition can now be detected by analysis of the amniotic fluid during pregnancy. A serum electrophoretic assay that distinguishes heterozygous from homozygous individuals has also been developed. This identifies carriers of the disease who have no symptoms.

Cystic fibrosis is treated using a high-calorie, low-fat diet, along with vitamin supplementation and replacement of pancreatic enzymes with commercial supplements (e.g., Viokase). Additional sodium chloride is needed to offset the great loss in perspiration. Respiratory therapy, utilizing mucolytic agents, such as acetylcysteine (Mucomyst), bronchodilators, and expectorants helps to keep the lungs more clear of mucus. Antibiotic therapy is often necessary for the recurrent respiratory infection seen in CF.

With careful medical management, many patients now survive into the 20- to 40-year-old age range or even longer. Life can be essentially normal for the CF patient with adequate treatment. Men are invariably sterile as a result of the characteristic deterioration of the vas deferens, which carries semen. Women, however, are usually fertile. The outlook for the CF patient is vastly better than it was even 10 years ago, largely as a result of a better understanding of the complexities of the disease and improved drug therapy of its complications.

DISEASES ESPECIALLY PREVALENT IN THE ELDERLY

As the average life expectancy of the combined male and female population in the United States exceeds 75 years, a number of diseases surface with greater frequency than in times when the average life span was only 40 to 50 years. Our ancestors were killed off early by pneumonia, epidemics of influenza, and diseases associated with occupational hazards (not only mining but also delivering the mail!). Those lucky ones who survived to old age often were not correctly diagnosed at the time of death, and many deaths were attributed to "heart trouble," "stomach trouble," or "bad blood," for want of a closer diagnosis. Without the laboratory techniques that have since become available, it was often impossible to arrive at a precise diagnosis. As many diseases were conquered or at least controlled, the life expectancy increased and, concurrently, the methods of diagnosis became more accurate. As a result, certain diseases are now noted more frequently in the elderly than in younger individuals.

Age As a Factor in Disease

With a constantly increasing percentage of older people in the general population, we find that age itself is a risk factor for disease development (see Chapter 1). The ability to prevent or overcome disease generally decreases with increasing age. Perhaps reduced immune response, increased frequency of mitotic errors, and attrition of organ function work in concert to undermine resistance to disease in the aged individual.

As we have noted in preceding chapters, heart disease, organic brain syndrome, and most forms of cancer are much more common in the elderly than in the younger population.

Cardiovascular Problems

Coronary artery disease and its complications of angina pectoris and myocardial infarction account for an increasing amount of morbidity and mortality with advancing age. The process of atherosclerosis, beginning at birth, continues until death. With luck, we escape its ravages because it progresses slowly enough that we live out our lives before it becomes clinically apparent. If we are unlucky, we die from a heart attack before our alloted time has elapsed (Chapter 10 describes ways by which we may slow the process.) Other forms of cardiovascular disease, such as congestive heart failure and hypertension, are more common in the elderly. However, with good medical care, these may be controlled for a very long time.

Organic Brain Syndrome

Organic brain syndrome (OBS) is seen frequently in the older person, presumably as a result of impaired cerebral circulation and/or deterioration of brain cells associated with aging (see Chapter 15). The disease processes that cause OBS move at dramatically different rates in different people. Some are senile at 60. Others have excellent mental function at an advanced age. I recall a professor of religious philosophy at the University of Houston who taught until age 92 and lived until the age of 96. He was intelligent, alert, and lucid all his life. Interestingly, as a young man he gave a eulogy following the assassination of President McKinley and much later gave a similar eulogy following the assassination of President Kennedy! I think that his lifetime of mental activity helped to prevent mental deterioration in old age.

Cancer

Most types of cancer, with the exception of certain childhood malignancies such as Wilms' tumor and acute lymphoblastic leukemia, are more common in the elderly. Perhaps this represents the results of a lifetime of exposure to carcinogens, along with a greater frequency of chromosomal errors and reduced repair or defense abilities in the older person. Again, though, there is a great difference among individuals. Some seem to have the extra "resistance factor" needed to avoid cancer for a long lifetime. Others succumb to the ravages of this complex disease before their proverbial "threescore years and ten" have been realized. As with many other diseases, the factor of luck seems to be operating. We can do everything possible to avoid developing cancer (see Chapter 21), but we must realize that this does not ensure a long lifetime without it. Nonetheless, our chances of avoiding cancer are much better if we make an effort to avoid exposure to carcinogens and to take advantage of the early diagnostic and treatment methods now available. Perhaps we should take advice from the old Pennsylvania Dutch saying: "Ve get too soon oldt und too late schmart" as we live from day to day.

SUMMARY

Infants and older people are different from the young to middle-aged adult population in a number of ways. Resistance to infection is often subnormal. The effects of drugs differ between these groups and the normal adult population, as well as between pediatric and geriatric populations themselves. The very young and very old suffer from diseases not common in adults of young to middle age: Hyaline membrane disease, sudden infant death syndrome, erythroblastosis fetalis, Down's syndrome, phenylketonuria, and cystic fibrosis threaten the infant population, while heart disease, organic brain syndrome, and cancer take their toll on the elderly. In many cases, it is not possible to prevent these disorders completely. However, with improved diagnostic and treatment techniques as well as knowledge of their causative factors, the devastation of these conditions can be minimized.

Questions

1. Explain why an anesthetic drug such as fluothane (Halothane), which is highly fat-soluble, would have a more pronounced effect on a full-term newborn that it would on a 2-year-old child if given in equivalent doses.
2. Why is hyperbilirubinemia often seen in premature infants, even though they do not have erythroblastosis fetalis or liver disease?
3. Do you think that a life-span of 150 years is possible with continued improvements in medical science? Does the body "wear out" from old age or can life go on indefinitely if geriatric diseases such as cancer and heart disorders are controlled?

Additional Reading

Bergman, H. D.: Drug use in the elderly patient. Southern Pharmacy Journal, 72:24, 1980. (*Overview of factors altering drug response in the elderly.*)

Georgakas, D.: *The Methuselah Factors: Living Long and Living Well.* New York, Simon & Schuster, 1981.

di Sant'Agnese, P. A., *et al.*: Cystic fibrosis in adults: 75 cases and a review of 232 cases in the literature. Am. J. Med., 66:121, 1979.

Kravitz, H., and Scherz, R. G.: The importance of the position of infants on the sudden infant death syndrome: A new hypothesis. Clin. Pediatr., 17:403, 1978. (*Hypothesis regarding the development of SIDS.*)

Samorajski, T.: Central neurotransmitter substances and aging: A review. J. Am. Geriatr. Soc., 25:337, 1977. (*Comprehensive coverage of the biochemistry of the aging brain.*)

Index

Page numbers in italics indicate illustrations; page numbers followed by (t) indicate tables.